PUBLIC HEALTH AND THE RISK FACTOR

Rochester Studies in Medical History

Senior Editor: Theodore M. Brown
Professor of History and Preventive Medicine
University of Rochester

Mechanization of the Heart:
Harvey and Descartes
Thomas Fuchs
Translated from the German by Majorie Grene

The Workers' Health Fund in Eretz Israel
Kupat Holim, 1911–1937
Shifra Shvarts

Public Health and the Risk Factor:
A History of an Uneven Medical Revolution
William G. Rothstein

PUBLIC HEALTH AND THE RISK FACTOR: A HISTORY OF AN UNEVEN MEDICAL REVOLUTION

William G. Rothstein

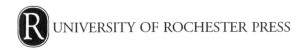 UNIVERSITY OF ROCHESTER PRESS

First published 2003
Transferred to digital printing 2008

University of Rochester Press
668 Mt. Hope Avenue, Rochester, NY 14620, USA
www.urpress.com
and Boydell & Brewer Limited
PO Box 9, Woodbridge, Suffolk IP12 3DF, UK
www.boydellandbrewer.com

ISBN-13: 978-1-58046-127-6 (hardcover)
ISBN-10: 1-58046-127-1 (hardcover)
ISBN-13: 978-1-58046-286-0 (softcover)
ISBN-10: 1-58046-286-3 (softcover)

Library of Congress Cataloging-in-Publication Data

Rothstein, William G./Public health and the risk factor: a history of an uneven medical revolution / William G. Rothstein
     p. cm. — (Rochester studies in medical history ISSN 1526-2715)
    Includes bibliographical references and index.
    ISBN 1-58046-127-1 (hardcover: alk. paper)
     1. Health risk assessment—History. 2. Health behavior—History. 3. Medicine, Preventive—History. 4. Coronary heart disease—Risk factors—History.
     [DNLM: 1. Public Health—history. 2. Risk Factors. 3. Coronary Disease—prevention & control. 4. History of Medicine, 20th Cent. 5. Life Style. WA 11.1 R847p 2003] I. Title. II. Series.

RA427.3 .R68 2003
362.1—dc21

2003001195

A catalogue record for this title is available from the British Library.
This publication is printed on acid-free paper.

To
James C. Mohr

CONTENTS

Part 4   Rick Factors and Coronary Heart Disease

TABLES

ix

PREFACE

Most laypeople, physicians, and other health professionals have a very different view of the relationship between personal behaviors and health and illness today than they did a century ago. At the beginning of the twentieth century, most people believed that their health was a matter of concern only when they were sick. By the end of the century, most people accepted the statistical evidence that specific behaviors and characteristics of healthy persons, called "risk factors," can increase the probability of developing disease, especially chronic disease. Most people also believe that making appropriate changes in their lifestyles, a concept associated with risk factors, can reduce the probability of the occurrence of disease. To facilitate this process, they expect health professionals, agencies concerned with public health, and the media to inform and educate the public about risk factors.

The acceptance of risk factors has produced changes in public health and medicine as profound as those that resulted from bacteriology and the germ theory of disease. The changes have been most evident in coronary heart disease, which was the major cause of death in the twentieth century and is the focus of this study. Yet the impact of the risk factor has been much more uneven than the germ theory. The risk factor concept has been controversial because of its statistical methodology, its multifactorial concept of disease etiology, and its effect on the economic interests of commercial, professional, and health organizations.

This study endeavors to explain in nontechnical language how one of the greatest revolutions in the understanding of health and disease could have produced such mixed outcomes. Although risk factors are a statistical concept, I have avoided all discussion of the mathematics involved. I have also refrained from using statistical terminology, although this has occasionally necessitated lengthier descriptions. Readers familiar with risk factor research will find that I have made little use of a popular statistical tool, meta-analyses. I believe that meta-analyses are based on the erroneous premise that methodological flaws in individual studies cancel each other when studies are combined. The history of the use of statistics in the social sciences, and I believe in medicine, provides convincing evidence to reject this assumption. Instead I have looked for agreement among studies that used the most rigorous methodologies.[1]

An anomaly of risk factor research is that many of the most useful quantitative studies are early ones. The early studies of the natural history of persons with risk factors occurred before medications were available and so provide the only longitudinal data on large numbers of persons with untreated risk factors. In studies of the treatment of risk factors, the protocols require that the experimental group receives the treatment being tested and the control group receives the standard available treatment. In the early studies of some widely accepted medications, the control groups received no treatment because there were no useful treatments. Today the control groups almost always receive an older treatment while the experimental groups receive the treatment being investigated. Today also, many members of both experimental and control groups are also being treated for other medical conditions. Consequently most persons in every group in these studies are receiving some kind of treatment and thus the studies have no true control groups.

Two other aspects of the statistics used in this study can be mentioned. Most historical epidemiological studies suffer from a paucity of trustworthy mortality and morbidity statistics. I believe that a major contribution of this study is the use of historical statistics of exceptionally high quality that are unknown to most scholars. In addition, erroneous reporting of cause of death has always been a major problem in coronary heart disease. However, studies have consistently found that reporting accuracy on death certificates is much greater for deaths below age 65, so I have focused on those age groups.

This study could not have been completed without the assistance of a number of persons. Professor James C. Mohr of the University of Oregon provided assistance in so many ways, including insightful readings of two drafts of the manuscript, that I cannot imagine its publication without his help. Doctor W. Bruce Fye of the Mayo Clinic explained the treatment and other aspects of coronary heart disease clearly and concisely and helped me avoid numerous errors. Edward Morman and the staff of the historical collections of the Welch Medical Library of the Johns Hopkins University were of great help in locating important historical materials. A journal article by Audrey Davis describing the influence of the life insurance industry on the practice of medicine provided the stimulus for this project, which grew in scope and depth as I realized its multifaceted implications.[2] I turned repeatedly to the writings of Rene J. Dubos, the great French-American bacteriologist, for enlightening explanations of multifactorial concepts of disease etiology. A grant from the Science, Technology, and Society program of the National Science Foundation enabled me to take a semester's leave of absence that was invaluable early in the study. A subsequent sabbatical leave from the University of Maryland, Baltimore County, was of equal benefit. Professor Theodore Brown of the University of Rochester and Tim Madigan and others at the University of Rochester Press provided friendly assistance far beyond their formal responsibilities. Last, I would like to express my gratitude to my family, friends, colleagues, and students for cheerfully tolerating my preoccupation with this research for so many years.

1

INTRODUCTION

> Scientific uncertainty is an unavoidable limit that is inherent in scientific knowledge and in the methods by which scientific facts are established. Because scientific knowledge is basically probabilistic rather than absolute and provisional rather than final, it can never be devoid of uncertainty or the possibility of inaccuracy or incompleteness.[1]

One of the fundamental transformations in twentieth century public health and medicine has been the widespread acceptance of a new concept of the causes of chronic and degenerative disease. This is the lifestyle theory, which holds that an individual's state of health is affected by specific aspects of the manner of living of that individual. In the same way that an individual suffering from a disease must follow a prescribed regimen to recover from that disease, a healthy individual must engage in continuous activities that are an integral part of daily life in order to maintain health. According to the theory, the behaviors involved in healthy lifestyles can increase or decrease the probability that an individual will develop particular diseases.

The idea that the maintenance of health requires continuous personal care and attention is an ancient one and a basic precept of the Hippocratic writings. Until the twentieth century, however, the behaviors prescribed for maintaining health were vague, ill–defined, and usually in the

1

form of aphorisms: moderation in all things; early to bed and early to rise; an ounce of prevention is worth a pound of cure. The recommendations were rarely enlightening because they were neither internally consistent nor based on scientific investigations. Most healthy persons did not believe that the maintenance of health required a specific lifestyle and lived without much concern about the effects of their daily actions on future health. Furthermore, many illnesses were considered an unavoidable part of the normal pattern of life and therefore beyond human control: the infectious diseases of infancy and childhood; women's deaths, diseases, and disabilities resulting from childbearing and housework; workers' deaths, diseases, and disabilities produced by hazardous, unhealthy, and arduous working conditions; and the infirmities produced by aging. Even if the diseases or deaths were preventable, the great majority of people lacked the financial and other resources to make the necessary changes in their lifestyles to avoid them.

The lifestyle theory was made possible by the invention of the risk factor, a quantitative concept based on statistics that was introduced into life insurance at the turn of the twentieth century. *A risk factor is a pattern of behavior or physical characteristic of a group of individuals that increases the probability of the future occurrence of one or more diseases in that group relative to comparable groups without or with different levels of the behavior or characteristic.* (Although it will not be discussed here because of differences in usage and historical development, a carcinogen is a risk factor for cancer.)

Risk factors need not be directly involved in the disease process. In many cases the etiological process is unknown but risk factors are used as proxies for the unknown causes because they have predictive value. Some risk factors are indicators that can be measured accurately, inexpensively, safely, or with simple instruments. These are great virtues that reduce the possibility of harm to the patient, the time and effort of the health professional, and the cost to society. An example is build, the relationship of body weight to height, one of the first and most useful risk factors discovered by the life insurance industry.

When the risk factor and its statistical methodology became accepted as a method of investigation in the health sciences about 1960, it provided a new basis for understanding the relationship between a disease and its causes: (1) multiple factors internal and external to the individual are involved in the etiology of every disease; (2) the inherent limitations of scientific methodology mean that all of the etiological factors can never be identified or measured precisely[2] and; (3) statistical analyses can determine the degree to which a specific factor by itself or in conjunction with others can increase or decrease the probability of occurrence of the disease. This approach is in striking contrast to the nineteenth-century doctrine of specific etiology, under which diseases were investigated as though they resulted from particular identifiable external causes, such as bacterial pathogens.

A social and intellectual revolution of this magnitude requires a number of basic discoveries and applications. The thesis of this study is that five historical innovations were necessary to produce the public health concept of the risk factor: (1) the development and adoption of probability and statistics as methods of quantifying the risk of death and disease and the benefits of treatment and public health measures; (2) the recognition that healthy lifestyles are essential to improve the health of the population; (3) the use of educational campaigns by public health departments to encourage the public to adopt healthy lifestyles; (4) the acceptance of probabilistic and multifactorial models of disease etiology; and (5) a disease, in this case coronary heart disease, that was so serious and prevalent as to warrant educational programs designed to change the lifestyles of the entire population.

Probability theory was devised in the seventeenth and eighteenth centuries as a technique for understanding the relative likelihood of alternative outcomes. Statistics developed in the eighteenth century as the quantitative and qualitative analysis of political entities such as states and cities. The two fields were brought together when probability theory was used to determine mortality rates for the population and for specific age and sex groups.

By the nineteenth century, convincing evidence existed that many social phenomena exhibited remarkable statistical regularities from year to year, including deaths, marriages, births, crimes, and suicides. These discoveries made it possible to apply the philosophy and methods of the natural sciences to study social phenomena quantitatively and contributed greatly to the development of public health and the social sciences. The life insurance industry was the first commercial enterprise to utilize this knowledge and developed mortality tables that placed life insurance on a sound financial basis. One basic actuarial principle was to adjust the premiums charged to specific groups, such as age and sex groups, to reflect statistical differences in their death rates. At the turn of the twentieth century, life insurance companies extended this principle to other characteristics, including occupations, build, and blood pressure, which they termed risk factors. Life insurance companies required physicians who examined their applicants to provide information on the applicants' medical risk factors, and the physicians soon applied this new knowledge to their private patients. The adoption of risk factors by physicians was hindered by the lack of treatments and the incompatibility with widely accepted models of disease etiology.

Meanwhile, a new public health program of disease prevention based on the education and active participation of the public was being applied to infectious diseases. In the late nineteenth century, bacteriological investigations found that bacteria that caused diseases in humans were also sometimes present in drinking water, milk, sewage, and foods. Public health programs thereupon endeavored to destroy the bacteria in these sources or prevent them from coming into contact with humans. By the early 1900s, many of these programs were found to be insufficient or ineffective. Public health departments thereupon began to educate the public to change their lifestyles to avoid contact with the bacteria and to maintain a level of health that would enable them to resist the harmful effects of the bacteria.

During the first half of the twentieth century, the major causes of death changed from infectious diseases to chronic diseases of the middle aged and elderly. Coronary heart disease became the single most important cause of death in all advanced countries. Chronic diseases have a latency period measured in years, are incurable, and are often degenerative. In investigating the causes of chronic diseases, medical researchers were unable to discover any specific etiological factors comparable to bacterial pathogens in infectious diseases. Instead, they adopted the risk factor approach of the life insurance industry, which quickly became the accepted etiological model for chronic diseases.

Public health agencies combined the risk factor model of disease causation with their educational programs to encourage the population to change their lifestyles to modify risk factors for coronary heart disease. Private health organizations and commercial businesses also adopted educational and advertising programs concerning risk factors. Public acceptance of risk factors was enhanced by the consumer movement and the widespread application of statistical risk analysis to environmental hazards.

Despite its many achievements, the risk factor model has inherent limitations that produce controversy and conflict. The outcome of any statistical analysis concerning the risks imposed by a risk factor is a set of probabilities whose interpretation requires a subjective judgment. The same numerical level of risk may be perceived as dangerous by one group and minor by another. Similarly, if a treatment of a risk factor reduces the probability of contracting a disease by a given amount, one group may conclude that the reduction is meaningful while another may consider it trivial.

Various interest groups have used this characteristic of risk factors to influence public policies by exaggerating or minimizing the benefits of particular preventive programs and treatments. The major interest groups are organizations that sell commercial products such as foods, tobacco, and pharmaceuticals or provide services such as medical care, health information, and medical research. These organizations include private businesses and corporations, government agencies, medical societies, voluntary health associations, and academic health centers.

As a result, risk factors, which were thought to be scientific decisions based on statistical analyses of research investigations, have become enmeshed in controversies resulting from different interpretations of the statistical findings. The disputes are magnified by the strong and conflicting economic interests of the groups and organizations involved. A study of the history of this process can contribute to an understanding of the determination of health policies, the evolution of the health sciences and professions, and methods of scientific inquiry.

PART I

The Invention of the Risk Factor

2

THE ORIGINS OF PROBABILITY AND STATISTICS

> Which was which he could never make out
> > Despite his best endeavor.
> Of that there is no manner of doubt—
> No possible, probable shadow of doubt—
> > No possible doubt whatever.
> > > (William S. Gilbert, "The Gondoliers")

Unlike many discoveries in public health and medicine, the concept of the risk factor had its origins in two disciplines unrelated to the study of health and disease: probability and statistics. The two disciplines were combined when probability theory was applied to the analysis of the population and mortality data being gathered by statisticians. The new quantitative statistical methods were soon recognized by some as useful for resolving medical controversies, but others considered them worthless or contrary to the goals of scientific medicine.

Probability

A probability, as applied to human behavior, is a ratio in which the numerator is the number of persons who experience events of interest and the

9

denominator is the total number of persons who are able to experience those events. For example, the probability that a person in a certain age and sex group will die is calculated by dividing the number of persons in the group who die by the total number of persons in the group. Probabilities are characteristics of groups rather than individuals. They also require at least two possible outcomes (in this case death and non-death). If only one outcome can occur, the situation is deterministic, not probabilistic. Probability theory was conceived by continental European mathematicians and scientists in the 1650s and 1660s. By 1700 they agreed on terminology and devised some fundamental mathematical techniques.[1]

Probability mathematicians from the seventeenth to the mid-eighteenth centuries were restricted to certain kinds of data for their calculations. Games of chance were particularly convenient because the numerical values of both the numerator and the denominator can be calculated by assuming symmetry. For example, a die has six sides and it can be assumed from symmetry that each side has an equal probability of coming up. Probabilities are much more difficult to obtain for events that require actual enumerations. The probability that a resident of a city will die during a specified time period requires counting both the number of deaths in the city during the period and the number of residents in the city who were alive at the beginning of the period. These numbers were rarely available until the mid-eighteenth century. The dependence of the early probability mathematicians on games of chance created doubts about the probity and social utility of the field that persisted for many years.[2]

During the eighteenth and nineteenth centuries, new kinds of quantitative data became available to probability mathematicians. They included astronomical observations, experiments in the natural sciences, and vital statistics. The mathematicians used these data to develop such important tools as the Gaussian or normal distribution, the binomial distribution, the Poisson distribution, the central limit theorem, and the use of the least squares methods.[3]

Most physical scientists renounced probabilistic reasoning until the twentieth century because of its rejection of determinism. The basic premise of probability is that no cause will produce precisely the same effect every time without fail. Based on the laws of Isaac Newton, physical scientists believed that it was theoretically possible to predict effects with absolute certainty. They willingly conceded their inability to make such predictions, but insisted that the solution was more and better research, not the adoption of uncertainty as a basic tenet of science. In the twentieth century physical scientists were forced to reject determinism and accept probabilities as a result of the Bohr model of the atom, the Heisenberg uncertainty principle, and quantum mechanics. Physicists now realized that it was theoretically impossible to predict the future motion and position of any individual atom in any specific location. The only practical approach was to use probabilities to predict the overall motions of large numbers of atoms.[4]

The new basic-medicine scientists of the nineteenth century aspired to the same goals of certainty and determinism as the physical scientists of that era. Some of them contended that human functions could ultimately be precisely explained by physical and chemical laws that governed each organ of the body and the microorganisms that entered the body. For example, the early bacteriologists conducted their research as though the human or animal body was a passive receptacle for bacterial pathogens. Eventually, biology and biomedicine also accepted probability, but not until the mid-twentieth century.

If natural scientists were adamant in rejecting probabilistic reasoning until the twentieth century, how did the discipline survive and expand until that time? Hacking has proposed that the progress of probability is not to be found in the "high sciences" of astronomy, physics, chemistry, or their emulators, including the biomedical sciences. Probability achieved its first success in disciplines that did not aspire to become true sciences at the time—demography, vital statistics, and insurance in the eighteenth and nineteenth centuries, and agriculture, business, and the social and behavioral sciences in the twentieth. Those disciplines believed that the limitations of their data were so great that only probabilistic models could be used to analyze them. Eventually, to everyone's astonishment, probability was adopted by all sciences.[5]

Statistics

Statistics originated in the mid-eighteenth century as a quantitative and qualitative description of social life. The term was coined in 1749 and for the next century encompassed descriptions of the social, demographic, economic, geographic, and political characteristics of a kingdom, region, or other political or geographic entity. After the middle of the nineteenth century, the term became restricted to descriptions using numerical data.[6] In the twentieth century it was further limited to two major methods of analyzing numerical data. Descriptive statistics include averages, rates, proportions, and other methods of summarizing data gathered from a number of individuals. Inferential statistics are based on probability theory and use data from samples of a population to make generalizations about the entire population. Descriptive statistics, especially vital statistics, became the primary source of data for public health, while inferential statistics were used to analyze epidemiological studies and clinical trials and had a greater impact on clinical and preventive medicine.

Among the earliest precursors of statistics were the bills of mortality, which were published records of deaths in a municipality. The best known and most influential of these, the London Bills of Mortality, began on an intermittent basis in London in 1562 to describe trends in plague deaths. Christenings were soon added, regular publication was begun in 1603, deaths from causes other than plague were listed after 1625, and the number of deaths for men and women were listed separately somewhat later. Age of death was not added until 1728. Similar listings were published later in other English cities and in newspapers in the American colonies beginning about 1700. Bills of mortality were published in Paris about 1670, but the French publication was not widely distributed or much used.[7]

The bills of mortality were effective for measuring short-term changes in deaths from specific diseases and births but of little value for other purposes. The London bills initially enumerated the number of burials each week, which provided useful information on whether an epidemic was beginning, intensifying, or diminishing. Plague was the epidemic disease of concern in the seventeenth century, smallpox in the eighteenth, and cholera in the early nineteenth. Although the total population of London was unknown, trends could be determined by weekly changes in the absolute number of deaths because the population of a city changes very little in the short run. However, ignorance of the size of the population made it impossible to calculate the proportion of the population that died each week, so that the severity of an epidemic could not be ascertained. The Bills of Mortality were also restricted to burials of baptized persons in Anglican cemeteries, Anglican christenings, and Anglican marriage ceremonies. Thus they excluded non-Anglicans, those who died before baptism, and the large numbers of the poor who were never baptized. In 1836, the government enacted legislation that required compulsory secular registration of all births, deaths, and marriages in England.[8]

John Graunt was the first person to apply quantitative analyses to the Bills of Mortality in his 1662 publication, *Natural and Political Observations Mentioned in a Following Index and Made Upon the Bills of Mortality.* Graunt estimated trends in mortality from the plague and other diseases, seasonal variations in morality, the size of London's population, and the rate of population growth in the city. His analysis has been acclaimed as the first identifiable epidemiological study, but its cavalier disregard of the many limitations of the data served as an unfortunate precedent for many subsequent analyses.[9]

As evidence of his indifference to methodological issues, Graunt estimated that less than one-half of the London population between 1650 and 1660 baptized their children, but he did not hesitate to use the listed births to make wholly unwarranted estimates of the growth of the population. He deliberately disregarded inaccuracies in the determination of cause of death, stating: "it matters not to many of our purposes, whether the Disease [reported by the searchers who inspected the corpses] were exactly the same, as Physicians define it in their Books. . . . if one died suddenly, the matter is not great, whether it be reported in the Bills, [as] Suddenly, Apoplexy, or Planet-strucken, etc." Graunt surely knew that unless all persons with the same symptoms were given the same diagnosis, the resulting enumerations were worthless. Had he restricted himself to total mortality, he would have avoided any problems. Instead he made such unequivocal and unwarranted statements about specific causes of death as: "The Diseases, which beside the Plague make years unhealthfull in [London], are Spotted Fevers, Small Pox, Disentery."[10]

Scientists of the period admired Graunt's statistical manipulations of the bills of mortality and showed little concern about the fundamental flaws in his methods of analysis. The Royal Society gave Graunt's tract to Christian Huygens (1629–1695), the Dutch mathematician and astronomer, who used it in 1669 to construct a mortality curve and calculate the mean and probable duration of life. Huygens was a skilled mathematics while Graunt was not, so his calculations were an important contribution to the concept of a life table, but the resulting statistics were meaningless.[11]

The limitations of Graunt's data and the errors of his analysis illustrate the many problems that statistics had to resolve if they were to contribute to public health and medicine. Progress in the development of mathematical formulas needed to be matched by progress in the methods of gathering and determining the accuracy and completeness of the data. In 1701, referring to Graunt and others, a mathematician conceded: "It is true, for want of good information, their calculations sometimes proceed upon erroneous suppositions; but that is not the fault of the art."[12] The belief that mathematical manipulations of data can be evaluated independently of the accuracy of the data has only grown stronger in the succeeding centuries.

The next major step in the statistical analysis of births and deaths was the calculation of a life table in 1693 by Edmund Halley (1656–1742), the famous English astronomer. Halley used 5,869 deaths between 1687 and 1691 in Breslau, then in Silesia, Germany (now in Poland and called Wroclaw), which had kept regular records of births and deaths from 1584. The data were superior to the London bills of mortality because they provided the ages of death, but no data were available on the size of the population. Halley estimated the size of the population using the number of births and the mortality rates at each age. He was forced to make the invalid assumption of a stationary population, with no migration into or out of the city. Migration affects not only the size of the population, but also its age distribution and birth and mortality rates, because most immigrants are healthy young adults in the prime childbearing ages. Halley developed the first modern life table, which began with the number of persons born and estimated the proportion surviving at each succeeding age up to age 84. Although the table was used by the first English life insurance company, it relied on so many dubious assumptions that it could never serve as the basis for the development of life insurance as an industry.[13]

Probability mathematicians soon realized that life tables provided a fruitful source of data. The risk of dying was in many respects analogous to the risks involved in gambling. Once population and mortality data were gathered periodically, it became possible to analyze the data in the same way as games of chance. In the eighteenth century governments asked mathematicians to apply probability theory to the annuities that they issued to raise money. The annuitant paid the government a sum of money (which the government treated as income) and received a fixed percentage of the amount plus interest as an annual payment thereafter. The earliest annuities had failed to consider such crucial factors as the age of the annuitants, often with financially disastrous results.[14]

The development of life tables for annuities and life insurance required that the mathematicians have skills other than computational ones. The problem is that unavoidable errors in the prediction of death rates have opposing consequences for life insurance and annuities. If the calculations overestimate the number of future deaths, fewer deaths will occur in practice and a life insurance plan will pay out less money in death benefits than was budgeted. If the same error is made for an annuity, fewer people will die and more people will be alive to collect their annuities. The annuity plan will therefore pay out more money than was budgeted, sometimes with financially ruinous consequences. Consequently a life insurance life table must overestimate the number of deaths to reduce its risk, while an annuity life table must underestimate the number of deaths for precisely the same reason. The mathematicians who constructed the life tables had to combine a knowledge of probability, statistics, the uses of the tables, and the commercial requirements of the life insurance industry. These conditions eventually produced the new profession of actuary.

Statistics and the Smallpox Inoculation Controversy

The smallpox inoculation controversy was the most striking medical application of mortality statistics in the eighteenth century. Smallpox replaced plague as the major epidemic disease in England in the late seventeenth and eighteenth centuries. Unlike plague, which practically disappeared between epidemics, smallpox was an endemic disease that flared up periodically in epidemics. In many respects smallpox was considered even more horrifying than plague: children were especially vulnerable; a few of the survivors suffered from gross disfigurement or blindness; and smallpox continued to infect the population between epidemics.[15]

It was well known that an attack of smallpox immunized the person against further attacks. This led to various methods of inducing mild cases in children, such as by inserting crusts from the pustules of smallpox victims into small incisions made in the arms of healthy individuals, later called inoculation or variolation. English visitors observed professional inoculators performing inoculations in Constantinople after 1700. This practice aroused great interest in inoculation among English aristocratic families, where smallpox was so prevalent that the survival of titled families was considered to be endangered. Under these conditions aristocratic families were willing to take risks with their children that middle-class families with less to lose might avoid.[16]

Interest in inoculation produced one of the first clinical trials in the history of medicine. With royal permission, in 1721 six male and female prisoners ages 19 to 36, who had been condemned to death, volunteered to be inoculated under the promise of pardons. The five prisoners who had not previously had the disease recovered from obvious cases of smallpox without incident. To verify the efficacy of the procedure, one of the women prisoners nursed hospital patients for six weeks at a town with a severe epidemic without contracting the disease. The following year, the Prince of Wales had his daughters inoculated safely, and other royal families followed his practice. By the end of 1722 more than 182 inoculations had been performed by fifteen inoculators, most of whom were physicians.[17]

Despite the royal imprimatur, inoculation became extremely controversial in England, which led to efforts to evaluate the procedure. Smallpox was a particularly suitable disease for analysis because the clearcut symptoms made the diagnosis of the victims straightforward. Most of the victims were young and otherwise in good health, so that few of them were suffering from other illnesses that could cause their deaths. In a country where the weekly bills of mortality had been analyzed, discussed, and cited in publications for over a century, statistical analyses appeared to be the obvious method of evaluating the efficacy of inoculation. In 1722 an English physician collected information on a number of smallpox cases and found deaths reported for 19 of 100 who contracted smallpox in the natural way compared to none of 61 who were inoculated. In 1721, Zabdiel Boylston, a physician in Boston, Massachusetts, inoculated patients during a local epidemic and found that 2 percent of the 247 patients whom he inoculated died compared to about 15 percent of those who contracted the disease naturally, based on statistics compiled by the Boston selectmen.[18]

In 1722, James Jurin, an English physician who was a student of Isaac Newton, published an analysis of the available statistics on inoculation, comparing the inoculation results in England and Boston to bills of mortality that listed death rates from smallpox before the introduction of inoculation. The percentage of those who died after contracting smallpox naturally was about 12% early in the century, rising to 15–20% in more recent epidemics, while fewer than 2% died as a result of inoculations. Jurin updated his reports annually with additional data until 1727, and a follow-up report by another physician in 1728 reported that only 17 of 845 inoculated persons reported (2%) died from smallpox.[19]

As statistical evidence of the benefits of inoculation accumulated, general agreement was reached among both physicians and laypersons that inoculation lowered mortality rates significantly. The consensus appears to have been reached jointly and not to have resulted from efforts of physicians to convince laypersons. By mid-century the major controversies among physicians had dwindled to the techniques of inoculation. Because inoculated patients could spread the more virulent form of the disease to others while they were ill, hospitals and other institutions began to perform inoculations and care for the patients until their recoveries.[20]

Attitudes toward inoculation varied among countries. Some places, like Holland and Geneva, adopted the practice readily. Others, like France, took decades to adopt it, with only the aristocracy using it in the early years. Jurin's report was translated into French in 1725 by an enthusiastic supporter, but critics contended that year-to-year variations in the severity of the disease made the statistics unreliable and that the English and French populations were not comparable. Oddly, given the eminence of French mathematicians, the French did not compile their own statistics but relied on the English data, perhaps because few French physicians were skilled in mathematics.[21]

Statistics and French Medicine

Pierre Charles Louis (1787–1872), a noted French physician, was among the first to urge the application of statistics to clinical medicine in the early nineteenth century. Louis claimed that therapeutics had failed to progress because of "the method pursued, or rather to the want of method." He proposed a numerical method that quantified the available facts, arguing that widely used terms like "more or less, rarely or frequently" lacked scientific precision. Louis's method consisted of taking two or more groups of patients and observing the effects of different treatments or no treatment on them. The survival rates of each group could be calculated and compared, which provided a statistical measure of the benefits of the treatment and enabled several treatments to be compared to each other.[22]

Louis recognized that the numerical method depended on groups of similar patients with the same disease. He admitted that it was extremely difficult to find cases of a disease that were "alike in every particular." It was equally difficult to find large numbers of patients who were similar in their personal characteristics and general state of health, which would affect the outcomes regardless of the treatment used. In his most perspicacious insight, Louis realized that this difficulty was the great advantage of statistical comparisons of groups of patients: "by so doing, the errors, (which are inevitable,) being the same in two groups of patients subjected to different treatments, mutually compensate each other, and they may be disregarded without sensibly affecting the exactness of the results." In other words, if large numbers of patients are placed randomly in different groups, the proportion of people with various personal characteristics—men and women, old and young, very ill and moderately ill—will be about the same in each group. Thus the two groups will be similar in all respects except the treatment, which must therefore be responsible for any differences in the rates of the various outcomes.[23]

Unfortunately, Louis failed to understand many of the complexities involved in the use of the numerical method. His samples of patients rarely exceeded a few dozen cases, which produced wide variations in outcome rates from study to study and frequent inconsistencies in findings. In addition, Louis could never be sure that the differences in outcomes between the groups were large enough to permit unequivocal conclusions. In one study he found that 18 of 41 cases (44%) who were administered bloodlettings during the first four days of their illness died, compared to 9 of 36 cases (25%) bled after four days. The small number of cases made it difficult to compare the proportions. Louis himself conceded that the numerical method could produce data that were "startling and absurd." His own conclusions were no more precise than those he decried from physicians who did not use the numerical method. Louis never provided any evidence, even of the most rudimentary kind, to support his contention that the numerical method was superior to other methods.[24]

Other French physicians who used the numerical method were also unable to demonstrate its advantages over other methods. Weisz examined the evaluation of new therapies in the debates of the Paris Academy of Medicine in the second quarter of the nineteenth century and found a growing use of statistics but no reduction in controversy. Critics of studies of new surgical procedures observed that survival rates were affected by choosing healthier patients for surgery and sicker patients for no surgery and by differences in surgical techniques. The physicians differed in their definitions of specific diseases and their criteria for cures. Many physicians rejected statistics and retained their belief in the uniqueness of each case of disease.[25]

Other physicians attacked the philosophical basis of statistics and urged scientific certainty as a goal for medicine. The most famous was Louis's countryman, Claude Bernard (1813–1878), a pioneer in the use of experimental methods in physiology. His 1865 treatise, *An Introduction to the Study of Experimental Medicine,* claimed that laboratory investigation enabled the new biomedical sciences and clinical medicine to achieve the same methodological rigor and deterministic conclusions that he erroneously believed characterized astronomy and other natural sciences.[26]

Bernard shared Louis's belief that progress in clinical medicine was impeded by the fact that individual patients experienced a disease in dissimilar ways and responded differently to treatment. Louis proposed that patients be grouped, and statistics, such as rates and averages, calculated for each of the groups. Bernard preferred to search for the factors that caused the individual differences. Once the causes of the differences were discovered, each patient's outcomes could be predicted precisely. Bernard stated that the physician must "try to learn the conditions of these variations, for there can be no effect without a cause. Determinism thus becomes the foundation of all scientific progress and criticism" (69–70).

While Bernard accepted certain kinds of mathematics, he opposed the use of statistics such as averages because "an average description . . . will never be matched in nature," inasmuch as each case differs from the average. Averages are artifacts that "confuse, while aiming to unify, and distort while aiming to simplify." Once the true causes were discovered, all statistics were unnecessary: "As soon as the circumstances of an experiment are well known, we stop gathering statistics. . . . The effect will occur always without exception, because the cause of the phenomena is accurately defined. Only when a phenomenon includes conditions as yet undefined, can we compile statistics. . . . we compile statistics only when we cannot possibly help it; for in my opinion statistics can never yield scientific truth" (134–37).

Bernard presented a medical example to apply his views to clinical medicine:

> A great surgeon performs operations for stone by a single method; later he makes a statistical summary of deaths and recoveries, and he concludes from these statistics that the mortality law for this operation is two out of five. Well, I say that this ratio means literally nothing scientifically and gives us no certainty in performing the next operation; for we do not know whether the next case will be among the recoveries or the deaths. (137)

Bernard's solution was conceptually straightforward: "In the patient who succumbed, the cause of death was evidently something which was not found in the patient who recovered; this something we must determine, and then we can act on the phenomena or recognize and foresee them accurately." Medicine treats individual patients, and "the law of large numbers never teaches us anything about any particular case. What a physician needs to know is whether his patient will recover, and only the search for scientific determinism may lead to this knowledge" (137–38).

Bernard failed to recognize the theoretical and practical impossibility of predicting the outcome of disease in each individual patient with total certainty. Although he realized that multiple factors affect the development of disease and the outcome of treatment, he refused to admit the impossibility of identifying and measuring every one of the factors. In addition, each factor has an influence on the others, so that each particular configuration of factors must be differentiated from all other configurations. As an example using only three factors, blood pressure level, body weight, and age, each affects the probability of developing coronary heart disease, but the effect of a particular blood pressure level is different at each age and each body weight. The number of factors plus the combinations of factors that affect disease are so large and so varied that each human being is effectively unique. Thus it is impossible both in theory and practice to have data from other identical individuals that can be used to make precise predictions about a particular case. Predictions based on probabilities are the only option.

In addition, medicine is evolving continuously and every new method of diagnosis and treatment creates uncertainty because it must be evaluated and compared to existing treatments. By the time many of these questions have been resolved, still newer methods of diagnosis and treatment have become available. Bernard witnessed but did not learn from the revolution in surgery of the late 1840s, triggered by the discovery of anesthetics, which created new uncertainties for surgeons that took decades to clarify.

Bernard also failed to address the issue of the surgeon's response to a patient with a kidney stone who arrived in his office immediately after he has calculated the mortality rate. Should the surgeon advise the patient to wait for greater knowledge, which might take years or decades? Bernard was trained as a physician and knew that the practice of medicine cannot wait for the discovery of all of the factors that determine the outcome of treatment. Decisions must be made when they are needed, using existing knowledge.

Bernard's belief in scientific determinism was closely associated with his methodology; he held that "the true sanctuary of medical science is a laboratory" where the physician will "achieve true medical science" by using experimental methods to understand disease in animals. Even though each experiment produced somewhat different findings, Bernard claimed that "we must . . . present our most perfect experiment as a type, which, however, still stands for true facts." (146–47, 135) Investigators today (and many in Bernard's time) reject the belief that perfect experiments are possible or that science should be based on experiments that do not exist in reality. Instead, variations among experiments should be analyzed using statistics.

Bernard conceded that statistics were useful as a temporary expedient, but insisted that the goal of science was to produce results so precise that all uncertainty was eliminated:

> I do not . . . reject the use of statistics in medicine, but I condemn not trying to get beyond them and believing in statistics as the foundation of medical science. . . . Statistics . . . apply only to cases in which the cause of the facts observed is still [uncertain or] indeterminate. . . . There will always be some indeterminism . . . in all the sciences, and more in medicine than in any other. But man's intellectual conquest consists in lessening and driving back

indeterminism in proportion as he gains ground for determinism by the help of the experimental method. (138–40).

Although Bernard's theories were accepted by many as the intellectual foundation for the biomedical sciences, few physicians in his lifetime considered scientific determinism to be a useful goal for clinical medicine. Bernard himself conceded: "I have heard old practitioners say that the words 'always' and 'never' should be crossed out of medicine." For these physicians medicine was based on the uniqueness of the individual patient, and they eschewed both determinism and statistics (70).

Thus medical statistics experienced two major difficulties in France in the nineteenth century: physicians like Pierre Louis, who accepted statistics, found that quantification did not resolve controversies; and medical scientists like Bernard opposed the use of statistics as antithetical to their deterministic goals for medicine. If support for statistics was so tenuous in France, where most of the world's greatest probability mathematicians lived or were trained, it was even weaker in other countries. Evidence of its benefits for medicine had to come from sources outside the medical community. As the English inoculation controversy demonstrated, many nonphysicians found statistics to be extremely useful and they assumed leadership in the movement to quantify both medical and nonmedical aspects of human behavior.

3

CENSUSES AND VITAL STATISTICS

Deaths, births, and marriages, considering how much they are separately dependent on the freedom of the human will, should seem to be
subject to no law according to which any calculation could be made
beforehand of their amount; and yet the yearly registers of these events
in great countries prove that they go on with as much conformity to
the laws of nature as the [seasonal variations] of the weather.

(Immanuel Kant, 1784)[1]

One of the greatest advances in modern public health and medicine was
the enumeration of mortality and disease rates and their longitudinal trends
for the total population and for age, sex, locality, and other groups. This
great innovation resulted from the discovery that statistics on births, deaths,
and other social behaviors in geographic regions showed striking regularities from year to year. The enumerations were soon recognized as being of
great practical value by governments. The United States government pio-
neered in developing the census while European governments assumed leadership in vital statistics.

Public health and medicine were held back for centuries by the inability to
obtain the most basic quantitative information: the proportion of the population that died each year; death rates by age, sex, and other characteristics;

death rates by cause of death; and birth rates. The lack of interest was based on two beliefs: with rare exceptions, deaths and births were private affairs of interest only to the families involved; and the rates varied so much from year to year that enumerations would be of little value.

In the late eighteenth and early nineteenth centuries, some European governments began to publish occasional statistics on births, deaths, and marriages. Observers were amazed to discover that the statistics were remarkably consistent from year to year. As examples, the number of suicides in France varied between a low of 1,542 and a high of 2,048 annually between 1827 and 1831, and accidental deaths varied between 4,478 and 5,048 annually over the same period. Yet each suicide results from a highly idiosyncratic individual decision and each accidental death is unpredictable by definition.[2]

In the 1820s the French courts began to publish annual statistical summaries of criminal actions brought before them and these also showed striking regularities. For example, the number of murders each year varied between a low of 205 and a high of 266 between 1826 and 1831, and the number of persons charged with crimes against persons varied between 1,666 and 2,046 between 1826 and 1831. Adolphe Quetelet (1796–1874), a pioneer in the statistical movement, observed in dismay: "Sad condition of humanity! We might even predict annually how many individuals will stain their hands with the blood of their fellow-men, how many will be forgers, how many will deal in poison, pretty nearly in the same way as we may foretell the annual births and deaths." Conviction rates of criminals were equally predictable, with guilty verdicts varying between a low of 54% and a high of 62% between 1826 and 1831.[3]

Although these data showed remarkable consistency, year-to-year variations of as much as 25% were common. Mathematicians and laypeople accepted these variations as fully compatible with a pattern of consistency. They recognized that random variations were inevitable in social statistics and did not diminish their utility. Unlike Claude Bernard and others, they did not believe that absolute precision was or should be the goal of the science of human behavior.

The discovery of regularities in social statistics had a profound influence on both the social and natural sciences. Many saw an analogy with the history of astronomy, the leading natural science. Astronomers described the predictable motions of stars and planets in the sixteenth century even though the phenomena remained unexplained until Isaac Newton formulated the laws of gravity in the next century. Yet the discovery was quickly applied with great success to assist maritime navigation. Social behavior was also highly predictable and social statistics had many practical applications in the absence of general laws. Even physics was influenced by social statistics. James Clerk Maxwell (1831–1879), who formulated the kinetic theory of gases, compared the statistical regularities of the motions of large numbers of molecules to the statistical regularities of the behavior of human groups and argued that both kinds of data were of great practical utility without being absolutely precise.[4]

Governments soon recognized the value of statistics as social and economic indicators to use in formulating public policies. Those nations capable of doing so began to gather systematic statistics about their populations and major social institutions.

The Census

The modern census was one of the most important social inventions of the nineteenth century and provided a multitude of social indicators of hitherto unimagined quality and scope. Censuses were particularly useful in placing mortality patterns in a meaningful context. Before censuses, the number of deaths in any time period from an epidemic or endemic disease could often be enumerated with some accuracy, but ignorance of the size of the population at risk made it impossible to know the severity of the disease. Population censuses enabled the number of deaths to be related to the size of the population.

Censuses had been used for thousands of years, with Roman censuses often cited as the first use. For many centuries census enumerations were used primarily as a basis for taxation and military conscription, which aroused public hostility and instigated widespread deception. The potential for civil disobedience at best and mass violence at worst discouraged all but the most ruthless governments from undertaking rigorous censuses. Furthermore, before the nineteenth century most governments consisted of small central bureaucracies and semi-autonomous local or regional governments. The central governments lacked the personnel and other resources necessary to conduct their own enumerations and were unable to compel the local governments to carry out the work for them.[5]

Governments were often wary of gathering statistics because other governments might learn facts about their nations that they did not want divulged, such as the size of key industries or the populations of sparsely populated border regions that were difficult to defend. The number of men available for conscription was an important military secret in an era when wars were fought by hand-to-hand combat. By the mid-eighteenth century, however, probability and statistics had progressed to a stage where any resourceful statistician could easily estimate many of these numbers using rudimentary statistics. For example, the number of births in a year could be used to estimate the number of women of childbearing age, which in turn could be used to estimate the number of men available for military conscription. Governments therefore made strenuous efforts to keep all statistical data concerning their populations from potential enemies. The practical impossibility of doing this made many governments realize that the best strategy was not to compile any statistics at all.[6]

As a result, during most of the eighteenth century population statistics, which was then called political arithmetic, was left to private individuals and groups. While many of those who gathered such data were well meaning and devoted to improving the condition of their countries, they lacked the resources to gather comprehensive and accurate data. Some also had strong ideological beliefs that influenced their analyses. George Rosen, the eminent historian of public health, concluded that in 1776 "Adam Smith probably expressed the opinion of many of his contemporaries with his statement: 'I have no great faith in political arithmetic.'"[7]

Late in the eighteenth century, governments began to recognize that statistical enumerations were so important that they outweighed the risks involved. Enumerations were undertaken for a variety of purposes, such as quantifying the production of goods and foodstuffs, but the most crucial information was the growth and characteristics of the population. Increases in agricultural and industrial production depended on increases in the labor force. Military power depended on the number of men available for conscription. Growing urbanization created the need to care for the unemployed, widows, orphans, and dependent groups like the insane and idiots. Enumerations of the total number of persons and the numbers in various geographic regions became essential to the operation of governments at all levels. The result was the development of the modern census during the early nineteenth century.

A population census of a community or a nation has several components. It is an enumeration of all individuals in a specified political jurisdiction on a specified date by their name, sex, age, locality, and possibly other characteristics. The enumerators ask a predetermined set of questions, so that variations in phrasings will not influence the responses. A central administrative office makes and standardizes all important policies and reviews and processes all completed questionnaires. A census is repeated at regular intervals, which enables governments to ascertain trends in the characteristics measured in the census. Statistics may be calculated for the country as a whole, for specific regions and localities, and for age, sex, and other groups.

None of the censuses undertaken in European countries during the eighteenth century had the characteristics specified above. Most of them utilized parish records gathered by clergy or information provided by heads of local or regional governments. The government thus did not obtain the statistics by direct enumeration but used third parties whose decisions and actions were not under its control. The enumerators omitted many persons and often did not obtain the same information from each individual.[8]

The United States was the first nation to undertake regular direct enumerations of its population. Before independence the British Board of Trade had requested periodic enumerations of the populations of the individual colonies. Although most enumerations were incomplete or inaccurate, a few went beyond simple population counts or estimates to include classifications by race, sex, age, and marital status. These censuses laid the groundwork for future enumerations.[9]

After independence, the census became one of the most important functions of the executive branch of the national government, which was responsible for carrying out the constitutional requirement that the number of representatives from each state in the House of Representatives be determined by a decennial census of the population. All residents were required by law to provide the necessary information to census enumerators, an indispensable requirement for an accurate and complete enumeration. The censuses from 1790 to 1810 were not censuses by modern standards because enumerators were told to ascertain the number of individuals in each family, but to list only the names of each family head.[10]

The 1820 census established an entirely new method of gathering census data. Enumerators were given written instructions and definitions of important terms so that they all used identical procedures, made similar decisions, and obtained comparable information. They were told to list the number of individuals in a family as of a specific date, regardless of the date of the interview, and to disregard changes in the family after that date. The enumerators were instructed to obtain the information "by an actual inquiry, at every dwelling house, or of the head of each family, and not otherwise." They were directed to record the name of the head of the family, who may be "a master, mistress, steward, overseer, or other principal person therein." They were to list the occupations of all persons in the family engaged in "agriculture, commerce, and manufactures" and warned that this "will not be without its difficulties because many persons will claim to be employed in all three simultaneously." The individual was to be the unit used to determine occupation, not the family (a common confusion in an era of family farms), and the occupation should be "the principal and not the occasional, or incidental, occupation of his life." Manufacturing workers were defined as both those who worked in "manufacturing establishments" and mechanics and others "whose labor is predominantly of the hand, and not upon the field" (133–36).

Further refinements were made in the next census in 1830. Each enumerator was given copies of questionnaires with the interrogatories printed at the head of columns and was told to fill out a single line for each family. The family (then the basic unit of enumeration of the census) was redefined by the exclusion of family members "whose usual abode was not in the family they are enumerating" on the census day (131, 140).

The most revolutionary changes occurred in 1850 and constituted a fundamental advance in the use of uniform definitions and detailed instructions. The unit of enumeration was made the individual rather than the family, which was fundamental to any analyses of population characteristics. Enumerators were given specific instructions concerning each question in the interview schedule. For example, the individual "dwelling house" was defined as a "separate inhabited tenement, containing one or more families under one roof" that could also be used for "a store, shop, or for other purposes." A family was defined as one or more persons "living together . . . upon one common means of support, and separately from others in a house or part of a house" (later called a household). Each person "whose usual place of abode" (place of abode being defined as "the house or usual lodging place of a person") on the census day was with a family was to be listed separately by name. Methods of enumerating sailors, students, and others temporarily away from home were explained (150–51).

The 1870 census made further progress by providing greater detail and more useful examples to the enumerators. Place of birth of the foreign-born was made more specific, for example Scotland rather than Great Britain. Enumerators were told that "it will not do to assume that, because a person can read, he can, therefore, write. . . . Very many persons who will claim to be able to read, though they really do so in the most defective manner, will frankly admit that they can not write." Occupation, which was called "one of the most important questions of this schedule," became a greater coding problem with the rise of factory labor. Enumerators were told to "make a study of it. . . . Call no man a 'factory hand' or a 'mill operative.' State the kind of mill or factory. . . . Do not call a man a 'shoemaker, 'bootmaker,' unless he makes the entire boot or shoe in a small shop. If he works in (or for) a boot and shoe factory, say so." Farm laborers were distinguished from farmers. A multitude of useful examples were provided, including cases where greater specificity was not desired. Enumerators were told that "the organization of domestic service has not proceeded so far in this country as to render it worth while to make distinction in the character of work." Enumerators were also told they were "under no obligation to give any man's occupation just as he expresses it. If he cannot tell intelligibly what he *is,* find out what he *does,* and characterize his profession accordingly" (154–59).

Census authorities also recognized that the demeanor and behavior of the enumerators affected the responses. In enumerating the "deaf and dumb, blind, insane or idiotic," enumerators in 1870 were instructed to exert "great care . . . so as at once to secure completeness and avoid giving offense." They were advised, in a concise description of the existing state of knowledge, that "the fact of idiocy will be better determined by the common consent of the neighborhood, than by attempting to apply any scientific measure to the weakness of the mind or will." The need to obtain the respondent's willing cooperation was emphasized:

> [Enumerators will] make as little show as possible of authority. They will approach every individual in a conciliatory manner; respect the prejudices of all; adapt their inquiries to the comprehension of foreigners and persons of limited education, and strive in every way to relieve the performance of their duties from the appearance of obtrusiveness. Anything like an overbearing disposition should be an absolute disqualification for the position. (158, 156)

In the 1880 census, the analyses and publications assumed major proportions. While the 1870 census was published in three volumes, the 1880 census encompassed twenty-two separate volumes totalling 21,000 pages and the final reports were not issued until 1888. The great increase was caused by the multiplication of questionnaires or schedules for individual industries, agriculture, husbandry, municipal governments, public and private educational systems, libraries, dependent populations, and mortality, an expansion that had begun in 1840. The total number of inquiries or detailed questions on all schedules combined increased from four in 1790 to 20 in 1820, 82 in 1840, 156 in 1870, and more than 13,000 in 1880 and 1890. Supervision of enumerators was much improved, tabulations were made more accurate, and experts were used to analyze data and write special reports (57, 68–69, 87).

Thus during its first century the census changed from being a crude enumeration of the population to a statistical inventory of the nation's population and resources. Some of the additional data were designed to be used in the care of the sick and dependent populations. As an example, in enumerating groups like the insane, "mentally and physically defective" (divided into specific categories), criminals, and institutionalized homeless children and paupers, the enumerators were instructed in 1880 and 1890 that "the object [is] not only for a complete enumeration of the insane, but for an account of their condition" (199–200 and passim).

During this same period the role of the census office in Washington was greatly expanded. The earliest publications simply printed the returns as received, with no effort to correct errors or to standardize information among states—for instance, some states listed populations by county while others did not. The 1830 census was the first in which the returns were revised and corrected in the central office in Washington. In that and subsequent censuses, the Washington office (in the Department of State up to 1840, and in the newly established Department of the Interior in 1850 and thereafter) assumed full responsibility for determining precisely how each census was to be carried out and reported. The entire census office was disbanded after each decennial census despite its growing complexity until 1902, when Congress established a permanent Bureau of the Census.[11]

European nations also began to undertake periodic censuses in the nineteenth century. In France the first census was undertaken in 1836 as a census of families and households, and the first census of individuals was undertaken in 1876, but only four censuses were completed between 1836 and 1901. The 1901 census was the first to be conducted by a central authority. On the other hand, the city of Paris conducted a well-planned and carefully organized census in 1817 and six more quinquennial censuses between 1831 and 1856. Beginning in 1821 a series of statistical publications (the *Researches Statistiques sur la Ville de Paris*) provided, according to the historian, William Coleman, "a collection of demographic data without parallel in its time and the model for many a subsequent census."[12]

In England the first decennial census was undertaken in 1801, when local officials were asked to provide statistical summaries (without names, addresses, or ages) of the population. This practice remained unchanged in 1811, 1821, and 1831. In 1837 the newly established General Register Office under William Farr assumed responsibility for the census. The 1841 census was the first to meet most of the criteria for a census, using the individual as the unit of enumeration and obtaining the ages of the respondents. Marital status was not included until 1851.[13]

Especially impressive early censuses were conducted in Belgium under the leadership of Adolph Quetelet. All of them showed care in questionnaire design and analyses, and provided cross-tabulations by characteristics like time, place, age, and sex. The 1846 census, which used the individual as the unit of enumeration and asked many useful questions, had a significant influence on the modifications made in the 1850 United States census.[14]

Thus by the mid-nineteenth century, censuses had adopted a methodology that permitted the collection of large amounts of quantitative data amenable to statistical analyses. Census officials focused on continual improvements in the accuracy and completeness of the data, not on mathematical techniques of analysis. They recognized that complete, accurate, and unbiased data were essential prerequisites for useful statistical analyses.

Vital Statistics

Vital statistics comprise records of births, deaths, and often marriages in a locality or a country. The original purpose of vital statistics was to verify names and dates of persons involved in births, marriages, and deaths in order to decide legal matters such as the heirs of estates or the legitimacy of offspring. In the nineteenth century the data were recognized as being equally essential for understanding the state of health of a nation.[15]

Because the need for legal records of births, deaths, and marriages antedated competent government bureaucracies, ecclesiastical authorities throughout Europe assumed responsibility for recording the events. By the end of the sixteenth century the established churches in England and France and the Council of Trent of the Roman Catholic Church required individual parishes to maintain records of baptisms, marriages, and burials. However, such records failed to enumerate the many newborn infants who died before baptism, those buried privately, usually on family farms, the unchurched, and those who could not pay the fees for the ceremonies. Furthermore, central church authorities were often unable to compel individual parishes to maintain accurate records or to submit them for compilation or analysis. During the eighteenth century the established church in France formally required individual parishes to maintain accurate records and submit them annually to a central authority, where they were occasionally compiled into national statistics.[16]

In the eighteenth century, as more persons adopted religions other than the established church of the country, they began to demand the right to register their births, marriages, and deaths. The demands produced a long period of agitation throughout Europe for the establishment of civil registration of vital statistics. In France, Protestants were provided civil registration in 1787, and civil records replaced religious ones in the early 1790s after the French revolution. However, municipal officials generally replaced parish priests as the initial recorders of vital statistics only in the 1820s. In England, after a long period of agitation and the courts' rejection of parish baptismal records as legal evidence by the 1830s, legislation in 1836 created the General Register Office as a national office to collect, maintain, and compile records received from local officials on births, deaths, and marriages. Death registration was made compulsory, but birth registration remained optional until 1874 in deference to sensitivities about illegitimate births.[17]

Despite the legal requirements, most countries did not compile accurate vital statistics for many years. Local officials often failed to maintain or transmit their records to the central authorities or to compel physicians and midwives to report all births and deaths. In England about 1900 it was estimated that more than 10,000 infant deaths went unrecorded in the large cities annually. The determination of cause of death was also a problem. Under the 1836 English law, anyone could report the cause of death, which rendered the data useless, but by 1870 physicians certified the causes of over 90% of all deaths and in 1874 medical certification was made compulsory.[18] This did not eliminate the problem completely, but it reduced the sources of error.

By the 1880s, an estimated 350 million people throughout the world, mostly in Europe, resided in areas where births and deaths were registered, compared to 100 million in the 1830s. Large cities were much better able to enforce civil registration of births and deaths than rural areas.[19] They had the resources to establish bureaucracies to gather and compile statistics and to compel physicians and midwives to report the births. The widespread use of cemetery burials in cities enabled municipalities to require undertakers to obtain death certificates prior to interment.

The gathering and compiling of vital statistics in the United States lagged decades behind that of every other western nation. In 1918, S. N. D. North, at one time director of the Bureau of the Census, complained: "It is humiliating to know that in vital statistics the United States stands at the foot of the nations of like rank in civilization." The problem was that each state bore sole responsibility for gathering its own vital statistics with, according to North, "total indifference on the part of the officials in most of them."[20]

Early in the nineteenth century some American cities required registration of deaths and sometimes births, but none of them enforced the laws. Official mortality statistics were published in New York in 1804, Boston in 1813, Philadelphia in 1825, Charleston in 1834, Baltimore in 1836, and Providence in 1841. Some northeastern and midwestern states enacted death registration laws in the 1840s and 1850s, but few were enforced and some were later repealed. In Massachusetts, the most progressive state with regard to vital statistics, registration laws were enacted in 1842, 1844, and 1849, but it was estimated that 13% of deaths and 20% of births went unrecorded in 1850. By 1870 practically all deaths in Massachusetts were thought to be reported, but only 90% of births. As late as 1910 the Secretary of the Commonwealth of Massachusetts complained that "a great many physicians neglect entirely to report the births at which they are present."[21]

The registration laws failed for several reason. The requirements were of no interest to working-class and rural persons, who had no legal need for them. Most residents of rural areas lived many miles from the registrars who recorded the information and often failed to report births and deaths. Many overworked registrars considered recording and compiling the information to be unnecessary burdens. The American Medical Association and most local and state medical societies were indifferent to or opposed reporting, stating that physicians should not be asked to bear the burden of completing and filing the necessary forms.[22]

The federal government began to enumerate mortality statistics in the 1850 census using a separate schedule that obtained personal information concerning all those who died in the past twelve months. The data were grossly inaccurate because respondents were often unable to recall the dates accurately and provide other information. In 1880 and 1890, in an effort to improve data on the cause of death, enumerators were instructed to list the "name of the primary disease," all complications, as well as the part of the body affected. They were warned to distinguish between typhoid, typhus, and typho-malarial fevers and to understand the differences between apoplexy, epilepsy, and paralysis. They were instructed to avoid terms like old age, intemperance, debility, or sudden death as causes of death. They were asked to visit each physician who attended the deceased for confirmation of the cause of death. Enumerators had neither the skills nor the time to devote to these tasks.[23]

In 1880, John S. Billings devised a new approach that eventually replaced enumeration. In Massachusetts, New Jersey, and twenty cities elsewhere (including the District of Columbia), all of which had registered at least 90% of their deaths, the 1880 census accepted state or local records instead of conducting its own enumerations. This produced the concept of a "death registration area" that was extended in the 1890 census to include eight northeastern states and eighty-four cities elsewhere. In that census 47% of all deaths reported by the census occurred in the death registration area, which contained only 31% of the United States population. This demonstrated that the use of a death registration area produced much more accurate and complete data than retrospective reporting by individuals. The system was expanded in the 1900 census and included the requirement that states be admitted to the registration area only when they adopted a standard death certificate and acceptable state registration laws.[24]

The 1902 legislation that created the Bureau of the Census formalized the concept of both death and birth registration areas. It permitted the bureau to determine which states and municipalities kept accurate death and birth statistics and to collect records from them. The bureau, in agreement with the American Medical Association, the American Public Health Association, and the National Association of Funeral Directors, stated in its 1907 report that experience had shown that accurate death reporting was possible only where undertakers and others responsible for the disposal of bodies were required to obtain burial permits from a central registration office prior to burial. This was practical only in towns and cities, because many rural residents were buried on private land. With regard to birth statistics, the bureau reported in 1907 that "there is at present no state or city in the United States which is accepted as having even fairly complete registration of births (90 percent)," with the result that a birth registration area was not established until 1915. In 1908 the bureau quoted with approval a statement in the *Bulletin of the American Medical Association*:

> It comes as somewhat of a shock to one to realize that in a nation where a record is made of every legal procedure, of every business transaction and commercial liability, no matter how insignificant, where millions are spent each year in recording and preserving all real estate transactions, . . . yet in more than half of the United States a human being can be born and can die without any record being made or official notice being taken of the fact. . . . Careful record is kept of acreage and crops, as well as all diseases of plant and animal life. . . . while in more than one-half of the United States it is even impossible to tell how many persons succumb during any length of time to [tuberculosis] or any other form of disease.[25]

By the early twentieth century the American public realized that the effective functioning of a modern society depended on compulsory registration of births and deaths. Evidence of death was indispensable for inheritance rights and payment of pensions and life insurance policy claims. Birth certificates were essential for public health programs, work permits, marriage licenses, school attendance laws, and military enlistment. Date of birth was required for criminal issues like statutory rape and whether an offender was a minor or an adult. Burial without proof of lawful death permitted the blameless disposal of victims of the most nefarious crimes. Professional societies and trade associations began to press states to improve their vital statistics, and by 1912 the Association of Life Insurance Presidents, the American Bar Association, the American Medical Association, and the American Public Health Association all supported universal registration of births and deaths. Urban public health departments wanted birth registration laws so that they could contact the mothers of the newborns to enroll them in programs to prevent infant deaths.[26]

The number of states included in the death registration area increased to twenty-one in 1910 (plus the District of Columbia and cities in other states), thirty-four in 1920, and all forty-eight states then in the union in 1933. However, demographers like Walter Willcox questioned the completeness of the data. The seven states with the lowest death rates in 1930 had been admitted to the death registration area within the previous decade, which suggested that their record-keeping was still deficient. In 1920, three sparsely populated counties in Colorado with 12,000 inhabitants reported a total of two deaths. Any examination of mortality statistics in many rural states and counties during the first few decades of the twentieth century suggested that eternal life was not only possible, but fairly common.[27]

Birth registration posed a much greater problem than death registration, because most births occurred in homes and many were not attended by physicians or professional midwives. Thus births lacked an event comparable to a cemetery burial for which a registration form could be required. Incompleteness of birth registration was more easily recognized, however, because the number of registered births in the year preceding a census could be compared to the number of children under one year of age enumerated in the census. If the number of children under one year of age enumerated in the census year equaled or exceeded the number of registered births in the previous year, not all births had been registered.

A birth registration area was established in 1915, comprising ten states, the District of Columbia, and a number of cities, all of which claimed that they registered 90% or more of their births. However, Willcox concluded that in 1920 no more than five states and the District of Columbia had "reasonably complete" birth registration. Although all forty-eight states were included in 1933, it was not until 1950 that concerns about incompleteness were put to rest by a study showing that 98% of births had been registered.[28]

Thus the history of vital statistics shows a persistent confusion between the legal and statistical uses of the data. Completeness of reporting and standard cause-of-death categories are essential for statistical purposes but not for legal ones. Statistical reports seek to group the individual with similar others to permit the aggregation of data. Legal records are designed to provide proof of the event and to distinguish the individual from all others in terms of factors such as parentage and residence. Place of birth or death is important for legal purposes, whereas domicile or permanent residence is more important for statistical analyses.

Vital statistics and censuses provided for the first time in history accurate periodic enumerations of both the number of births and deaths in a locality or country and the size and composition of its population. It was now possible to compute death rates for the total population and for groups of different ages, sexes, and localities. Birth and death rates and their trends over time could be determined for the total population and particular groups and localities, and, for death rates, specific causes of death. This information revolutionized nineteenth-century public health and medicine and produced greater acceptance of the benefits of statistics.

4

STATISTICAL ANALYSES OF MEDICAL AND SOCIAL DATA

> The greater the number of individuals observed, the more do individual peculiarities, whether physical or moral, become effaced, and leave in a prominent point of view the general facts, by virtue of which society exists and is preserved.
>
> (Adolphe Quetelet, 1835)[1]

The discovery of regularities in social statistics led to efforts to use them to better understand the health and social conditions of the population. Physicians analyzed hospital and patient records and other investigators carried out social surveys of communities. Two investigators were especially effective in using statistics to understand health and disease. A physician, John Snow, used statistics to demonstrate the relationship between polluted water and the spread of cholera, and a statistician, Adolphe Quetelet, developed important new methods of categorizing and analyzing social and health data.

Hospital and Asylum Statistics

The discovery of regularities in social statistics and the researches of Pierre Louis soon led to statistical studies in many of the hospitals, dispensaries, and insane asylums established during the nineteenth century. These institutions brought together in one location large numbers of patients who were seriously ill and reasonably homogeneous because most were poor and urban. Hospitals were especially useful because the patterns of diseases among the poor in their communities could be measured by examining admissions and mortality rates and their trends for particular diseases and personal characteristics of the patients. Treatments could be evaluated because the patients could be retained in the hospital until the outcomes were certain and, if necessary, autopsied to determine the cause of death.

Many American physicians compiled hospital statistics and published them in medical journals and hospital annual reports. Although they believed they were providing quantitative descriptions of the health of the population, their methods were unsystematic and the samples inappropriate. The data were usually presented without explanations of their significance or comparisons with other hospitals or types of patients. Furthermore, hospital patients were atypical in that they were the urban poor in an era when most of the population was rural. They were in poor health because they were malnourished and lived in unhygienic conditions. They were very sick because most sought hospital care only when they could no longer be cared for at home.

The superintendents of insane asylums were among the most enthusiastic compilers of institutional statistics. A number of public and private insane asylums were constructed in the first half of the nineteenth century under the belief that proper asylum care could restore most mentally ill patients to health. With the goal of demonstrating the benefits of institutional care, the superintendents made their annual reports veritable statistical compendia of data concerning admissions, discharges, length of institutionalization, deaths, personal characteristics of patients, and types of illnesses. The statistics rarely demonstrated the conclusions that superintendents drew from them. Many annual reports showed high discharge rates, which superintendents considered cures. The rates, however, usually included discharges due to factors other than recovery and did not consider subsequent rehospitalizations of the patients. Most asylum superintendents were administrators who were ignorant of these and other statistical and methodological pitfalls. A few knowledgeable superintendents exposed the errors, which only reinforced the beliefs of many physicians that statistical data were more polemical than scientific.[2]

A few studies of asylums and other kinds of patients had a major impact on public policy. Massachusetts and other states had built insane asylums in central locations in order to serve the entire state. In 1850 Edward Jarvis (1803–1884), a psychiatrist who became president of the American Statistical Association and a consultant to the Census Bureau, carried out statistical analyses showing that the patients in Massachusetts insane asylums tended to have their homes near the asylums. Hence asylums located in different parts of the state would better serve the needs of the population than centralized ones. Jarvis's findings influenced asylum construction throughout the nation for many decades.[3]

Frank Hamilton (1813–86), an American physician, used statistics from community patients to influence the legal system. In the 1840s and 1850s malpractice suits increased steadily against physicians whose treatment of bone fractures resulted in shortening, imperfect alignment, or other deformities. Hamilton used statistics to disprove the claim that perfect healing was a reasonable expectation. His analysis of fractures of the femur (thighbone) can be used as an example of his method. He cited leading physicians throughout the centuries who considered shortening of the femur after a fracture to be the norm. He showed that shortening was often difficult to detect because a given amount of shortening produced a perceptible limp in some patients and none in others. Accurate measurements of the length of the two limbs required care and expertise and casual measurements could easily overlook a shortening of more than an inch.[4]

Hamilton had studied in France in the 1840s and was influenced by Louis's numerical method. He meticulously compiled and evaluated reports on many hundreds of fractures of different bones and obtained information on the age and sex of the patients, the length of time to recovery, and the outcomes, complications, and treatment. Hamilton conceded that his personal standards produced many fewer cases of "perfect" healing than other surgeons claimed, but asserted that if he had used less rigorous criteria, the surgical "art would have been less scandalized, but . . . truth would have been less faithfully vindicated."[5]

Unfortunately, Hamilton's meticulous data-gathering was not matched by his statistical expertise. He compiled 83 reports of cases of fractures of the shaft of the femur. In describing the ages of the cases, he reported only the range of ages (1 to 55 years) and the average age (17 years), but not the number of cases in specific age groups. He found that the average shortening was about 0.6 inches in 56 cases without serious complications. In the 47 of these cases with some amount of shortening, the average shortening was just over 0.75 inches and the maximum shortening was 3 inches. Hamilton provided no data on the number of cases with shortening of various lengths (e.g., less than 0.5 inches, 0.5 to 1 inch, etc.) and did not analyze shortening in different age groups, which was essential because children were much less likely than adults to experience permanent short-ening. Despite the limitations of his methods, Hamilton's study made him famous both as an author and a defense witness in malpractice suits. His statistics became obsolete with the introduction of plaster of Paris casts in the 1870s.[6]

Other statistical analyses by physicians were hampered by excessively rigid theories. Edward Jarvis, who was as methodical and meticulous as Hamilton, undertook a complete census of all of the insane in Massachusetts, a truly enormous undertaking for a single individual. He canvassed physicians, asylum superintendents, clergymen, local officials, jailkeepers, and others, as well as institutions in other states that might house insane residents of Massachusetts. Jarvis received replies from over eight hundred respondents and carefully checked the replies for problems such as duplicate names. Although he gathered data on characteristics such as age, sex, and place of residence, he discussed only two characteristics that he claimed were the predominant social causes of insanity: poverty and nationality, measured by place of birth. He found that there were 2.72 insane persons per 1,000 foreign-born population compared to 2.25 insane persons per 1,000 native-born population. This was far from a convincing difference, and would have been even smaller had children been excluded from the two populations, because the native-born population contained more children. The inclusion of children in the population increased the size of the native-born population compared to the foreign-born population and reduced its insanity rate. Critics also noted that incorrect diagnosis of many foreign-born adults who were actually mentally retarded exaggerated the number of foreign-born insane.[7]

Jarvis's statistical study of the prevalence of mental illness in an entire state did have considerable influence because it was addressed to policymakers, not the medical profession. It was intended to help determine the need for new insane asylums and other kinds of care. In trying to influence public policies, Jarvis was emulating an approach that had progressed much further in Europe than in the United States.

English Social Surveys

English investigators were the primary users of statistical research to understand the social and economic impact of industrialization and to influence public policy. Beginning in 1833, laypersons and government officials organized statistical societies in London and at least six other English cities and created a statistical section in the British Association for the Advancement of Science. An analysis by Abrams of 511 "themes treated in papers read" to the Statistical Society of London from 1838 to 1888 found that 25% concerned economic matters, ranging from finance to trade and industry; 19% concerned vital statistics; and 18% involved social conditions, including "poverty, crime, illiteracy," and other social problems of the poor. Only eleven papers, or 2%, concerned statistical methods.[8]

The English statistical societies carried out the first social or community surveys, which became the primary method of examining urban living conditions, including housing, rents, schools, food supplies, crime, health, medical care, and sanitation. Questionnaires were sent to local experts, such as members of school boards, government officials, and employers. Observers from the society visited the communities and gathered data through informal interviews, personal observations, and government statistics. The multiple measures of social conditions enabled the investigators to validate the usefulness of their statistics. For example, one study of the educational system in Manchester concluded that attendance statistics were "a very imperfect criterion" of the city's educational system because of the poor quality or lack of education provided in many schools.[9]

Another type of social survey was the neighborhood surveys of the London society, which examined problems like sanitary conditions and housing. Neighborhood surveys were primarily descriptive and evaluative rather than statistical, often with sweeping conclusions, such as the London neighborhood that was described as "a disgrace to a civilized society."[10]

John Snow and the Epidemiology of Cholera

Most early nineteenth-century statistical analyses described general disease patterns and trends but did not test hypotheses about the relationships between the diseases and their causes or modes of transmission. At that time methods for testing hypotheses or measuring relationships were in their formative stages. Laboratory experiments were just beginning to be used systematically. Statistical comparisons, such as the smallpox inoculation controversy and Pierre Louis's evaluations of treatments, were considered inferior to laboratory investigations. Nevertheless, a physician, John Snow, used statistical methods to carry out a brilliant and innovative investigation of the mode of transmission of cholera in London.

John Snow (1813–1858), who was the first English physician to specialize in the administration of anesthetics, shared the widespread interest in the periodic outbreaks of cholera that had replaced smallpox as the great epidemic disease. Three great cholera pandemics and numerous smaller outbreaks struck Europe, North America, and other parts of the world in the early and middle years of the nineteenth century. Using the research findings of his contemporaries, Snow concluded that human beings were the vector for spreading the disease because cholera always appeared in a country first at seaports and never attacked ship crews coming from countries free of the disease until they had contact with the shore of a country with the disease. Direct person-to-person transmission was not the primary means of transmitting the disease because the disease often did not develop among persons present in a room with a patient but did spread to many persons who had no contact with cholera patients.[11]

By reviewing research on cholera patients in the 1831–32 and 1849 English epidemics, Snow concluded that the first symptoms of cholera occurred in the "alimentary canal" or gastro-intestinal tract. Snow then reasoned that the matter producing cholera "must be introduced into the alimentary canal—must, in fact, be swallowed accidentally, for persons would not take it intentionally; and the increase of the morbid material, or cholera poison, must take place in the interior of the stomach and bowels." In a brilliantly prescient observation before bacteriology, Snow realized that the so-called "period of incubation . . . is, in reality, a period of reproduction, as regards the morbid matter; and the disease is due to the crop or progeny resulting from the small quantity of poison first introduced."[12]

Snow reasoned that the cholera "poison" spread from the victim to others through the evacuations of the victims and the "want of personal cleanliness, whether arising from habit or scarcity of water" among those caring for the patients. Their hands become soiled with the vomitus and excretions of the patient and unavoidably:

> they must accidentally swallow some of the excretion, and leave some on the food they handle or prepare, which has to be eaten by the rest of the family, who, amongst the working classes, often have to take their meals in the sick room; hence the thousands of instances in which, amongst this class of the population, a case of cholera in one member of the family is followed by other cases; whilst medical men and others, who merely visit the patients, generally escape. (16–17)

If personal contact was the only means by which cholera spread from person to person, the disease would be restricted to the poor. Snow concluded that it spread to the rest of the community when the cholera evacuations mixed with the family's waste water and permeated the water supply by soaking through the ground into wells or entering sewers that emptied into the rivers that supplied drinking water to the cities (22–23).

Thus Snow formulated two hypotheses concerning the spread of cholera as a water- borne infectious disease. He now searched for ways to verify: (1) that the "morbid matter" that caused cholera was present in the water supply; and (2) that those who drank the contaminated water were more likely to contract cholera than those who did not drink it. Snow had a microscopist examine some water that he suspected to be a cause of cholera. The microscopist "found a great number of very minute oval animalcules in the water," as had others. Because the germ theory was unknown at the time, Snow interpreted this as "of no importance, except as an additional proof that the water contained organic matter on which they lived." A few decades later, Robert Koch and others produced evidence that the "comma-shaped" bacillus was the bacterial etiological agent in cholera (52).

Snow was more successful in demonstrating that those who drank contaminated water were more likely to contract cholera than those who did not. In his search for a source of contaminated water, he excluded wells and other confined water supplies because they could produce limited outbreaks but not widespread epidemics. The most likely source of polluted water as a cause of widespread epidemics was the Thames River that flowed through London and provided most of its water supply. During summers, lack of rain reduced the Thames water flow and led to the accumulation of sewage that contained the evacuations of cholera patients (95).

At the time Snow was writing, most London houses obtained their water from underground pipes installed and owned by several private water companies, each of which drew its water supply from a different source or a different location on the Thames River. The remaining residents used pump-wells or drew water directly from the Thames River. Snow found that the highest death rates from cholera during the 1849 epidemic occurred in the districts served by one company that drew its water from a particularly polluted location on the Thames. The high death rates, however, could have been produced by other characteristics of the districts or their residents, such as their social classes (61–70).

During the 1854 epidemic, a unique opportunity presented itself to Snow. Due to previous competition for customers, the houses in one area of London south of the Thames were served by underground water pipes from two different water companies. In response to recently enacted legislation, one of the companies, the Lambeth company, had relocated its water works, "obtaining a supply of water quite free from the sewage of London" (68). The other, the Southwark and Vauxhall company, had not yet relocated its water works and continued to draw water from an area where raw sewage emptied into the Thames. The houses supplied by the two companies were distributed almost randomly in the district:

> [T]he mixing of the supply is of the most intimate kind. The pipes of each Company go down all the streets, and into nearly all the courts and alleys. A few houses are supplied by one company and a few by the other, according to the decision of the owner or occupier at that time when the Water Companies were in active competition. In many cases a single house has a supply different from that on either side. Each company supplies both rich and poor, both large houses and small. (74–75)

Here then was a unique opportunity for a natural experiment that divided a large number of people into two groups by essentially random decisions unrelated to social class or other obvious factors:

> The experiment . . . was on the grandest scale. No fewer than three hundred thousand people of both sexes, of every age and occupation, and of every rank and station, from gentlefolks down to the very poor, were divided into two groups without their choice, and, in most cases, without their knowledge; one group being supplied with water containing the sewage of London, and, amongst it, whatever might have come from the cholera patients, the other group having water quite free from such impurity. (75)

Snow obtained the names and addresses and personally visited the houses of every person who died from cholera in these districts during the first seven weeks of the epidemic. In cases where renters or others did not have verifiable knowledge of their water companies, Snow found that the sodium chloride content of the Southwark and Vauxhall water supply was much higher than that of the Lambeth water supply. A simple chemical test of a sample of the water from the house enabled him to obtain conclusive evidence of the water's source. Snow did not know the number of individuals living in the houses, but he did know the number of houses served by the two companies in the previous year and assumed that the average number of persons per house was about the same for the two companies. As a result he calculated the cholera death rates on a per-house basis rather than a per-person basis (77–78).

During the first seven weeks of the 1854 epidemic in twenty-one districts served by the two companies, Snow found by personal inquiry that 507 deaths occurred in 16,038 houses served by the Southwark and Vauxhall Company, which used polluted Thames River water, compared to

98 deaths in 20,554 houses served by the Lambeth company, which used unpolluted water. This corresponded to rates of 31.6 deaths per 1,000 houses served by the Southwark and Vauxhall Company and 4.8 deaths per 1,000 houses served by the Lambeth Company. Snow estimated the average number of residents per house in each subdistrict of the district and calculated that 4.7 cholera deaths occurred per 1,000 persons in houses supplied by the Southwark and Vauxhall Company, compared to 0.7 cholera deaths per 1,000 persons in houses served by the Lambeth company during the seven week period (183).

Snow's research was brilliant in its conceptual rigor, careful delineation of hypotheses, meticulous attention to detail in gathering the data, and thorough analyses. However, Snow became famous for an entirely different and inappropriate reason: the number of deaths from cholera dropped near a particular well after he had the pump handle removed.[13] The removal of the handle proved nothing, because no comparisons were made with deaths at other wells. It has appealed to many physicians and others because it falsely indicated that simplistic cause-and-effect relationships exist in medicine.

One striking finding of Snow's analysis was that many thousands of people drank the contaminated water but never contracted the disease. Snow explained this by saying that the "cholera-poison" was not present in every glassful of water. This is an unacceptable explanation because every person drank many glassfuls of water during the epidemic. The only acceptable explanation, which Snow did not discuss, was that cholera has multiple causes. The great majority of persons exposed to the bacterial pathogen did not contract cholera because they did not have other factors that produced the disease.[14]

Snow's other striking finding was that the group who drank the polluted water had only 0.4 more cholera deaths per hundred persons than the group who drank the unpolluted water. Such a small difference was hardly overwhelming support for his theory. Furthermore, the numbers resulted from the particular features of Snow's study: it was conducted for seven weeks in a specific district. Had Snow used more or fewer weeks or another district, each of the two death rates would have been different and the disparity between them would probably have been smaller or larger. It was therefore quite possible that the actual disparity was even less than 0.4 deaths per hundred. Snow was unable to test this possibility because the necessary statistical techniques were not devised until the twentieth century. Given the limitations of his study and the lack of support for statistical methods, it is not surprising that Snow's theory was not accepted until bacteriology verified the existence of the cholera bacillus.[15]

Other medical innovators also discovered that medical statistics could produce controversy rather than agreement. Joseph Lister (1827–1912), the great English surgeon, claimed in the late 1860s that his new antiseptic surgical techniques were superior to older ones and provided statistical evidence that compared his mortality rates to those obtained with non-antiseptic techniques. Other surgeons soon presented statistics showing that their non-antiseptic techniques produced equal or even lower mortality rates than Lister's. Lister's antiseptic techniques were still rudimentary and the other surgeons used equally sterile techniques without consciously applying the principles of antisepsis. Lister thereupon ceased making statistical comparisons.[16]

The Statistical Analyses of Adolphe Quetelet

Adolphe Quetelet (1796–1874) was the outstanding analyst of social statistics before the end of the nineteenth century. He was the first to apply descriptive statistics like averages and rates systematically to make comparisons among groups. He was the first to use this technique on a substantial scale to demonstrate that many important medical and social phenomena had multiple causes.

Quetelet was born in Belgium when it was still part of France, studied and later taught mathematics in Brussels, and became the astronomer at the Royal Observatory in Brussels in 1832. He was greatly influenced by French probability mathematicians, with whom he studied in 1823. Quetelet was called upon to direct the first Belgian census in 1829 and until his death was responsible for most Belgian government statistics, which became internationally renown under his leadership. Quetelet organized and became the first president of the International Statistical Congress in 1853. He acquired great fame during his lifetime, but his renown diminished in the twentieth century, probably because his most lasting contributions were improved methods of data analysis, not new statistical techniques or sociological theories.[17]

Quetelet is best known for the concept of the average man, or *l'homme moyen,* by which he meant the use of statistical averages to describe characteristics of groups. He believed that averages eliminated individual idiosyncrasies, which confused and distorted the general patterns. The concept was of elementary importance because it permitted meaningful comparisons among groups. With regard to directly measurable "physical qualities" like "weight and stature," Quetelet wrote, "we might then say that the Englishman is of greater height and larger size than the Frenchman or Italian" in the same way that we already say the average temperature of London differs from the average temperature of Paris and Rome. Another type of average comprised "non-material measures" like "average duration of life for any particular nation." Comparisons of the average duration of life at different times and places were extremely useful because "the laws which relate to the social body are not essentially invariable; they change with the nature of the causes producing them." By understanding and modifying the causes, the average length of life can be increased. At Geneva, statistics showed a steadily increasing life expectancy, which Quetelet attributed to a higher standard of living.[18]

Another useful type of comparison, especially in clinical medicine, was between the level of a characteristic in an individual and the average level of the characteristic in a group. In evaluating the condition of a sick person, "it is almost impossible to judge the state of an individual without comparing it to that of another imagined person, regarded as being in a normal condition." Ideally, the physician would like to know the pulse, respiration, and other characteristics of the same person in both health and illness, but that is often impractical. Therefore, "the physician is obliged to have recourse to the common standard, and compare his patient with the average man."[19]

Quetelet's goal as a social researcher was to compile an inventory of all that was known about social phenomena "nearly as physical science brings together the phenomena appertaining to the material world." For each phenomenon he studied, from average heights to average numbers of crimes, he endeavored to describe how it was affected by "regular and periodic causes" (7). Quetelet was particularly interested in causes that could be altered by human intervention. If socially important phenomena like deaths and crimes were found to be determined by modifiable causes, that knowledge "would form some of the noblest and most interesting results of human research" (9).

In his 1835 book, *A Treatise on Man and the Development of His Faculties,* Quetelet summarized a number of his previous publications that presented rates and averages for a wide range of human phenomena: births, deaths, heights, weights, pulse rates, respiration rates, intellectual eminence, insanity, intemperance, suicides, and crimes. Some of his statistics were taken from Belgian vital statistics, others from French statistics, and still others from studies by researchers throughout Europe. Each human characteristic was related systematically, whenever possible, to a host of factors, including age, sex, season, climate, nationality, social class, occupation, and education.

One of Quetelet's greatest contributions was his recognition of the need to explain outcomes using several causal factors simultaneously, today called multifactorial or multivariate analysis. For example, comparisons of urban and rural residents in the early nineteenth century always showed that urban residents had higher mortality rates than rural residents. Residence, however, may not have been the causal factor; urban and rural residents may differ on two other factors known to affect mortality, sex and age. To show that residence was the cause, urban and rural mortality rates had to be compared for each age and sex group separately. Quetelet therefore constructed a four-variable table with mortality rates for each age, sex, and rural or urban residence group based on Belgian vital statistics over a three-year period in the 1820s or 1830s. He found that each of the three factors affected mortality rates independently of the others: urban mortality rates were higher than rural rates for each sex at every age; death rates were highest among infants and the elderly for both men and women in both urban and rural areas: and men had higher mortality rates than women at all ages in both urban and rural areas. This type of analysis has become universal in epidemiological and social science research, but it was a brilliant innovation in Quetelet's lifetime (30–31).

Quetelet was one of the first to recognize that many human characteristic were so complex that they were not adequately described by any single measurement. He examined the impact of social and economic status on mortality using several different measures. Regardless of the type of measurement used, his statistics supported earlier findings that groups with lower social and economic status had higher mortality rates than the upper groups in all age groups (37–41).

Quetelet's most ingenious analyses involved what he called "moral qualities," particularly crime. Quetelet believed that crime was a social phenomenon because of the regularity of crime rates, and that crime rates could not be reduced "without the causes which induce them undergoing previous modifications." In a deterministic conclusion which he later regretted, Quetelet wrote: "society prepares crime, and the guilty are only the instruments by which it is executed" (108).

Quetelet's analysis of criminal activity was based on French statistics of those formally indicted for committing crimes. He could not compare crime rates for specific groups because he did not know the total number of persons in each group in the French population. He therefore devised several ingenious measures to make other types of comparisons. For example, he examined the relationship between type of crime, whether against persons or against property, and education, measured using an innovative four-point scale: "could not read or write," "could read and write but imperfectly," "could read and write well," and "had received a superior education." Quetelet compared the ratio of property crimes to crimes against persons for groups of criminals with each of the four education levels and found that the least educated group of criminals had a higher ratio of property to personal crimes than the most educated group. Thus a higher proportion of the crimes committed by the lower classes were property crimes than those committed by the upper classes (84).

Quetelet made similar comparisons concerning male and female criminals. He found that the ratio of men to women criminals was greatest among the best educated and lowest among the least educated. The male-female ratio was also higher for crimes against persons than for property crimes. In other words, female criminals were more likely to be found among the worst- than the best-educated groups and among those committing property rather than personal crimes. He performed similar analyses for age groups of men and women and concluded: "women, compared to men, are rather later in entering on the career of crime, and also sooner come to the close of it" (90–93).

Quetelet also compared conviction rates among different groups of criminals. Criminals who committed property crimes were more likely to be convicted than those who committed crimes against persons, which he attributed to the excessive severity of punishments for personal crimes that deterred juries from convicting defendants. He also compared conviction rates for different education, sex, age, and other groups. He summarized his findings by saying that the "most advantageous position an accused person can possibly be in [to avoid conviction], is to be more than 30 years of age, a female, to have received a superior education, to appear under an accusation of a crime against person, and to come when cited, previously to being taken into custody" (104).[20]

These analyses are astonishingly innovative and many could hardly be improved by a creative modern sociologist or criminologist. The state of statistical knowledge made it impossible for Quetelet, like Snow, to deal with the variations in rates that would have occurred had he used other time periods or countries, but he came surprisingly close to applying modern methods even to this problem.[21]

Quetelet's other major contribution was to apply the normal distribution to characteristics of human beings. The normal distribution is a particular kind of symmetrical distribution of data points around an average or mean, such as the heights of a group of men. The largest number of men have heights very close to the mean, with the numbers dropping off rapidly with greater distance from the mean in both directions (shortness and tallness). The normal distribution is most closely associated with the mathematician Karl Friedrich Gauss (1777–1855), after whom it is called a Gaussian distribution in the natural sciences. The statistician, Francis Galton (1822–1911), called it the normal distribution or curve, the name that is used in the social sciences.[22]

By the 1830s the normal distribution was being applied to some human characteristics and in 1846 Quetelet compared the actual distribution of the chest measurements of 5,700 Scottish soldiers and the heights of 10,000 French conscripts to the theoretical distributions of the measurements predicted by the normal distribution. He found that both sets of measurements approximated a normal distribution, although he did not demonstrate this mathematically, and he concluded that many human characteristics were normally distributed. The application of the normal and other mathematical distributions to describe human characteristics or behaviors for medical and social purposes has became a major method of statistical analysis.[23]

Thus during the early nineteenth century the study of statistical regularities moved beyond simple descriptions of groups. Researchers used statistics to test hypotheses by relating the personal and social characteristics of persons to death rates and other medically important outcomes. This new method of medical research was first used on a large scale by the life insurance industry, with results that had immediate applications to public health and clinical medicine.

5

LIFE INSURANCE AND THE RISK FACTOR

In tracing the evolution of the concept of normal blood pressure in clinical medicine, it is surprising to find that the definition of its normality depended largely on the results of statistical studies by life insurance companies. (1952)[1]

Most of the pioneer studies of blood pressure were done by and for insurance companies, and the tables are still accepted in all textbooks as the basis of blood pressure levels. Insurance statisticians did not set out to make contributions to human physiology; they were interested in the range of blood pressure in which they could establish a profitable insurance premium. (1939)[2]

Life insurance companies devised a fundamentally new statistical approach to predicting chronic disease as they improved the process of selecting policyholders. They discovered that the risk of premature mortality was increased by specific personal characteristics that could be determined by analyses of policyholder mortality rates. Once the characteristics were identified, the companies required the physicians whom they employed as medical examiners to measure them in their medical examinations of applicants.

Life insurance was the one field of commercial endeavor that was totally and irreversibly committed to mathematical statistics. Life tables based on statistical analyses of policyholder mortality rates were used to predict the proportion of policyholders who would die every year. Because the predictions were not completely accurate, the companies maintained financial reserves to protect themselves against years with unusually high mortality rates. Other kinds of statistical analyses enabled the companies to estimate the amount of variation in annual mortality rates and select their financial reserves rationally. Statisticians recognized the industry's commitment to statistics, and Quetelet, for example, devised several mortality tables beginning in 1826 to provide a basis for life insurance in Belgium.[3]

By contrast, few physicians and public health officials knew anything of statistics. Because of recent discoveries in bacteriology, medical education was placing increasing emphasis on the laboratory sciences and students were required to learn experimental techniques.[4] Few if any medical school graduates had any knowledge of statistics. Public health officials were preoccupied with the exacting task of improving the accuracy and completeness of enumerations of births and deaths. Their efforts were devoted to determining the sources of error and improving reporting, not to more sophisticated methods of analyzing the enumerations.

Most physicians obtained their first knowledge of the value of statistics for medicine from life insurance companies. In 1911 an estimated 80,000 of the approximately 150,000 physicians in the United States and Canada were medical examiners of applicants for life insurance policies.[5] These physicians practiced in practically every town and city in America. Given normal turnover, the great majority of American physicians served as medical examiners at some time during their careers, often when they were young and receptive to new ideas. As medical examiners, they were required to administer the tests and measurements specified by the life insurance companies. In this way many thousands of physicians learned about important innovations in diagnosis. They often applied this knowledge to their private patients as well.

Development of Life Insurance

England became the innovator in life insurance in the eighteenth century as a result of its international leadership in marine and fire insurance in the preceding centuries. Life insurance was first used by creditors to insure the lives of their debtors, but it soon became popular among gamblers, who insured the lives of celebrities in ill health, betting that they would die before the policy expired. Gambling on the lives of others became so widespread that most European nations banned life insurance. The industry was transformed in England in 1774, when legislation made a policy valid only if a meaningful relationship existed between the beneficiary and the policyholder, such as wife and husband. This led to a new type of life insurance company that sold thousands of small policies that were held for decades by policyholders distributed over a large geographic area. The large number of policyholders enabled the companies to use statistical methods to predict their mortality rates. They also minimized the impact of a single death or a local epidemic on the companies' financial reserves.[6]

Life insurance for the poor was provided by English workingmen's friendly societies, which collected weekly premiums and paid small sums to defray the burial costs of deaths in the families of their members. Friendly societies were legalized in England in 1793 and grew rapidly to 9,672 societies in 1802 and 925,000 members in 1815. Most of the societies were small and restricted to a town or village. They often became insolvent due to high mortality rates produced by local epidemics or industrial accidents, lack of actuarial expertise, and incompetent or dishonest officials.[7]

The commercial life insurance companies gradually devised several basic principles. One was to use the premiums of all of the policyholders with a particular type of policy in a given year to pay all of the death benefits in that year. The strategy of balancing yearly income and expenses depended on the "law of large numbers," a term coined by the statistician S. D. Poisson in 1835 to describe an older concept. As used in life insurance, it held that the proportion of policyholders who will die in a given year becomes more predictable as the number of policyholders increases. Once a company had a sufficient number of policyholders, it could predict its annual death benefit payments with considerable accuracy. The other basic principle was to vary premiums with the age of the policyholder, because age affects death rates more than any other factor. In order to prevent the premiums from rising to unaffordably high levels over the life of a policy, companies charged a level or fixed premium and invested most of the premiums received from policyholders when they were young and healthy to earn interest income that helped pay the death benefits when they grew older and had higher death rates.[8]

The first English life insurance companies, which began in 1762, were hampered by untrustworthy life tables of mortality rates by age. This forced the companies to charge very high premiums to avoid defaulting. As a result, by 1845 commercial life insurance was owned by only an estimated 100,000 persons in a country of 25 million inhabitants. The industry's problems were compounded by the gross mismanagement and outright fraud of many companies through the 1860s.[9]

In the United States, the first life insurance companies in the early nineteenth century sold policies only to specific groups, such as clergymen, thereby making mortality rates more predictable. In 1843 two commercial life insurance companies were organized and 35 others, most short-lived, followed within a decade. A reliable American life table was constructed in 1868 and the number of companies increased from 43 in 1860 to 59 in 1880 and 84 in 1900. The face value of the life insurance policies in force grew from $173 million in 1860 to $1.5 billion in 1880 and then surged to $7.6 billion in 1900.[10]

Throughout this period the American industry suffered from policy provisions that were unfavorable to the policyholders, and from unsound management practices, duplicity, and fraud. Policies were originally sold by direct application to the company office, but later by independent contractors who had little interest in the integrity or welfare of the company. The policy provisions excluded some common causes of death. Premiums were excessively high and dividends were often given to the few stockholders rather than returned to the policyholders. Policies did not accumulate cash value, so that forfeited policies were a major source of company profits. Companies often voided policies for late payments, travel, trivial or outdated errors on the application form, and changes of occupation or residence. Companies sold "participating" policies in which dividends were to be paid to policyholders out of surpluses. The surpluses actually resulted from inflated premiums, but the companies often retained and misused the funds for years before paying dividends to the small number of surviving policyholders, a classic Tontine scheme.[11]

Toward the end of the century the public began to appreciate the benefits of life insurance and demanded government regulation of the industry. Previously life insurance had been of little importance to most middle- and upper-income families because their wealth consisted of land or property, which could be sold or used to obtain income after the death of the owner. By the end of the nineteenth century the major source of earnings of most heads of families was an occupation that provided regular earnings. When death occurred, the earnings ceased and the family was left without a source of income. The change from property to earnings as the major source of income created a great need for financial protection for the family in the event of the untimely death of the breadwinner.

Around the end of the century, state governments enacted consumer protection laws that regulated an insurance company's right to void policies, limited agent commissions, and required the use of certain life tables. Most important in the long run, states obtained the right to regulate a company's policies in every other state in which it did business on the grounds that losses elsewhere put the state's policyholders at risk, even if the company did not have its headquarters in the state. New York, the nation's most populous and wealthiest state, performed the functions of a national government and actively regulated practically all major life insurance companies for many decades.[12]

The life insurance statistical studies that had the greatest relevance to public health and medicine concerned the selection of applicants. Life insurance was most appealing to those who were seriously ill, employed in a hazardous occupation, or otherwise had a high risk of dying. This strong bias toward "adverse selection" needed to be offset if life insurance companies were to remain solvent. The problem was exacerbated by several other factors: life insurance agents worked on commissions and wanted to sell as many policies as possible; the companies needed large numbers of policyholders to benefit from the law of large numbers; and medical diagnosis was accurate only in the later stages of most diseases.

In order to avoid adverse selection, the companies established both nonmedical and medical selection criteria. The nonmedical selection factors, primarily age, occupation, geographic residence, race, and sex, were based on statistical studies that compared the long-term mortality rates of groups of policyholders and rejected applicants. Age was surprisingly difficult to measure because compulsory birth registration did not exist in most states until the 1920s and many immigrants had no evidence of their date of birth. Many occupations had high mortality rates and were grounds for rejection. Geographic region was a key selection factor and by 1914 each county in the nation was placed in one of 22 classes based on the mortality rates of its inhabitants. A more qualitative selection factor was evidence of the applicant's financial status and social and moral qualities.[13]

Race and sex were important selection factors in the nineteenth century. Blacks had much higher mortality rates than whites so practically all companies either refused to insure them or insured them at higher premiums. As a result, a number of black-owned life insurance companies were formed and became the largest minority-owned businesses in America during most of the twentieth century. Few women applied for life insurance before the end of the century and most were adverse risks, which led to a general bias against them. As more women entered the labor force and sought life insurance, companies became more receptive to selling them insurance. Josephine Baker, the noted New York City public health administrator, reported that about 1900, she and another woman physician convinced two major life insurance companies in New York City to employ them as medical examiners for women applicants who wanted a woman physician, which "brought us a steady stream of profitable fees and opened up that whole field of medical activity for women."[14]

The original medical criteria used in the selection process provided few quantitative measurements that could be related to mortality rates using statistics. The Mutual Life Insurance Company of New York, one of the first and most influential companies, appointed local physicians to examine applicants and in 1869 employed 3,500 medical examiners nationwide. Most companies, including the Mutual, at first permitted applicants to use their personal physicians or physicians chosen by the agents, but they soon discovered that these physicians favored the applicants and so appointed their own medical examiners. In 1860 Mutual Life required its medical examiners to complete a questionnaire that provided information on certain previous diseases and family longevity. The medical information gradually became more detailed in terms of both the applicant's own medical history and that of the family and asked about both infectious and chronic diseases. The medical selection criteria were accurate enough to exclude applicants with serious medical conditions and describe the applicant's overall health.[15]

The selection process was surprisingly effective in reducing short-term mortality rates, the only practical goal. Evidence of its value was shown as early as 1876 by "select" and "ultimate" life tables, which compare mortality rates for persons of the same ages who have been insured for different lengths of time. The tables found that, for a group of policyholders of the same age, those who purchased life insurance recently had lower mortality rates than those who purchased the policies a few years earlier. This demonstrated the effectiveness of the selection process because those who were insured earlier had a longer time after the medical examination in which to develop illnesses and die. A major study of American life insurance companies from 1900 to 1915 found that 24 year-old male policyholders in their first year as policyholders had a mortality rate of 2.91 per 1,000, those of the same age in their second year as policyholders had a mortality rate of 3.80 per 1,000, those of the same age in their third year as policyholders had a mortality rate of 3.99 per 1,000, and those of the same age in their sixth year as policyholders had a mortality rate of 4.43 per 1,000. The selection effect almost always disappeared before ten years had elapsed.[16]

Industrial Life Insurance

Industrial life insurance was one of the most important social innovations in life insurance. It provided life insurance for millions of persons who could neither afford nor qualify for "ordinary" life insurance. It forced life insurance companies to adopt a completely new approach to evaluating the health of their applicants. It produced a new occupation, the industrial life insurance salesman, who would play a significant role in providing health education to the public.

Industrial life insurance was devised as a method for offering inexpensive policies to low income families to provide small funds for burial and other expenses. The earliest ordinary life insurance companies refused to sell to low income people because of their high mortality rates, low earnings, and frequent periods of unemployment. Low income families also had difficulty amassing enough money to mail in the quarterly, semi-annual, or annual premiums of ordinary policies, as a few ordinary companies discovered when they tried to sell low-cost policies.[17]

The development of industrial insurance was made possible by the growing expertise of life insurance workers in sales, underwriting, premium collection, claims processing, investing, marketing, and advertising. The actuarial profession originated in England in the eighteenth century and the term actuary came into general use in the 1820s. The first American life insurance companies in the 1840s used English life tables constructed by English actuaries, but American actuaries soon devised life tables based on American populations, the most important one in 1868. The profession grew slowly and the Actuarial Society of America had only 38 charter members at its founding in 1889. Actuaries were not simply mathematicians, because they needed to estimate future interest rates, determine desirable levels of surpluses and profits, and consider the policies sold by competing life insurance companies.[18]

Industrial insurance required completely new methods of operating a life insurance company. Liberal underwriting standards were necessary to make policies available to low income men, women, and children. In order to minimize defaults, agents collected the premiums, which were as low as a few cents, each week at the homes of the policyholders. Each agent was assigned a small geographic territory in a city, called a "debit" (industrial insurance was often called debit insurance), within which he was responsible for sales, premium collection, and bookkeeping for all of the company's industrial insurance policies. Debits provided new agents with immediate earnings in the form of commissions on the premiums of existing policies. All agents, who walked their debits, were expected to become familiar with the residents and the community and use the relationships to sell new policies. The high cost of collecting weekly premiums at the homes of policyholders was offset by the inexpensive underwriting procedures and the use of the agent, rather than the home office, to record all premium payments in a booklet kept by the policyholder. The need for agents to walk their debits made industrial life insurance practical only in densely populated cities.

Industrial insurance originated in England in the mid-nineteenth century, when some friendly or burial societies expanded into large regional organizations that collected premiums periodically at the homes of members, but that system failed because of faulty actuarial methods. In 1854, the year after a committee of the House of Commons urged the study of appropriate forms of life insurance for lower income groups, the Prudential Assurance Company of London began to sell industrial insurance policies with considerable success. This was due largely to its willingness to pay death claims immediately and its decision in 1858 to offer insurance on the lives of children.[19]

In the late 1870s three small, recently organized American life insurance companies began to sell industrial life insurance: the Prudential Insurance Company in 1875, and the Metropolitan Life Insurance Company and the John Hancock Life Insurance Company in 1879. All three modeled their operations after the London company and Prudential even borrowed its name. Industrial insurance was an immediate success: in 1880 all American ordinary life insurance companies combined sold 72,000 ordinary policies, while the Metropolitan alone sold 214,000 industrial policies. Although other companies (including black-owned companies) also sold industrial insurance, Metropolitan and Prudential dominated the rapidly growing market, with John Hancock third. In 1900, 11.2 million industrial policies were in force. In 1913, 29.2 million industrial policies were in force worth $4 billion, with Metropolitan having 44% of the total number of policies, Prudential having 38%, and John Hancock 8%. In 1924, 66.4 million industrial policies were in force, with Metropolitan having 43% of them and Prudential 37%.[20]

Industrial life insurance became a fixture of urban American working class life. Robert Chapin surveyed poor and working class families in New York City in 1909 and found that 60% of the 318 families with incomes between $600 and $1100 owned industrial life insurance policies. The families averaged five persons, and about two persons per family had insurance. The premiums varied from about 10¢ to 25¢ per week, and death benefits provided $100 for adults and $50 for children. Chapin observed that "provision for the expenses of the last sickness and burial constitutes an essential part of the American standard of living, and . . . most families will go without many comforts in order to keep up their insurance." However, only 25% of the 25 families with incomes of $400–599 had life insurance. Policies were considered essential for children as well as adults and Josephine Baker reported: "A dead baby always meant a neat little white funeral because, no matter how poor the families were, they always insured their babies."[21]

The significance of burial insurance to working class families is indicated by a 1916 description of a visiting nurse in Chicago about the death of a baby in a poor family:

> The baby got very, very ill. I did my best for it, but the poor home and hot weather and not the best sort of care and never the right kind of food did its work, and the baby died. When I went there one morning hoping that we had pulled the baby through, I found what all of you are familiar with, that the little form was covered with an old sheet and dressed in what clothing the mother could get for it. She was frightfully distressed because it was warm weather, and the child had to be buried that day. I went out to see what I could do, and came back in about an hour overjoyed to think that I had the promise of a grave from one friend and a funeral from another. I was met by the distracted mother, who told me that some one from the Public Health Department had called and taken the baby from her. That poor mother cared just as much for her baby as any mother cares for hers, but it was buried in Potter's Field. From that day to this I have been favorable to Industrial insurance, and particularly to the insurance of children. I know it is hard to meet the premiums. . . but nevertheless it is infinitely harder to meet times of that sort.[22]

Industrial life insurance was especially popular among the growing numbers of eastern and southern European immigrant groups who had traditions of sickness and burial societies in Europe and organized similar ones in American cities. W. I. Thomas, a sociologist, found that mutual aid societies were "the basic institution" in immigrant communities and that death benefits were important because immigrants wanted to die "decently, ceremoniously, and socially." A Chicago study about 1920 located 313 local mutual benefit societies, and an analysis of 161 of them found that 78% provided death benefits, 60% funeral benefits, and 58% sickness and accident benefits. Dues for these types of organizations varied from 35¢ to 75¢ per month, with death benefits varying from $15 to $250 and sickness benefits of $2.50 or more per week. The societies often failed due to mismanagement, competition from other societies, and the movement of members to other neighborhoods.[23]

Many immigrants turned to industrial life insurance as alternatives or supplements to burial societies. The companies in turn recognized that the immigrants, who lived in densely populated urban neighborhoods, were ideal candidates for industrial life insurance. The companies emphasized their size and security: Prudential used the Rock of Gibraltar as its symbol and Metropolitan's motto was "the light that never fails." They issued publications in numerous languages and employed agents who were immigrants or spoke languages in addition to English. In the 1890s two-thirds of all Metropolitan agents were born outside the United States.[24]

Industrial insurance was so successful that by 1909, just three decades after its introduction, Metropolitan had a larger amount of life insurance in force than any other life insurance company in America and Prudential was third. Metropolitan and Prudential were so large that they used multiple life tables based on the experiences of their own policyholders, which greatly improved the accuracy of their mortality predictions.[25]

Several other factors were also responsible for the success of industrial insurance. According to Louis Dublin, a Metropolitan statistician, Metropolitan, Prudential, and John Hancock "were managed with high integrity and skill," which prevented a repetition of the duplicitous early history of many ordinary life insurance companies. As evidence of the quality of management, when the Metropolitan decided to sell industrial insurance, its president visited England and recruited several hundred experienced English industrial insurance agents to emigrate to the United States at the company's expense. These agents became the managers of district offices, set up company operations and procedures, and trained local agents. Under their leadership, the agency force grew from 130 agents in three offices in 1879 to 8,000 agents in 146 offices in 1893. Turnover was high in the early years; the average Metropolitan agent survived for only four months in the 1880s.[26]

The Metropolitan and other companies recruited their industrial insurance agents from the same social classes and nationality groups as their policyholders. This gave them a reputation of being sympathetic to the immigrant communities, in sharp contrast to most other major industries. Foreign-born agents had opportunities for advancement in their companies at a time when many industries discriminated against immigrants from eastern and southern Europe. Annual earnings for agents were about $600 in 1905 and $950 in 1909, somewhat above manufacturing workers, who earned an average of about $600 per year in 1909, but below all workers in finance, insurance, and real estate, who earned an average of $1,260 in that year.[27]

The companies greatly simplified their underwriting and claims procedures to meet the needs of poorly educated families with immediate financial needs and no savings. At first the Metropolitan required medical examinations for applicants, but soon based its decision on a recommendation from the agent and an application form used by their underwriters to evaluate the health of applicants. The companies paid all death claims promptly and contested extremely few. In 1912 the Metropolitan rejected only 441 of 147,000 claims, and some of those were later paid.[28] Although industrial insurance was designed for low income groups, it was also used by higher income persons who had been denied ordinary policies for occupational and other reasons.

Policy provisions were gradually liberalized. In 1891 Metropolitan industrial policies combined high expenses with narrow and rigid policy provisions. In the next year Metropolitan began giving paid-up life insurance to policyholders who lapsed (discontinued payments) their policies after five years, and in 1897 both Metropolitan and Prudential began paying dividends on policies in the form of reduced premiums. Improvements continued at a steady rate thereafter. The major barrier to more liberal provisions was the expenses of selling industrial insurance: in 1905 Metropolitan agents had to make 7,000 sales to produce one million dollars worth of industrial life insurance compared to 400 sales to produce an equivalent amount of ordinary insurance.[29]

Critics of industrial insurance pointed to the enormous waste that occurred because so many policyholders lapsed their policies. In 1891, about two-thirds of policyholders of the three leading industrial companies lapsed their policies in the first three years, most of which occurred in the first six months at a financial loss to the company. The Metropolitan lapse rate declined to 58% in 1904, 46% in 1914, and 30% in 1919, but lapse rates in some companies were as much as 20% higher than for ordinary policies. The critics claimed that the federal government could provide equivalent death benefits at a small fraction of the overall cost using tax revenues, but this proposal was not put into effect until Social Security provided death benefits for covered workers in 1935. The Metropolitan tried to lower premiums by using an intermediary, such as a labor union or mutual benefit society, to collect the premiums. The reduced expenses to the company were passed on as lower premiums to the policyholders. The plans, which were instituted in 1909, almost all failed.[30]

Among the most important aspects of industrial life insurance was the role of the agent. Industrial insurance agents had a frequency and intimacy of contact with tens of millions of Americans that was unique among business organizations. They entered the homes of policyholders every week and learned about deaths, births, marriages, job changes, and family achievements. They were often taken into the confidence of families in matters of unemployment, serious illness, and other family misfortunes. As will be shown subsequently, these relationships enabled agents to educate policyholders in new ways of thinking about health and illness.[31]

The Invention of the Risk Factor

Industrial life insurance proved to be both a challenge and an opportunity for the ordinary life insurance companies. The enormous success of the leading industrial companies, which also sold ordinary insurance, posed a competitive threat to the ordinary companies. At the same time, the actuarial soundness of industrial insurance demonstrated that ordinary companies had completely misunderstood the objective of selecting policyholders. Their strategy had been to insure only applicants whom they believed were healthy and at low risk, whereas they should have graded the risks of the applicants and adjusted the premiums to the level of risk. This innovation would lead to new statistical criteria in the selection process that would ultimately be of great significance to medicine and public health.

The original purpose of evaluating applicants was designed to decide whether to accept or reject the applicant for a standard policy. An insurance historian wrote in 1905: "To most [ordinary life insurance] companies there were only two classes of people in the world; one was entitled to all the privileges and benefits of life insurance; the other was entitled to nothing. . . . It had come to be considered a mark of superiority in a company to advertise—'None but first-class lives accepted.'" Yet he also observed that "medical directors did not themselves agree as to what constituted a first-class risk." Applicants rejected by one company were often insured by another because the standards varied widely from company to company. One actuary stated that the person responsible for selection "reviews each factor, giving it a value in accordance with his impressions, the existing medical statistics, the custom of his company, the tradition of his department and so forth." He "mentally determines that a case has so many favorable points and so many unfavorable features and, after balancing these in his mind," accepts or rejects the applicant. The evaluator "who is inclined to be stout, [for example,] looks with favorable eyes on people with the same tendency." Another basic flaw of the process was that rejections were expensive because of the cost of the medical examination and the time wasted by the agent and underwriters.[32]

In order to reduce the number of rejections, ordinary life insurance companies devised a new system that graded applicants by their level of risk and varied the premiums or the death benefits accordingly. The very first life insurance company, the Equitable in England, had charged extra premiums in 1762 for applicants with gout, hernia, and no history of small-pox, and the general approach was used sporadically thereafter. More than a century later, life insurance companies placed this approach on a sound actuarial basis by constructing new life tables for persons with various kinds of risks. In 1890 the New York Life Insurance Company began to compile statistical data on the twenty-year mortality experience of accepted and rejected applicants with different occupations, personal and family histo-ries of disease, physical characteristics, and habits. In 1896 the company constructed and used life tables to insure many previously unacceptable men by selling them policies with the same premiums but smaller death benefits. The same approach was also used with women until their favor-able mortality rates led companies to eliminate the higher premiums. Other companies followed New York Life in the next decade, with the Metropolitan offering both sub-standard ordinary and industrial life insurance policies.[33]

The applicant's medical condition was among the most difficult fac-tors to grade. Major differences existed between the thinking of physicians in private practice and life insurance medical examiners. Physicians in pri-vate practice prefer to delay a diagnosis until it can be made with reason-able confidence. Life insurance medical examiners must make a report when the applicant seeks life insurance, even though the physician may be uncer-tain about the presence of disease. Life insurance companies differ from patients, who want unequivocal statements concerning the effect of a medical impairment on their survival. The companies group large numbers of poli-cyholders with a particular medical impairment and use statistics to esti-mate the number of extra deaths in the group over a specified time period. They do not need to know which of the policyholders will die.

The medical criteria used in the selection process were determined by company medical directors, physicians employed in the home office who appointed and supervised the local medical examiners. By 1889 enough companies employed medical directors so that they organized the Associa-tion of Life Insurance Medical Directors.[34] The medical directors were much more knowledgeable than actuaries and underwriters about the medical examination. They standardized its content and met regularly with medi-cal examiners in the field to oversee their activities. They also introduced diagnostic innovations on a company-wide basis and made sure that the examiners had the skills to use them.

The greatest innovation in the life insurance medical examination in the late nineteenth century was urinalysis. The presence of sugar in the urine as an indicator of diabetes mellitus had been known since antiquity, but in the early nineteenth century Richard Bright (1789–1858) demonstrated that albumin in the urine, which could be detected by a simple chemical test, was associated with kidney disease. Because kidney disease and diabetes were important causes of death among adults, medical directors made urinalysis a standard part of the insurance medical examination after 1885. By contrast, most physicians, according to an 1896 article in the *Journal of the American Medical Association,* did not perform one "unless absolutely compelled by consultation, or by life insurance companies." About 1905 the New York Life Insurance Company, concerned about the poor quality of urinalyses, devised a method for preserving urine, provided examiners with bottles and preservative, and required them to mail the samples to the home office for chemical analysis. Other companies soon adopted the practice.[35]

Urinalysis was a revolutionary advance in life insurance medicine. It predicted the development of life-threatening chronic diseases in apparently healthy applicants. It was inexpensive, could be obtained by even the least competent physician, and produced reasonably accurate results. If necessary, the test could be easily repeated. Statistical differences in levels of risk could be calculated by comparing the survival rates of groups with different test results.

In 1889 the newly organized Actuarial Society of America began a study to determine the feasibility of expanding the number of policyholders by insuring applicants with health impairments or adverse family histories. The study, which was published in 1903 as the *Specialized Mortality Investigation,* was based on the pooled experience of 98 classes of risks in 38 companies. It confirmed the feasibility of insuring persons at above average risk, who were called "impaired lives" or "substandard risks," by constructing life tables that quantified the risks of factors such as build, occupation, medical history, and residence. According to a life insurance historian, the *Specialized Mortality Investigation* "provided the spark which touched off a veritable explosion of biostatistical investigations, the foundation of our present system of life insurance medicine."[36]

The success of the study led the associations of actuaries and medical directors to organize a Joint Committee on Mortality in 1909 that published seven influential studies between 1912–14 and 1939. These established the preeminence of American research on life insurance medical selection and changed the practice of medicine everywhere. The studies identified several new medical factors that increased the risk of mortality and removed many nonmedical factors, including numerous occupations.

They enabled life insurance companies to develop a range of substandard, standard, and preferred risk policies using a simple numerical rating system invented in 1919. The state of each risk factor for an applicant was assigned a number, the numbers for all factors were summed, and the total score was compared to a scale developed by the company that assigned applicants to specific risk categories.[37]

The most unexpected finding of the original 1903 study was the discovery of a strong relationship between mortality and "build," a construct that combined height and weight. Using industry data gathered between 1909 and 1928 for all male policyholders ages 40 to 49 and taking 100 as the average mortality rate, those who were at least 25% overweight for their height had a relative mortality rate of 141, those of average weight had a relative mortality rate of 86, and those who were 5% to 14% underweight had a relative mortality rate of 77. Policyholders who were very much underweight had higher than average mortality rates, primarily from tuberculosis. The low mortality rates of slightly underweight policyholders astonished physicians who were busy treating gaunt patients sick or dying of tuberculosis, the "wasting disease." They viewed ruddy and rotund persons as the epitome of good health and underweight ones as suspect. Although the medical directors had no theory of disease etiology that explained the statistical relationship, they accepted it unequivocally and made it a key factor in selection.[38]

The discovery of build constituted a revolution in prognosis. Physicians had treated overweight and underweight patients for hundreds of years without recognizing any relationship between build and mortality other than a few specific diseases. They failed to do so because clinical observations of small numbers of patients could not elucidate this kind of relationship. Only the life insurance industry's statistical expertise and information on the mortality rates of many thousands of persons over long periods of time could determine the medical significance of build. Furthermore, physicians searched for the presence of disease, while overweight was neither a disease nor a sign of ill health. It was a characteristic of healthy persons that increased the risk of a variety of diseases.

The life insurance industry readily accepted build because it was interested in predictors of mortality, not causes, and especially predictors that were inexpensive, accurate, consistent, and simple to measure. By contrast, most medical scientists insisted that predictors be incorporated into causal models and tested experimentally with laboratory animals, as was being done with bacterial pathogens. The receptivity of the life insurance industry to prognostic factors from any source is illustrated by an experience of

Edward Trudeau (1848–1915), one of the first Americans to investigate the tubercle bacillus. In 1890 he diagnosed tuberculosis in a young man who insisted that he was in perfect health because he had just been approved for policies by medical examiners from two leading life insurance companies. Trudeau wrote:

> This brought a letter from one of the insurance companies asking me on what I based my diagnosis. I answered that the symptoms were very suspicious, but that the presence of the [tubercle] bacillus, in my mind, was irrefutable evidence of the presence of a tuberculous process as their cause. An interval followed, then a very nice note came from the insurance company asking me whether, if they sent up one of their doctors, I would show him my method of detecting the bacillus and making such a diagnosis. The doctor arrived. I showed him how to find the bacillus and he departed the next day. Within a couple of days I received a nice note of thanks from the insurance company and a check for one hundred dollars. The patient died several years later of tuberculosis.[39]

At the same time, the industry's single-minded focus on the prediction of mortality had serious limitations. It led to the perpetuation of many outdated beliefs, such as the role of heredity in disease etiology, and restricted the scope of factors in the medical examination. Louis Dublin, chief statistician of the Metropolitan Life Insurance Company for many years, observed that when he joined the company about 1909, the company's statistics were "constructed for financial purposes primarily, and for checking on the rates of premiums charged. There was little, if any, interest in the social data on the death certificates, on the causes of death, on the occupations, and on other factors which might have precipitated the death."[40]

By 1911, life insurance companies had identified a number of appropriate medical and nonmedical risk factors and quantified the statistical risk of excess mortality associated with each. These included build, family history of diseases, insanity, stroke, premature death of parents and siblings, physical condition, personal and medical history and habits, occupation, residence, and moral hazard (dubious reasons for obtaining insurance or a specific amount of insurance).[41]

Risk factors were a remarkably useful, although not ideal, solution to the problem of substandard risks. They were applied to many thousands of applicants, so that any unsatisfactory risk factors were soon identified and discarded. As the mortality patterns of the population changed, obsolete risk factors were eliminated, new ones added, and the weights attached to others modified. Yet only about one-tenth of an average company's business consisted of substandard policies. Consequently the companies lacked sufficient experience with each class of risk to construct sound actuarial tables for that group and did not have enough insured persons in each risk class to be confident that the law of large numbers would prevent unanticipated deviations from actuarial predictions.[42]

Blood Pressure

Blood pressure became the risk factor besides urinalysis and build that was most closely associated with life insurance. Throughout the first half of the twentieth century, practically every discussion of blood pressure in the medical literature referred to the central role of the life insurance industry in this major discovery. The industry determined the levels of blood pressure that were associated with health or disease, educated the medical profession about its importance, and trained physicians in the use of the sphygmomanometer.

Throughout medical history a few diseases had been associated with a strong pulse, but interest in the subject was limited by the inaccurate methods of measurement. The radial artery in the wrist was compressed with a finger until the pulse, felt with a second finger placed below the first, disappeared. The subjectively estimated pressure required by the first finger determined the strength of the pulse. During the nineteenth century efforts were made to improve blood pressure measurements without cutting an artery, and in 1876 Ritter von Basch invented the first practical sphygmomanometer, which consisted of a water-filled cushion attached to a mercury column. The physician pressed the cushion against the radial artery at the wrist until the pulse could no longer be felt by a finger placed below the cushion, and the systolic blood pressure was measured by the height of the mercury column. The instrument was too imprecise to be of value to practicing physicians.[43]

Meanwhile, other physicians were studying the medical significance of high blood pressure. In 1836 Richard Bright found high blood pressure in some cases of kidney disease. In the 1870s Frederick Mahomed, another English physician, and others discovered the presence of high blood pressure in the absence of kidney disease, which led Mahomed to conclude that it constituted a pre-symptomatic stage of the disease. Investigators soon discovered that the great majority of persons with high blood pressure never developed kidney disease, and termed the condition essential (unknown origin) hypertension. The finding was of little significance because of the lack of a reliable and convenient method of measuring blood pressure or knowledge of its consequences.[44]

In 1896 Scipione Riva-Rocci, an Italian physician, revolutionized the measurement of blood pressure by inventing a prototype of the modern sphygmomanometer that was soon improved and made more accurate, reliable, and portable. Riva-Rocci used a rubber tube or "cuff" that was wrapped around the upper arm of the patient and inflated with air using a bulb squeezed by the physician. A narrow tube was attached from the cuff to a mercury column, which measured the pressure of the air in the cuff. The physician placed his finger on the radial artery at the wrist and inflated the cuff until the pulse could no longer be felt. At that point the pressure of the air in the cuff just exceeded the pressure of the blood in the artery and could be used as a measurement of the systolic pressure. The ease of use and accuracy of this invention led Theodore Janeway to observe in 1910: "five minutes' trial will convince the most skeptical that his previous judgments, based on his supposedly trained sense of touch, were often fallacious. High tension was certainly recognized before the introduction of the sphygmomanometer, but so was fever before the days of clinical thermometers."[45]

In 1905, Nicholai Korotkoff, a Russian physician, reported on his development of a new auscultatory method that was much more accurate than the palpatory method and only slightly more difficult to use. The bell of a stethoscope was placed over the brachial artery on the inside of the elbow and a Riva-Rocci cuff was inflated until the blood flow ceased. As the cuff was slowly deflated the resumption of blood flow produced a series of distinct audible sounds, each of which could be associated with a pressure reading observed on the manometer. The manometer pressure reading at which blood resumed flowing through the artery, called the systolic blood pressure, was the only one used initially. Use of the diastolic, or minimum, pressure was delayed because of disagreement over the appropriate sound, but the issue was gradually resolved.[46]

The first application of the new sphygmomanometer was to detect low blood pressure, or hypotension, during surgery. Anesthesia and asepsis had greatly increased the use of surgery and lengthened the duration of operations, which made shock during operations a more common medical problem. It was discovered that a fall in blood pressure during the operation could be used to detect the onset of shock. In 1903, Harvey Cushing reported that Riva-Rocci's sphygmomanometer had enabled him "to anticipate and ward off severe conditions of surgical shock, and indeed in some instances to save lives." He also discovered that chloroform, an anesthetic that had become popular because it reduced the likelihood of hemorrhage, did so because it lowered blood pressure. This strengthened the existing popularity of ether in America and resolved an international debate concerning ether and chloroform. The successful use of the sphygmomanometer in surgery helped convince physicians that it was an important innovation in medicine.[47]

The adoption of the auscultatory method of measuring blood pressure occurred quite slowly. A 1910 edition of a book on blood pressure by Theodore Janeway, the foremost American investigator, did not mention Korotkoff or the auscultatory method. A medical director of a major life insurance company reported a study of over 150,000 blood pressure readings taken by the company's New York City medical examiners from 1907 to 1919. The palpatory method (using a cuff) was employed during the early years, but "nearly all" the readings taken since 1916 used auscultation, at which time diastolic pressures were first measured. New York City physicians, however, were far above the national average in their use of auscultation and other new developments in medicine. In 1930 and even as late as 1951 textbook authors recommended that physicians take blood pressure measurements using a stethoscope and then check them using the palpatory method.[48]

Although most physicians had little interest in blood pressure, the life insurance industry quickly recognized its utility in diagnosing kidney disease and predicting premature mortality. Blood pressure could be measured easily and inexpensively in any physician's office. High blood pressure was prevalent in the age groups of many applicants. The levels could be readily applied to the companies' numerical rating systems.

The first step in investigating the significance of blood pressure was for the companies to order their medical examiners to provide blood pressure readings on applicants. Most companies originally required readings on a few types of cases and then extended it to others. A 1910 survey that received replies from thirty-two medical directors found that 22 companies used blood pressure readings in "certain cases," 10 not at all, and none in all cases. Ten companies required readings for policies above a certain amount, 14 for applicants above a certain age, and some for applicants with specific medical conditions. Only 10 companies of 24 replying to the question rejected applicants for high blood pressure. The companies delayed requiring readings from all medical examiners because many examiners did not own an instrument or were unable to take accurate readings. The companies also disagreed as to the definition of normal blood pressure, which ranged up to 170 mm Hg systolic.[49]

Another step was to improve the accuracy of the blood pressure readings submitted by the medical examiners, which was discussed at annual meetings of the Association of Life Insurance Medical Directors. Some medical directors required blood pressure measurements on all applicants primarily to give their examiners experience in using the instrument. One reported in 1914 that for the previous two years "blood pressure [was] taken in every instance, irrespective of the amount of application, or the age of the applicant. . . . [B]esides giving us these interesting facts it is in a way a training to the examiners to make them proficient in this rather important portion of our examination." The percentage of his company's applications that included blood pressure readings increased from 85% in 1911 to 97% in 1914.[50]

The need for greater accuracy led the medical directors to try to influence the methods used by medical schools in teaching the techniques of taking blood pressure readings. A Blood Pressure Committee appointed in 1922 by the Association of Life Insurance Medical Directors surveyed eleven "leading internists and teachers" in medical schools and concluded: "different instructors in the same school and in different schools are teaching varying and often contradictory methods which may in part at least explain the deplorable confusion of both examiners and practitioners in regard to many simple and important clinical and laboratory procedures." Nine of the eleven preferred the auscultatory method, but five believed that it should be checked by palpation. The committee made several recommendations, including the sound to be used for diastolic blood pressure.[51]

The discussions in the annual meetings also revealed that many medical examiners objected to the medical directors' insistence on blood pressure measurements. One director said in 1913 that when an examiner complains that "he cannot afford to buy a sphygmomanometer to be used in connection with insurance examinations, I tell him . . . that the instrument will be an invaluable aid to him in his regular practice as well as in our work, because there are so many degenerative conditions that he will not be able to detect in any other way than by taking a blood-pressure reading." Another director expressed a similar view in 1912: "We are going to ask each Examiner to have an instrument in his possession, as we expect him to use it in his private practice, and then the use of the instrument will be compulsory in making examinations for our Company." Other directors were less insistent because they were dubious of the accuracy of the blood pressure readings provided by small town physicians whose medical knowledge was not abreast of the times.[52]

Medical directors also dealt with the problem of poor quality sphygmomanometers. They evaluated specific models of sphygmomanometers and found that instruments with mercury tubes were too fragile for portable use and those with spring-operated gauges were unreliable. O.H. Rogers, Medical Director of the New York Life Insurance Company, invented an aneroid sphygmomanometer that became the standard instrument for many years.[53]

The directors instructed their medical examiners about the specific procedures to use in taking blood pressure readings. In the 1921 meeting a speaker observed that "apparently a very large majority of the companies represented here" require their examiners to take the diastolic pressure by the auscultatory method. The medical directors prepared and distributed pamphlets for their examiners. One director observed in 1913:

> The circular we issue to our Examiners calls particular attention to the fact that blood pressure should be taken when the pulse returns and not when it disappears [i.e., as the cuff is being deflated, not inflated]; that the man should be put in a comfortable position and that the test should not be taken the first thing, as he enters, but perhaps after the examination is finished and he has been put at his ease; that it should be repeated two, or better, three times, at intervals of half a minute or so, in order to get it right.[54]

Physicians in turn had to educate their patients about the sphygmomanometer because it was soon discovered that blood pressure readings could fluctuate markedly from moment to moment. One 1914 book cautioned physicians to "discard the result of the first reading, using it simply to demonstrate the harmless and painless character of the procedure; and when possible make subsequent readings after some little time has elapsed." The book also advised physicians to "avoid making blood-pressure estimations when the subject is excited, anxious or worried, as a result of the examination, etc." It recommended that the physician take "several consecutive readings and if they correspond more or less closely, take the arithmetic mean."[55]

Once the life insurance companies accumulated the necessary data, they related blood pressure levels to mortality rates using both rejected and accepted applicants. The Northwestern Mutual Life Insurance Company analyzed its experiences between 1907 and 1910 and grouped the applicants into three blood pressure levels. One group of 2,661 policyholders with an average systolic blood pressure of 142 mm Hg had a mortality rate about equal to the company average. Another group of 525 policyholders with an average systolic pressure of 152 mm Hg had a mortality rate 30% above the company average. A third group of 1,082 rejected applicants with an average systolic pressure of 161 mm Hg and no other impairment listed on their application forms (an extremely important consideration that reduced the likelihood of other causes of death) had a mortality rate that was more than twice the company average. High blood pressure readings occurred in 6.5% of applicants who were rejected for policies.[56]

Many physicians believed that life insurance companies exaggerated the importance of hypertension. Most did not consider it to be either a disease, because it was typically asymptomatic, or a symptom, because overt disease did not appear for years or often at all. They viewed blood pressure as affecting the mortality rates of older patients at a time when tuberculosis and some other infectious diseases were more important causes of death in all age groups. Consequently medical examiners were often charitable in reporting blood pressure measurements of life insurance applicants. Two observed: "few physicians will deny a person insurance because of a reading of 5 mm or so of mercury. . . . He gives the patient the benefit of the doubt." The companies complained that medical examiners did "not realize that a small increase in the number of deaths each year means a great difference to life insurance."[57]

Medical examiners were also confronted by demands from life insurance agents to report blood pressure readings that enabled their applicants to qualify for insurance. In most cities agents could chose from an approved list of company medical examiners and often selected the most liberal ones. In 1950, two physicians complained: "Any physician who has ever done any examining for insurance companies knows that unless he is willing frequently to read low, the agent who patronizes him will soon seek elsewhere for someone who is more complaisant."[58]

When clinicians began to take blood pressure readings of their personal patients, they wanted a specific blood pressure level that constituted hypertension. The life insurance companies had divided blood pressure levels into several groups for rating purposes and had no need for a simple dichotomy between normal and high blood pressure. A widely publicized early study of 7,782 blood pressure readings by two clinicians, Edward and Theodore Janeway, proposed a level of 160 mm Hg systolic for hypertension. The Association of Medical Directors of Life Insurance Companies and the Society of Actuaries undertook a major multi-company study of 707,000 policyholders of twenty-six leading companies that was published in 1925. This led to a definition of hypertension as a systolic level of 140 to 150 mm Hg or higher and a diastolic level of 90 to 95 mm Hg or higher.[59]

As the measurement of blood pressure became more widespread, the life insurance industry corrected misunderstandings of physicians about its significance. Early in the century most physicians believed that high blood pressure was a progressive, fatal disease, because the palpatory method detected only cases with extremely high blood pressure levels. In a 1904 book on blood pressure, Theodore Janeway reported that "the more common readings in high tension cases lie in the neighborhood of 200 to 220" mm Hg. Like others he believed that the outcome of the condition was fatal and often rapid: "Death may come suddenly in an anginal seizure, or an attack of cardiac asthma or pulmonary oedema; or it may be the result of gradual asystole." Life insurance statistical investigations demonstrated the falsity of this belief. Studies in the 1920s using the auscultatory method, which permitted finer gradations in blood pressure measurement, showed that many persons with hypertension, even with levels much above the average, lived unexceptional lives and died at or close to their normal life expectancy. Nonetheless, many physicians continued to believe that hypertension was a progressive and fatal disease.[60]

Another issue was hypotension, or low blood pressure. The traditional clinical perspective concerning medical factors like blood pressure was that average levels were healthy and that all deviations from the average, whether high or low, were unhealthy. Theodore Janeway wrote in 1910: "Abnormally low blood pressure must lead to an accumulation of blood in the veins and a slowing of the current in the arteries, if it be progressive." Once again the life insurance industry provided the necessary statistical evidence, as three company physicians noted in 1943: a "finding of extreme interest, which has been noted previously in actuarial studies, is that the . . . life expectancy in subjects with blood pressure below average values is decidedly better than the life expectancy of the average population and that fewer deaths from cardiovascular disease occur in this group." They concluded that "hypertension should not properly be defined by departures from the average pressure but that the lowest arterial pressure compatible with normal physiologic function is the optimal one."[61]

In the 1880s and 1890s, a number of physicians discovered that high blood pressure was associated with arteriosclerosis, a buildup of plaque within the inner lining of the wall of an artery that reduced its blood flow and elasticity. If an artery supplying blood to the brain was blocked sufficiently, the reduction in blood flow could produce the death of brain cells (stroke or apoplexy). A similar blockage in an artery supplying blood to the heart could lead to the death of tissues in the heart muscle (myocardial infarction or heart attack) or to sudden death. The buildup process was often lengthy and many persons with arteriosclerosis never developed either disease. Furthermore, most cases of both diseases occurred in persons with average blood pressure levels. The precise relationships could be determined only by long-term statistical studies of thousands of people with different blood pressure levels. Only the life insurance industry had the statistical expertise and thousands of policyholders required for such investigations.[62]

As life insurance companies discovered more risk factors and accumulated statistics on each of them, the role of the medical examiners changed significantly. Companies increasingly required examiners simply to send their findings, together with urine specimens that required laboratory analyses, to the home office. In 1915, the president of the Association of Life Insurance Medical Directors of America noted with disapproval in his presidential address that "some of our companies have of late shown a tendency to eliminate the question formerly asked almost universally of the Medical Examiner, 'What is your opinion of the risk? Good, bad, first-class, second-class, or not acceptable?'" Formerly the physician evaluated the applicant; now the physician provided the data and the company made the decisions based on statistical expertise that the physician did not possess.[63]

As a result, company medical directors became much more cognizant of the statistical aspects of life insurance, according to the same presidential address:

> The majority of our Medical Directors were clinicians first, Medical Directors second. They had not then learned to view life insurance from the actuarial standpoint, nor had they then appreciated the profound meaning of the study of the class, of groups, of individuals, of selected lives, and noted what the combination and grouping and classification of these varied human units into such groups would show when the mortality was thoroughly worked out. If we as Medical Directors have progressed at all in the past twenty years, it is, I think, in the realization of the fact that we no longer deal as Medical Directors with the individual, but with the class, that we must think in the language of the actuary and not in that of the physician.[64]

Actuaries also changed their views as quantitative medical data became more available, according to an insurance official in 1911:

> Until a few years ago it was almost a universal custom to confine the actuary strictly to the mathematics of the business, and the Medical Director to the selection of risks. That was unavoidable when statistics regarding mortality among the different classes of risks were very scanty, and when selection was therefore largely based on the judgment and experience of the medical man. With the advance in knowledge of the mortality under different conditions and with the increase in competition, it became necessary for the Medical Director to have a knowledge of statistics, and for the Actuary to learn the views of the Medical Director in order to properly compile statistics bearing on the selection of risks.[65]

Throughout the first half of the century, life insurance companies continued to innovate in medical diagnosis. They conducted research on improving the accuracy and reliability of urinalyses and adding blood sugar measurements. Insurance companies were among the first large-scale users of chest X rays for tuberculosis in the 1920s and electrocardiographs for heart disease in the 1920s and 1930s.[66] By requiring their medical examiners to use the tests, insurance companies educated tens of thousands of physicians about new developments in diagnosis.

Thus the life insurance industry used medical statistics to make important discoveries in disease etiology and prognosis and educated their medical examiners about them. As a result of the educational process, most physicians gradually accepted the concept that asymptomatic personal characteristics could increase the long-term risk of developing disease.

PART II

Health Education for Healthy Lifestyles

6

CULTURAL AND ENVIRONMENTAL INFLUENCES ON URBAN MORTALITY RATES

> [In my study of ten blocks of tenements in New York City, the] comparison . . . has proven most surprising, for while in certain blocks [populated by one nationality group] there is a very high [infant] death rate, in certain other blocks [populated by a different nationality group], half a mile away . . . the [infant] death rate is only one-half as great as the average death rate of the city, . . . yet in the latter district there is a greater population, the tenement houses are taller, and the general sanitary conditions are worse. (New York City physician, 1908)[1]

The invention of the actuarial risk factor was one of two major innovations required for the formulation of programs to promote healthier lifestyles. The other was the concept of educating the public that personal behaviors can affect health. The discovery that some lifestyles were healthier than others emerged from findings that nationality groups with similar incomes and living conditions varied widely in their total and infant mortality rates.

One of the major uses of vital statistics in the early twentieth century was to compare the health status of different population groups. Nationality groups were the most important groups in the northeastern and midwestern cities teeming with immigrants and their children. Federal, state, and local governments regularly gathered information on place of birth and the place of birth of both parents. Individuals were categorized as "native born," "foreign born," and "foreign stock" (native born with at least one foreign born parent).

Nationality groups were useful categories because they constituted genuine communities. They shared languages, neighborhoods, occupations, cultures, churches, and fraternal and mutual aid societies. Their members had high rates of marriage within the group. Group solidarity was strengthened by language barriers, discrimination, and mutual hostilities with other nationality groups.

The foreign born and their children were also considered the source of most social and health problems. In his 1870 book, *The Dangerous Classes of New York,* Charles Loring Brace, a pioneer in the social welfare movement, stated that "an immense proportion of our ignorant and criminal class are foreign born; and of the dangerous classes here, a very large part, though native-born, are of foreign parentage." He cited statistical tabulations of prison populations as evidence. About 1900, the journalist Hutchins Hapgood observed in the first analytical description of an immigrant community:

> The Jewish quarter of New York is generally supposed to be a place of poverty, dirt, ignorance, and immorality—the seat of the sweatshop, the tenement house, where "red-lights" sparkle at night, where the people are queer and repulsive. Well-to-do persons visit the "Ghetto" merely from motives of curiosity or philanthropy; writers treat of it "sociologically," as a place in crying need of improvement.[2]

Immigrant Nationality Groups

An understanding of the health and social problems of the foreign born and their children requires some description of their patterns of migration and experiences in America. Although early twentieth-century America has been considered a refuge for impoverished and subjugated groups in Europe, most immigrants were continuing a long European tradition of migratory work. Throughout the seventeenth and eighteenth centuries, many of the rural poor in Europe sought periodic employment away from their farms to supplement their incomes. The women found jobs such as domestic servants and seamstresses in the pre-industrial European cities and the men worked as farm laborers and migratory workers. Few came to the United States because of the cost and dangers of ocean travel in the small sailing ships and most of those who did were permanent settlers.[3]

Changes in European life during the nineteenth century forced many rural Europeans to become migratory workers. The population of Europe grew from 187 million in 1815 to 468 million in 1913, excluding 52 million persons who emigrated from Europe. The population growth increased family size in rural areas far beyond the capacity of the farms to support them. Many European farmers also could not compete with the low-priced wheat, corn, meat, other foodstuffs, hides, tallow, and wool brought by steamships and railroads to European cities from North and South America and Australasia. The products of European rural cottage industries were displaced by the goods manufactured in European and American factories.[4]

Travel to other countries for migratory work was facilitated by the low cost and speed of railroad and steamship travel. Italians who had once gone to France and other nearby countries in the fall to help harvest crops now traveled by steamship each fall to Argentina, where they worked as agricultural laborers during the Argentine summer and returned to Italy for spring planting. Many migratory workers traveled to American or European cities each spring to work on construction projects and returned to their home countries in the fall. Agents of steamships lines toured Europe promoting the opportunities abroad, the inexpensiveness of the voyages, and the ease of returning. They helped provide rail travel to seaports (sometimes in sealed railroad cars that traveled across borders without inspections), assisted the travelers in obtaining passports, and aided them in passing through customs at their destinations.[5]

The major cities of America and Europe needed thousands of migratory workers and immigrants to construct the infrastructures required for their rapidly growing populations. The cities were constantly building roads, railroads, dams, bridges, tunnels, reservoirs, water and sewerage systems, subways, elevated railroads, and buildings. Port cities were adding filled land and improving their harbors, piers, and shipping facilities. Each major construction project, undertaken in an era with little machinery, required hundreds or thousands of skilled and unskilled workers for several years. Because most native born workers had more secure employment, the projects required a large and mobile international labor force that was willing to travel to cities in Europe and North America.

American industry employed many thousands of migratory and immigrant workers. Large mills and factories required a constant flow of new workers to offset their high turnover rates, caused in part by migratory workers returning to Europe. New and expanding factories needed an ever-growing supply of workers. Once again, most native-born Americans had better alternatives, so the factories relied on immigrant workers and asked them to recruit their friends and relatives at home. The experienced workers assisted the newcomers with travel arrangements and housing in ethnic neighborhoods and socialized them in the ways of the factory, including acting as translators.[6]

This vast back-and-forth international migration is demonstrated by Italy, a country of 33 million inhabitants in 1900 with reliable statistics and a long tradition of migratory work. Between 1876 and 1915, Italians made 14.0 million trips abroad, with about 45% to other countries in Europe and the rest to North and South America. The number of trips to the United States increased from 770,000 from 1876–1900 to 3.4 million from 1901–1915. Between 1901 and 1915, the Italians who came to the United States made approximately 2.7 million return trips to Italy. Cinel has estimated that about 60% of Italian immigrants to the United States between 1908 and 1923 returned to Italy within a few years. A survey of those who left Italy in 1909 for all destinations reported that 80% said that they did not plan to stay abroad indefinitely.[7]

Migratory workers who came to America followed a predictable pattern. Workers already in America provided prepaid passage and often other forms of assistance to an estimated 60% of the immigrants from southern and eastern Europe in 1908–9. Many of those who remigrated to Europe returned to the United States to obtain additional earnings, sometimes more than once. From 1899 to 1906, 12% of all incoming Europeans had been to the United States previously.[8]

Migratory workers had very specific needs and goals. Between 1900 and 1914, most Polish, Russian, Italian, and German immigrants arrived with funds averaging from $13 to $41 and so were forced to take any available work immediately. According to contemporary observers, "After a few years of work and privation, [the immigrant] hopes to accumulate enough money to enable him to return to his native land and purchase a farm, remove a mortgage from property he already possesses, or to improve his economic status in some other way. . . . He wishes to earn as much as he can within a limited time, and by living upon a basis of minimum cheapness to save the maximum amount possible." These goals required hard work from the immigrants, and most acknowledged that they worked harder in the United States than they ever did at home.[9]

Many immigrants settled in America. They found long-term jobs, married, and established communities with their fellow immigrants. Some immigrant groups arrived intending to settle: the propertyless urban poor whose handicraft trades were eliminated by machine production; the rural landless, primarily the Irish; and the persecuted, including eastern European Jews, Socialists, Communists, and anarchists.

The foreign-born and their children dominated the populations of America's largest cities. In 1910 New York City, which was the port of entry of 74% of all European immigrants between 1890 and 1919, had 4.8 million inhabitants, of whom 40% were foreign born and 38% of foreign stock. Chicago had 2.2 million inhabitants, with 36% foreign born and 42% of foreign stock. About 28% of the foreign-born population of the United States lived in these two cities and Philadelphia, Boston, Detroit, and Cleveland. In most other cities with more than 50,000 inhabitants in the Northeast and Midwest, between 50% and 80% of the inhabitants were foreign born or of foreign stock. Only cities in the Far West and the South were inhabited primarily by native born citizens of native born parents.[10]

The countries of origin of immigrants became more diverse from the mid-nineteenth to the early twentieth centuries. Of the 6.7 million foreign-born in 1880 (13% of the total U.S. population), 29% were born in Germany, 28% in Ireland, 26% in Great Britain (England, Wales, and Scotland), and 11% in Canada. These four groups comprised 94% of the foreign-born population and about 60% of them spoke English as their native language. The groups arriving after 1900 were more diverse, as shown by their native languages. In 1910 only 25% of the 13.3 million foreign-born (now 15% of the population) spoke English, whereas 21% spoke German, 10% Italian, 8% Yiddish or Hebrew, 7% Polish, 5% Swedish, and 10% other eastern European languages. Altogether 27 different languages other than English were spoken by at least 20,000 foreign-born immigrants.[11]

The mix of nationality groups varied widely among cities, with Jews and Italians more prevalent on the east coast and Germans and Poles in the Midwest. Of the 2 million foreign-born in New York City in 1920, 26% spoke Yiddish, 20% Italian, 16% English, 13% German, and 4% Polish. Of the 805,000 foreign-born in Chicago, 18% spoke German, 17% Polish, 14% English, 11% Yiddish, and 7% Italian. Philadelphia and Boston were similar to New York City, while Detroit and Cleveland resembled Chicago.[12]

One of the most salient differences among immigrant groups was their literacy levels, work skills, and incomes. About one-third of the immigrants from eastern and southern Europe were illiterate, compared to about 3% of those from northwestern Europe. Farming predominated as the homeland occupation of the Irish and eastern and southern European groups, including Greeks, Italians, and Slovaks, with less than 15% having worked in manufacturing. About one-half of the Jews and the English had worked in manufacturing and very few on farms. The Germans were in between, with about 30% having experience in manufacturing and a similar proportion in farming. Because of these differences, northwestern European immigrants had higher earnings than those from southern and eastern Europe. A study of male workers by place of birth in the 1920s found the following annual earnings: Swedes $692, Germans $613, native-born whites $595, Bohemians and Moravians $538, Irish $535, Russian Jews $461, native-born Negroes $441, northern Italians $425, southern Italians $368, and Poles $365.[13]

Each national group tended to enter the same occupations and industries. Often the first workers from a European region had particular skills that provided a labor force for a particular industry and enabled it to grow. These workers informed their fellow villagers or townspeople in Europe with the same skills, who soon followed. Employers grouped workers who spoke the same language to facilitate communication and avoid traditional European national and ethnic rivalries. An observer noted in 1912: "The Pole and the Lithuanian, the Slovak and the Magyar, the Italian and the Austrian, the Turk and the Armenian, the Hebrew and the Pole, will not, if they can help it, work together."[14]

Remigration was strongly affected by gender and nationality. Men left their wives and families in Europe while women came to America with their husbands and families. Between 1899 and 1909, men comprised more than 85% of the immigrants from east of the Adriatic, including Greece and Bulgaria, as well as 79% of the Italians and 69% of the Poles. A sociologist reported in a 1925 study: "The new immigration is in no sense an immigration of families, but of men, either single men, or married men who have left their wives on the other side." Most of these men remigrated within a few years. On the other hand, men comprised only about 60% of the immigrants who were Jews or came from the British Isles and Germany. About 90% of the Irish and the Jews remained in the United States, as did about 80% of the English, Scandinavians, and Germans.[15]

Childbearing rates varied considerably among nationality groups, as shown by a study of women under age 45 who were married for 10 to 19 years and lived in Rhode Island, Cleveland, and Minneapolis about 1910. Between 13% and 18% of native-born couples of native parentage had no children, compared to 6% to 7% of the foreign-born couples. The average number of children born to the native groups varied from 2.4 to 2.5 in the three cities, while the range for the foreign groups was 4.0 to 4.7. Between

7.6% and 11% of the couples born in Ireland, Germany, and England were childless, compared to 4.9% of those from Italy and 3.0% of those from Russia (mostly Jews). The Italians averaged 4.8 children and the Russians 5.2, compared to 3.2 for the English, 3.7 for the Germans, and 4.4 for the Irish. Married couples of foreign stock were between the foreign- and native-born groups.[16]

The First World War constituted the great turning point in migration between Europe and the United States. From 1914 to 1918 few immigrants entered and many men remigrated to enlist in the armies of their homelands. Immigration dropped from about 1.2 million persons annually in 1913 and 1914 to 111,000 in 1918. The number gradually rose to 707,000 in 1924 but a new immigration law curtailed the annual rates from 1925 to 1930 to 300,000 or fewer, and more than one-third of those entered from Canada or Mexico. The depression of the 1930s and World War II continued the low rates of immigration until after mid-century.[17]

Immigrant Health and Living Conditions

Most early-twentieth-century immigrants were healthy young men when they arrived. Men comprised more than 60% of all immigrants entering in every decade between 1861–70 and 1911–20. Persons ages 15 to 40 constituted over 70% of all immigrants entering in 1880, 1890, 1900, and 1910. Unhealthy immigrants were legally excluded by restrictions in 1882 that barred the mentally ill and in 1891 sufferers from "loathsome or dangerous" contagious diseases. Even considering lax enforcement, very few of those disembarking were unhealthy. In 1907 only 4,400 of 1.3 million immigrants were denied entrance for physical and mental diseases and in 1911 11,000 of 1.2 million immigrants were turned back. In 1917 a federal law fined shipping firms for transporting aliens who were debarred for physical or mental reasons, which led the firms to undertake health inspections of their passengers at the ports of embarkation.[18]

Once in America, the health of immigrants declined significantly. Migratory workers endured the least expensive and poorest quality living conditions because they wished to save as much money as possible. Many lived four to a room in boarding houses, where they paid a few dollars per month for lodging, meals, and laundry. Most other migratory workers boarded with immigrant families, who badly needed the extra income. A study about 1920 of 15,000 families of immigrant industrial workers found that 33% kept one or more boarders, compared to 10% of native white families. The boarders usually slept in the same rooms with family members or on cots in the parlor or kitchen.[19]

Immigrant families lived under primitive and unhygienic conditions. In New York City most lived in tenements, which housed 2.4 million of the city's 3.4 million inhabitants in 1900. Apartments in the newer "dumbbell" tenements had a window in each room while the older ones usually had some rooms with no windows. Much of the housing for immigrants in other cities consisted of large private homes that were subdivided into apartments, many with windowless rooms. The newer buildings had toilets and faucets in the hallways for common use while the older buildings had outdoor privies. The communal toilets and faucets transmitted infectious diseases from person to person. The lack of running water or hot water in many apartments made cleanliness an arduous task. The small apartments made it impossible to isolate the sick from other members of the family. Overcrowded neighborhoods led to the rapid spread of childhood diseases. Most immigrants were ignorant of methods of protecting themselves. Family life in rural Europe took place in both the house and the surrounding yard and garden, with easy access to pure fresh water, outdoor privies that were used only by members of the family, and convenient and safe disposal of garbage.[20]

Working conditions were another source of disease. Michael M. Davis, a leader in the health movement, observed that on the farm in Europe, the immigrant had "dealt with materials and processes which involve little risk of accident or disease. He has not been used to machinery. His new job may necessitate quick motions, there may be poison in the materials to be handled, danger in the processes to be performed." Many immigrant workers ran high risks of contracting infectious diseases in crowded, unhygienic, and poorly ventilated workshops. W. Gilman Thompson, the author of the first American medical text on occupational diseases in 1914, observed:

> In New York City, a hotbed of tuberculosis is found in the so-called "sweat shops," where so much ready-made clothing is manufactured. If a man comes to my Cornell [University medical school] Out-Patient Clinic and gives his occupation as a "tailor's presser," I always ask him at once how long he has had a cough. He is almost certain to have worked in a densely crowded unventilated room, dusty from the lint of clothing. . . . He has had long hours of work and poor food. Thus, anemic, ill-nourished and fatigued, his body is an ideal condition for the development of the germs of tuberculosis, which one of his comrades is tolerably certain to pass on to him in the sweat-shop.[21]

Other deaths resulted from the nature of outdoor work, as described by the New York City Department of Health in 1906: "The greater prevalence of [pneumonia] among the Irish and the Italians is due to the more usual occupation of these people. In New York, at the present time, . . . the Irish are largely employed as truck, cab, or car drivers, motormen, bricklayers, etc., while the Italians are very largely laborers. All these occupations are attended with considerable exposure to inclement weather."[22]

In many cases occupation and low earnings combined to increase the risk of disease. Louis Dublin, Alfred Lotka, and Mortimer Spiegelman, Metropolitan Life Insurance Company statisticians, observed that "heavy physical labor and poor pay often go together. When earnings are small, the worker and his family suffer privations of many kinds. . . . Food and clothing are apt to be inadequate and their living quarters crowded and unsanitary. . . . Economic pressure is powerful enough to keep men on the job after common sense and sane medical judgment would suggest medical attention."[23]

Nationality Differences In Mortality Rates

Recognizing the hazards of immigrant life, public health officials frequently gathered statistics on the mortality rates of the various nationality groups. Analyzing the data presented a major statistical problem because the native born population included many more children than the foreign born, which invalidated comparisons of overall mortality rates. Considering the white population of cities of 250,000 or more population in 1920, among the 35% who were native born of native parentage, 32% were under age 15, 63% were ages 15–59, and 6% were ages 60 or over. Among the 27% who were foreign born, only 4% were under age 15, 84% were ages 15–59, and 12% were ages 60 and over. Large numbers of young children were found among the 38% who were of foreign stock: 40% were under age 15, 57% were ages 15–59, and 4% were ages 60 and over.[24] A new statistical technique called "age adjustment" equalized the age distributions of all nationality groups and permitted accurate comparisons of group mortality rates.

One outstanding study comparing the mortality rates of nationality groups was carried out by Louis Dublin, an eminent epidemiologist and statistician, and Gladys Baker. They analyzed mortality rates in New York and Pennsylvania, two populous states that maintained accurate vital statistics. In 1910 the white population of New York State was 9 million, of whom 30% were foreign born, and that of Pennsylvania was 7.5 million, of

Table 6.1: Age-Adjusted Mortality Rates by Place of Birth and Sex: Pennsylvania and
New York State, 1910

| | (Whites ages 10 and over per 1,000 population) | | | |
| Place of birth | Pennsylvania | | New York State | |
	M	F	M	F
Native born, native parents	12.8	12.3	13.8	12.4
Native born, foreign or mixed parents	18.8	16.3	19.5	15.5
All foreign born	17.5	16.0	17.3	16.2
Austro-Hungary	14.4	13.5	14.3	12.4
Russia	13.7	12.7	13.1	12.3
Italy	14.5	12.6	12.9	13.7
Germany	17.0	14.2	17.9	14.4
England, Scotland, Wales	16.1	15.1	16.6	15.8
Ireland	23.6	20.5	25.9	23.5

Source: Louis I. Dublin and Gladys W. Baker, "The Mortality of Race Stocks in Pennsylvania and New York, 1910," *Quarterly Publications of the American Statistical Association* 17 (1920): 13–44.

whom 19% were foreign born. The nationality groups listed in Table 6.1 constituted 93% of the foreign-born population in Pennsylvania and 87% of the foreign-born population in New York State. The study used age adjustment and limited their analyses to persons ages 10 and over, which removed infants and young children with their very different causes of death. However, state-wide data include both urban and rural residents, and urban death rates were much higher than rural death rates. All of the foreign-born groups were predominantly urban, while the native born of native-born parents were primarily rural.

Dublin and Baker found that the native born of native-born parents had significantly lower age-adjusted mortality rates than both the foreign born and those of foreign stock (Table 6.1). The differences were greater for males than for females and for older age groups than younger groups (not shown). These findings were consistent with the urban-rural differences of the groups and the disparities in living and working conditions.

When the mortality rates of the individual nationality groups were analyzed separately, the results confounded all expectations (Table 6.1). Immigrants from southern and eastern Europe were expected to have higher mortality rates than those from northwestern Europe because of their lower incomes, lesser education, language deficiencies, insalubrious living arrangements, more hazardous jobs, and lack of familiarity with urban living.[25] Yet the foreign born from Austro-Hungary, Russia, and Italy had age-adjusted mortality rates comparable to the native born of native-born parents and lower than the foreign born from Germany, Ireland, and Great Britain. According to Dublin and Baker, the Russians and Austro-Hungarians were predominantly Jews.

In order to understand this surprising finding, Dublin and Baker examined age-adjusted mortality rates for specific diseases for each foreign born group and for the entire native-born group (disregarding parent's place of birth). Using New York State as an example (Table 6.2), tuberculosis of the lung was a major cause of death among men and women ages 25–44 and 45–64 in all nationality groups. Immigrants from southern and eastern Europe were considered especially vulnerable to tuberculosis because of their rural backgrounds and living conditions. Yet men and women who were born in Italy, Russia, and Austro-Hungary had no higher and often lower death rates from tuberculosis than those born in America, Germany, Ireland, and Great Britain. The Italians and Jews also had lower or as low death rates from most other major causes of death in the 45–64 age group, the youngest age group with significant mortality rates from individual diseases.

A number of explanations were advanced for the lower mortality rates of Italians and Jews. Some observers claimed that eastern and southern European immigrants had low mortality rates in America because they returned to Europe when they developed tuberculosis or other diseases. This was not true of Italians and Jews. Between 1903 and 1923, only about 375 persons returned to Italy annually with tuberculosis[26] and Jews had very low remigration rates.

Another possible explanation was childhood nutrition, which may have been superior among Italians and Jews. Malnutrition can increase the risk of many diseases, such as tuberculosis and rheumatic fever, that reduce adult lifespans. Probably the best measures of childhood nutrition are adolescent weight and height. One study examined 5,393 boys and 4,650 girls of different nationalities between the ages of 14 and 16 who were granted employment certificates in New York City from July 1914 to April 1915. Certificates were granted only to children who were in sound health, achieved normal development for their age, and completed six years of elementary school. These criteria excluded children suffering from the effects of severe malnutrition, but this condition was rare. This analysis will examine children ages 14.0 to 14.5, the largest of the four age groups, but the other age groups have similar patterns.[27]

The heights and weights of the children in the various nationality groups were so similar that nutritional factors could not explain nationality differences in mortality rates. Native-born boys of native parentage aver-

Table 6.2: Mortality Rates for Selected Causes of Death, by Sex, Age, and Place of Birth: New York State, 1910

(Per 1,000 persons)
Ages 25–44

		Males			*Females*
Place of birth	All causes	Pulmonary tuberculosis	Violence*	All causes	Lung tuberculosis
U.S.	10.1	3.5	1.1	7.4	1.9
Austro-Hungary	6.7	1.8	1.2	5.8	1.4
Russia	5.1	1.2	0.7	5.3	1.1
Italy	6.6	1.0	1.6	7.0	1.6
Germany	10.0	2.5	n.l.	6.3	1.3
England, Scotland, Wales	8.7	2.4	1.4	7.6	1.7
Ireland	18.5	6.6	2.8	12.0	3.5

Ages 45–64
Males

Place of birth	All	Pulmonary tuberculosis	Cancer	Organic Heart disease	Pneumonia	Kidney disease	Violence*
U.S.	22.1	2.6	1.5	3.2	1.9	2.7	1.3
Austro-Hungary	21.0	3.0	2.6	2.4	2.3	3.0	1.1
Russia	20.1	2.5	2.8	2.5	2.3	2.4	0.8
Italy	19.3	1.7	1.2	2.5	3.9	1.7	1.7
Germany	27.7	3.5	2.9	3.3	2.7	3.3	n.l.
England, Scotland Wales	24.6	2.7	2.4	2.7	2.5	2.9	1.8
Ireland	46.3	6.8	3.4	5.8	6.0	6.6	3.2

Ages 45–64
Females

Place of birth	All	Pulmonary tuberculosis	Cancer	Organic Heart disease	Pneumonia	Kidney disease
U.S.	16.6	1.1	2.9	2.5	1.3	2.1
Austro-Hungary	18.2	1.2	3.9	2.2	1.7	2.4
Russia	16.0	0.8	2.9	2.4	1.6	2.8
Italy	17.9	1.2	2.4	3.7	2.5	2.1
Germany	18.4	1.1	3.3	2.9	1.4	2.5
England, Scotland, Wales	21.0	0.9	3.6	3.0	2.0	2.4
Ireland	40.7	2.5	4.3	6.6	5.2	6.4

*excluding suicide

n.l. not listed

Source: Louis I. Dublin and Gladys W. Baker, "The Mortality of Race Stocks in Pennsylvania and New York, 1910," *Quarterly Publications of the American Statistical Association* 17 (1920): 13–44.

aged 61.4 inches and 100.8 pounds and the girls averaged 62.1 inches and 104.4 pounds. Native- and foreign-born boys of parents born in Germany averaged 61.7 inches and 102.0 pounds and the girls averaged 62.4 inches and 106.9 pounds. Native- and foreign-born boys of parents born in England, Scotland, and Ireland averaged 61.2 inches and 98.8 pounds and the girls averaged 61.7 inches and 101.0 pounds. Native- and foreign-born boys of parents born in Italy averaged 60.5 inches and 100.3 pounds and the girls averaged 60.2 inches and 103.2 pounds. Native- and foreign-born boys of Jewish parents averaged 61.4 inches and 104.0 pounds and the girls averaged 60.9 inches and 105.1 pounds.[28]

A last explanation for the differences in mortality rates to be examined here is working conditions. Dublin and Baker measured work-related deaths in New York and Pennsylvania using the cause-of-death category, "violence (excluding suicide)," which consisted primarily of industrial accidents. Lower death rates from this category did not explain the lower overall mortality rates of Jewish and Italian men. In Pennsylvania, with its many mines, mills, and hazardous industries, violence (excluding suicide) was the primary cause of death of foreign born men ages 25–44 and a major cause of those ages 45–64. Italian and Jewish men were particularly likely to die from this cause, as indicated by death rates per 1,000 males ages 25–44 by place of birth: Austro-Hungary 3.6; Italy 3.2; Russia 3.1 (mostly Jews); Ireland 2.6; Great Britain 2.2; and United States 1.3. In New York, with its different mix of industries, violence was a less important cause of death, but Italian and Jewish men died from that cause at rates similar to those of other nationalities (see Table 6.2).

Another method of examining the relationship between nationality and mortality rates is to compare infant mortality rates, defined as the number of infants under one year of age who died in a year divided by the number of live births in that year. Infant mortality rates were considered to be the best indicator of a society's health status because they were affected by so many social and environmental conditions. Those born in the United States and northwestern Europe, with their higher incomes and better living conditions, were expected to have lower infant mortality rates than those born in southern and eastern Europe. Yet once again this expectation was not supported.

Useful data on infant mortality are available for New York City, which had the nation's largest foreign-born population and maintained among the best vital statistics (see Table 6.3). The city's infant mortality rates for 1913, 1916, and 1917 showed higher than average rates for children of parents born in the United States, Ireland, and Germany, slightly above average rates for children of parents born in Italy, and well below average

Table 6.3: Infant Mortality Rates by Nativity of Parents: New York City, 1915–1917

Nativity of both Parents	Births Reported			Infant Mortality Rate		
	1915	1916	1917	1915	1916	1917
All*	141,256	137,664	141,564	98	93	89
U.S.	36,992	37,590	37,555	106	106	111
Italy	29,717	29,011	28,989	103	101	92
Russia-Poland	24,432	23,016	24,099	78	75	64
Austro-Hungary	11,797	10,613	10,377	80	92	75
Ireland	5,027	4,662	4,752	119	115	113
Germany	1,903	1,764	1,704	116	109	100
England	486	443	669	138	99	40
Sweden	550	463	567	66	99	72

*including mixed nativity and other groups

Sources: New York City Department of Health, *Annual Report for the Calendar Year 1915* (New York: 1916), 182; Ernst C. Meyer, *Infant Mortality in New York City* (New York: 1921), 135.

rates for children of parents born in Russia-Poland and Austria-Hungary (primarily Jews). Rates for parents born in England and Sweden fluctuated widely from year to year because of the small number of cases.

Very similar nationality differences were found in a study of deaths in the first *month* of life in the 1917–21 United States birth registration area, primarily the northeastern states with their large immigrant populations. Children of mothers born in the United States, regardless of the place of birth of their mothers, had a death rate per 1,000 live births in the first month of life of 46 for males and 36 for females. Children of mothers born in the following countries had higher or similar rates for males and females respectively: French and English Canada (55 and 43), Poland (55 and 42), Ireland (51 and 39), Austria (51 and 39), Germany (46 and 36), and Great Britain (44 and 36). Children of mothers born in the following countries had lower rates: Denmark, Norway, and Sweden (41 and 32), Russia (39 and 28), and Italy (37 and 29). These comparisons worked to the disadvantage of urban nationality groups such as the Italians, Poles, and Russians because groups with members in rural areas benefited from the lower mortality rates in those areas. A 1911 death registration area study found an infant mortality rate of 136 per 1,000 live births in the cities compared to 94 in rural areas. The disparity occurred throughout the first year of life and for every major cause of death.[29]

More sophisticated analyses were employed in one of the most brilliant of all American epidemiological studies: an investigation of infant mortality by Robert M. Woodbury and the U.S. Children's Bureau.

Woodbury studied 23,000 live legitimate births to mothers from 1911 to 1916, 60% of them residents of Baltimore, Maryland, and the rest living in seven smaller cities in the Northeast and Midwest. The cities were chosen because they were industrial cities with large foreign born or, in the case of Baltimore, black populations. All participants were interviewed personally and each infant was followed from birth to its first birthday or earlier death, which enabled Woodbury to calculate the true probability of dying in the first year of life.[30]

Woodbury found a strong relationship between nationality or race and probability of dying in the first year of life that was similar to data from New York City (see Table 6.4). Extremely high mortality rates occurred among the Portuguese and French-Canadian immigrants; high rates among the Polish immigrants and native-born "colored" group; moderate rates among the native-born white group and the German and Italian immigrants; and a very low rate among the Jewish immigrants. Deaths due to conditions in early infancy, including prematurity and congenital debility, exhibited less variation among nationality groups than those due to gastro-intestinal diseases (mostly diarrhea and enteritis) and respiratory diseases (primarily pneumonia and bronchitis). Congenital causes of death are considered to be less influenced by environmental factors.

Table 6.4: Death Rates in the First Year of Life by Nativity of Parents: Selected Cities, 1913–1916

| Nativity | Number of live births | *Death rates per 1,000 live births* | | |
		All causes	Gastro-intestinal	Respiratory	Early Infancy
Native-born					
White	12102	94	25	13	36
Colored	1457	154	28	45	52
Foreign born					
Italian	1426	104	22	27	34
Jewish	1233	54	11	9	23
French-Canadian	1074	171	64	25	45
German	776	103	27	18	31
Polish	1226	157	64	33	39
Portuguese	669	200	102	51	21

Source: Robert M. Woodbury, *Causal Factors in Infant Mortality: A Statistical Investigation based on Investigations in Eight Cities,* U.S. Children's Bureau Publication No. 142 (Washington: U.S. GPO:

Woodbury then carried out a number of multifactorial analyses to determine the role of causal factors other than or in addition to nationality or race. Two such factors were the number of births and the spacing of births, because death rates were higher for later order births and for closer spacing of births. Woodbury compared the actual infant death rates of each group to the rates that would have occurred if the birth order and spacing of births had been the same for all groups. He found that the adjusted rates maintained the nationality differences in infant death rates. Woodbury also examined the proportions of births to women below age 20 and above age 35 and found that the small differences among the groups could not have affected the infant death rates.[31]

Another factor was the employment status of the mother. For the whole sample infants born to mothers employed away from home either during pregnancy or in the infant's first year of life had much higher mortality rates than infants whose mothers did not work or worked at home. Thirteen percent of the births occurred to mothers who worked away from home during pregnancy. Although this varied greatly by nationality, a statistical adjustment that equalized the employment rates for each nationality did not alter the relative infant death rates of the groups significantly. Eight percent of all births were to mothers who worked away from home in the first year of the infant's life. The rates also varied greatly among nationality groups, but similar statistical adjustments did not materially change the relative infant death rates of the nationality groups (119–21).

Housing congestion has often been cited as an important factor in infant death rates. Woodward found that infant death rates increased significantly as the number of persons per room increased. Because crowded housing was more common among low income families, Woodward used statistical adjustments and found that within the low income group those who lived in more congested housing had higher infant death rates than those who lived in less congested housing. He also found that the various nationality groups differed in the proportion who lived in congested housing, but that adjusting the data for the variations in housing congestion did not significantly alter the rankings of the groups (116–17, 125–29).

Two other factors of great importance were type of feeding and father's income. At every month of life, death rates for the entire sample were much higher for artificially fed than breast-fed infants. Death rates for the whole sample were also inversely related to father's income. Woodbury combined both factors and calculated the ratio of actual to expected deaths (expected being the overall death rate for the total sample) for each nationality group. If a nationality group's ratio was more than 100, factors other than type of feeding and father's income were raising the death rate; if a group's ratio was less than 100, other factors were lowering it. The ratios were: Polish 150; Portuguese 141; French Canadian 128; native-born "colored" 118; German 97; native-born white 89; Italian 87; and Jewish 49. Clearly eliminating the effect of socio-economic status and type of feeding did not equalize infant mortality rates among nationality groups (124, 137).

Woodbury found that some of the causal factors were interrelated. For example, breast feeding reduced infant mortality rates compared to artificial feeding in lower income families, but not in higher income families. Woodbury offered this explanation: "artificial feeding was fraught with greater dangers to the baby's health in the lower-earnings groups. Doubtless such feeding as practiced in the families with larger incomes was accompanied by safeguards that were not employed to the same extent in the poorer families. These safeguards probably included the use of pure milk, the practice of proper sterilization of bottles and nipples, [and] the advice of a competent physician" (90–95, 163).

A possibility that Woodbury did not consider is that nationality differences in infant mortality rates simply matched the patterns in the home countries of the immigrants. The infant mortality rate per 1,000 live births in the 1920 birth registration states in the United States was 95 for males and 76 for females. Using data between 1909 and 1920, much higher infant mortality rates were found in Italy (175 and 158), Germany (144 and 118), Austria (171 and 142), Hungary (282 and 245), and Russia (265 and 237). Lower rates existed in Ireland (90 and 75), England (90 and 70), and Sweden (77 and 63). Infant mortality rates among French-Canadians in Montreal were extremely high, much above those of other groups in the city.[32]

These statistics show only a slight relationship between infant mortality rates of the groups in their home countries and in America. Italy and Germany had very high infant mortality rates, but Italians and Germans in America had rates that were close to the United States average. Ireland had among the lowest infant mortality rates in Europe, but Irish immigrants had above average rates in the United States. Two groups had similar patterns their homelands and in America: French-Canadians had very high infant mortality rates in both Canada and the United States and studies of Jews found that they had low infant mortality rates in the United States and in numerous cities and countries throughout Europe.[33]

Still another possible explanation is that the nationality groups differed in their total numbers of births, because later births had higher mortality rates. However, fertility differences among nationality groups were very small. For most of the United States birth registration area in 1920, the total number of children ever born to women 45–49 varied from a low of 8.2 to a high of 10.0 for the following countries of birth: United States (both whites and blacks), Austria, Hungary, Canada, Denmark-Norway-Sweden, Great Britain, Ireland, Germany, Italy, Poland, and Russia.[34]

A last possible explanation to be considered here is the levels of personal and household cleanliness of each nationality group, which were especially important at a time when infectious and gastro-intestinal diseases were responsible for most infant deaths. Contemporary observations show little relationship between a nationality group's cleanliness and its infant mortality rates. A study in the early 1920s examined the overall condition of the apartments of immigrants. It rated three-fourths of those of Swedes and Germans and two-thirds of those of Bohemians and Moravians as "good," compared to about one-half of those of Northern Italians and Jews and one-third of those of Southern Italians. Josephine Baker (1873–1945), who spent her career in and headed the children's bureau of the New York City Department of Health, described her experiences with several groups:

> The Germans were the cleanest; that was axiomatic. The Italians came next; not only would the front room of an Italian family usually be moderately clean but there would have been some pathetic attempt at brightening the place up with paper flowers, religious pictures and a fancy bedspread. . . . [The colored] district contained the densest population in town . . . but they managed to stay decent in spite of that inhuman handicap. The houses were clean in a sad poverty-stricken fashion and the children were kept so clean that I often wondered how it was done. . . .
>
> The Irish and the Russian Jews vied for the distinction of living in the most lurid squalor. The Irish did it . . . out of a mixture of discouragement and apparent shiftlessness, but they were happy people too and soon pulled themselves up out of the ruck. The Russian Jews did it out of thrift. . . . While [one of the children] was being educated [to help support the family after graduation] the whole family worked like mad under sweat-shop conditions and skimped incredibly on food, clothes and rent, not to mention soap and sunlight. Then, when the chosen son started making money, they moved out and followed his rising fortunes uptown.[35]

Thus consistent differences were found in total and infant mortality rates among nationality groups that could not be explained by the many factors examined here.[36] The most likely explanation is that the disparities were due in part to unidentified differences in the cultures of the groups. This suggested that public health programs should focus on education to change the knowledge and beliefs of immigrants.

7

THE GERM THEORY AND HEALTH EDUCATION IN DIPHTHERIA AND TUBERCULOSIS CONTROL

The successors to Pasteur and Koch were not always sufficiently broad to appreciate that with the discovery of the infectious agent, the epidemiology of a disease was not always explained. . . . Epidemiology is not bacteriology, nor is it applied immunology. The genesis of infectious disease and of epidemics is more than a simple reaction between man and his parasites.

(John E. Gordon, 1953)[1]

The tubercle bacillus, although being the "sina qua non" of tuberculosis, is after all practically, especially from a prophylactic or hygiene point of view, a minor element in its multitudinous etiological factors.

(Early twentieth-century physician)[2]

The contrast between public health programs based on the germ theory and those based on public education are exemplified by controversies over the effectiveness of diphtheria antitoxin and tuberculosis control. Evaluations of antitoxin treatment concentrated on the diphtheria bacillus and disregarded the patient, resulting in inaccurate and conflicting findings. Early tuberculosis control programs also emphasized the tubercle bacillus, but the lack of success led to greater concern with patient education and community involvement.

95

The Development of Urban Public Health Programs

Federal, state, and local governments undertook different types of public health activities in the first decades of the twentieth century. The federal government gathered statistical data, conducted many useful and some outstanding research studies, occasionally distributed limited funding to states, and provided some health care for veterans and merchant seamen. State governments operated mental hospitals, tuberculosis sanatoria, and similar facilities for specific groups, but undertook few health programs for the general public. States were unable to resolve the conflicts between their cities, which wanted public health programs, and their rural areas, which sometimes opposed even compulsory birth and death reporting as government intrusions into the privacy of citizens. Many states undertook local health initiatives only in response to conflicts among towns or cities, such as the pollution of one town's water supply by another town's sewage. State governments employed physicians, engineers, and bacteriologists in the 1880s to monitor the drinking water and sewage disposal of local governments, but forty years later only two-thirds of the states required state approval of all municipal water supplies and sewerage systems.[3]

The nation's major cities therefore conceived and shaped the first modern public health movement. They devised popular programs that could be delivered efficiently to their densely populated communities. The cities had the skilled public health, medical, nursing, and other professional personnel and the bureaucracies necessary to devise and implement the programs. Although the states had ultimate authority over the cities, they usually acceded to the wishes of the localities because of the long tradition of local self-rule.[4]

The earliest sanitary and public health initiatives of nineteenth century cities—water supplies, garbage collection, sewerage systems, and birth and death registration—were intended only in part to improve the health of the public. Water supplies were constructed both to meet the demands of fire insurance companies for better methods of fighting fires and to provide water for consumption. The water, while plentiful, was unfiltered, contained sediment and organic matter, and was sometimes unsafe to drink. Garbage collection was primarily an opportunity for political patronage, as demonstrated by the frequent scandals and the mounds of rotting garbage ubiquitous in city streets. Municipal sewerage systems often discharged untreated sewage into rivers, lakes, or the ocean. Birth and death registration were designed for legal rather than public health purposes and seldom enforced systematically.[5]

The emergence of new kinds of urban public health programs at the end of the nineteenth century was a response to the public health dangers posed by the enormous influx of immigrants. The youthful immigrant population created unprecedented demands for housing, schools, and medical care for their large and growing families. Their overcrowded neighborhoods, insalubrious housing, and ignorance of urban living made infectious diseases endemic among them and a danger to the remainder of the population.[6]

The modern public health movement received its greatest impetus from the combination of bacteriology and vital statistics. Bacteriology provided the first practical method of tracing disease from the victims to the source of the bacterial pathogens and of modifying the source to prevent future cases of the disease. Birth and death registration and vital and hospital statistics provided the information required for decision making. For example, the reporting of a case of typhoid fever by a hospital could produce an investigation that discovered bacteriological evidence of contaminated milk. The health department could then take legal action against the milk vendor or dairy. If vital statistics indicated an excessive number of cases of typhoid, the department was often able to convince the municipal government to enact appropriate ordinances.[7]

This study will use the New York City Department of Health as a prototype for the emergence and evolution of public health programs. The human and financial resources available in America's largest city enabled the health department to serve as a national standard. The department's impressive staff of administrators, physicians, and nurses drew upon the city's expertise in public health, medicine, nursing, social work, education, business, life insurance, and even entertainment. By the 1920s the department's responsibilities included: infant and maternal care; birth, death, marriage, and midwife registration; school medical inspection and dental and ophthalmic care; patients with tuberculosis and other diseases; specialized hospitals and a tuberculosis sanitorium; a bacteriological laboratory for diagnosis and the manufacture of diphtheria antitoxin and other serums and vaccines; food and milk inspection; sewage disposal; mosquito control; work permits for children; and industrial hygiene, including smoke and noise abatement. Water and sewerage systems were the responsibility of other municipal departments that had the necessary specialized skills. The level of implementation of the health department's programs fluctuated widely depending on its budget and political support. For that reason, this analysis will emphasize the basic policies of the department.[8]

The health needs of children and young adults were the focus of the department's efforts at the turn of the century. In 1900 78% of New York

City's population was under age 40, including 22% who were under age 10 and 18% who were ages 10–19. The diseases of greatest concern were childhood infectious diseases and tuberculosis. Evidence of ongoing improvement in the city's health was provided by the crude death rate per 1,000 population, which declined steadily from 31 for the 1.25 million residents in 1880 to 21 for the 3.4 million residents in 1900.[9]

The Diphtheria Antitoxin Statistical Controversy

Control of diphtheria was revolutionized at the end of the nineteenth century by the discovery of the diphtheria bacillus and an antitoxin that could cure patients with the disease. Diphtheria is predominantly a children's disease of the larynx spread by personal contact. For centuries it was confused with croup, a much milder condition, and was not given its modern name until the 1820s. During the nineteenth century, diphtheria was one of the most serious endemic diseases of children in densely populated cities and occasionally flared up in deadly epidemics that varied unpredictably in severity. The diphtheria bacillus was discovered during the 1880s, but the highly variable mortality rates were explained only decades later with the identification of three types of the bacillus with different levels of virulence. In New York, Baltimore, Boston, Pittsburgh, and Philadelphia from 1880 to 1895, diphtheria produced 1–2 deaths per 1,000 population annually with occasional higher or lower rates. In New York City in the 1890s the deaths were about equally divided among children under age 2, ages 2–4, and over age 4. Because the crude death rate included all age groups, it greatly understated the severity of the disease in young children.[10]

The verification of the bacillus in 1890 made it possible to diagnose diphtheria bacteriologically using cultures produced from throat swabs, the only part of the body where the bacilli resided (a toxin produced by the bacilli circulated in the bloodstream). Largely to improve the diagnosis of diphtheria, in 1892 the New York City health department established the nation's first municipal bacteriological laboratory. A study by the laboratory of 5,611 suspected cases of diphtheria in 1893–94 found ample justification for bacteriological diagnosis: many patients diagnosed clinically with croup actually had diphtheria, and others with no symptoms had the bacillus present in their throats and could transmit the virulent disease to others. In 1893 the department established collection stations in local pharmacies where physicians could obtain kits for taking throat cultures and then deposit the cultures for daily pick-up and examination. Up to one-half of the cultures produced no evidence of diphtheria, sometimes due to the difficulties of swabbing the throats of patients.[11]

The discovery of diphtheria antitoxin in 1894 provided the first effective treatment for a major bacterial disease. Because antitoxin was made from the serum in blood drawn from horses, pharmaceutical firms had no expertise in the process and were not interested in producing antitoxin. The New York City health department established the first American diphtheria antitoxin production laboratory in 1894 using both public and private funds. The antitoxin was sold to local physicians for patients who could afford to pay, given free to physicians for poor patients, and administered by department physicians to other poor patients without cost, sometimes at the request of the attending physician. The surplus was sold to other cities and constituted a source of income to the department for years. The laboratory served as a model for other cities that produced their own antitoxin.[12]

Studies undertaken to evaluate the antitoxin brought about the first modern statistical controversy in clinical medicine. The controversy resulted from several striking characteristics of diphtheria: the substantial year-to-year variations in mortality rates; the much lower mortality rates in older than in younger children; and the greater benefits of antitoxin at earlier than later stages of the disease. The early hospital studies of the antitoxin produced contradictory findings because they disregarded some or all of these characteristics. At one extreme, in Boston City Hospital from 1891 to 1895 1760 cases were treated without antitoxin with a mortality rate of 43%. From September 1895 to May 1896, 1359 cases were treated with antitoxin with a mortality rate of 13%. At the other extreme, an American hospital study of 164 cases showed an insignificant decline in mortality rates from 32% to 27% and a Berlin study of 562 cases treated with antitoxin produced a mortality rate of 15% compared to a practically identical mortality rate of 17% in 282 cases not given antitoxin.[13]

Critics recognized the methodological weaknesses and attacked all hospital statistics as untrustworthy. A New York City physician, J. E. Winters, pointed out that the mortality rate from diphtheria in the hospital in Basel, Switzerland was 34% in 1876 and 6% in 1886. If a treatment had been introduced in that hospital in 1886, it would have been considered a great triumph. He stated: "Why have the reports from the French and German hospitals so moved the medical world for the antitoxine treatment of diphtheria? Because the advocates of this treatment have ingeniously compared the lowest death-rate of the present with the highest death-rate of the past. They have not told the whole truth."[14]

The benefits of antitoxin were equally difficult to demonstrate in community medicine, again due to disregard of the personal characteristics of patients. Prior to antitoxin treatment, many physicians had reported cases of diphtheria only after the death of the child and had never reported the many mild cases. When antitoxin was introduced, health departments required all cases to be reported. The additional mild cases lowered death rates and gave the false impression that the decline was due to the antitoxin. In addition, many physicians were reluctant to administer the antitoxin early in the disease when it was most effective because of its cost or the fear of adverse effects, thereby diminishing its benefits.[15]

Supporters of the antitoxin did not deny the validity of many of the criticisms of statistical studies and referred to other types of evidence. Hermann Biggs (1859–1923), a physician who was the effective head of the New York City health department, stated that "the strongest evidence" comes "not so much from clinical investigation, as from the results of experimental work." He urged physicians to disregard statistics and accept the findings of laboratory research. He also asked physicians to use the treatment under the proper conditions:

> All that is required to convince any skeptical observer of the efficacy of the serum is that he may watch the results in one single, severe, uncomplicated case of diphtheria, when the remedy is administered on the second day or the beginning of the third day. They are sometimes most extraordinary, and seem to me to approach the miraculous more nearly than anything which has previously come under my observation in medicine.[16]

Proponents of antitoxin treatment conducted systematic clinical trials, including hospital studies that emulated the methods of laboratory research. Patients were divided according to some method of randomization into two groups, a treatment group that received antitoxin and a control group that did not, and their outcomes compared. Because the patients were admitted to the hospital without regard to their participation in the study and received similar care, any meaningful differences in survival rates between the two groups could be attributed to the antitoxin. An 1896 study administered antitoxin to every other patient admitted to a New York City municipal hospital while the intervening patients received standard care. At the end of six weeks, according to William Park, the chief investigator and head of the New York City bacteriological laboratory, "the difference in the outcome of the cases was so great that we decided to discontinue the observations. We believed that although we had lost a few lives by it, we had gained a certainty as to the value of the antitoxin which we would not otherwise have obtained, and this enabled us to persuade the members of the medical profession much more rapidly than if we had not carried out the experiment."[17]

A similar study was carried out in 1896 in Denmark because a consistent trend toward milder cases of diphtheria made it impossible to use historical comparisons to evaluate the effectiveness of the antitoxin. In this 365–day study, only patients admitted on alternate days were given the antitoxin. The untreated control group of patients experienced steadily declining mortality rates during the study, which made it difficult to detect any differences between the two groups that might have produced an early termination of the study. At the end of the year, the investigators found that 2% of 204 diphtheria patients treated with antitoxin died, compared to 7% of 201 patients not treated.[18]

Both studies had significant methodological limitations because of their disregard of the characteristics of the patients. The studies provided no statistics to show that the age distributions of the treatment and nontreatment groups were similar or that they received the antitoxin at the same stage in their illnesses, even though the importance of both factors was well known. Indeed, neither study described the patients or compared them to the general population.

Another difficulty resulted from the difficulty of generalizing from the samples to the general populations. Different samples of patients or time periods would have altered the mortality rates of both the control and treatment groups. Those samples would probably have produced smaller or larger differences in mortality rates between the treatment and control groups. It is possible that, by chance, the samples in these two studies produced unusually large differences in mortality rates. In the 1950s, after methods were devised to evaluate this possibility, the Danish data were re-analyzed and indicated a reasonable probability that the difference in mortality rates could be explained by chance variations.[19]

In 1896 the American Pediatric Society established a committee headed by L. Emmett Holt to investigate the effectiveness of antitoxin treatment in community medicine. The committee conducted three analyses: 3,384 cases collected from information supplied voluntarily by 613 individual society members, 28% of whom were treated on the fourth day or later; 942 confirmed cases treated in New York City tenements by public health department physicians, 40% of whom were treated on the fourth day or later; and 1,468 confirmed cases treated in Chicago homes by public health department physicians, 25% treated on the fourth day or later. Once again the primary focus was on the bacillus, not the personal characteristics of the patients.[20]

The committee's findings generally supported the use of antitoxin. The most surprising finding was the small difference in the death rates of the 4,837 cases diagnosed by throat cultures (11%) and the 957 cases diagnosed clinically (16%), which suggested that throat cultures did not identify as many mild cases as physicians had thought. Mortality rates in the three studies combined rose from 5% for the 996 cases treated with antitoxin on the first day to up to 35% for the 690 cases treated on the fifth day or later. The committee concluded that antitoxin was important but not essential in all cases and deemphasized bacteriological diagnosis: "antitoxin should be administered as early as possible on a clinical diagnosis, not waiting for a bacteriological culture. However late the first observation is made, an injection should be given unless the progress of the case is favorable and satisfactory."[21]

Although the study lacked control groups of patients who did not receive the antitoxin, the committee measured the benefits of the treatment by comparing those who were treated earlier and later in their illnesses. The value of the antitoxin was so limited when administered late in the illness that those patients could legitimately be considered a control group. The strikingly lower mortality rates of patients who received antitoxin early in their illnesses satisfied the committee.

Despite the controversies generated by the clinical studies, the earlier laboratory evidence had convinced leading physicians, medical educators, public health departments, and community leaders, and their views were widely publicized by the media. The publicity and successes of antitoxin treatment soon won over many physicians and the public. One general practitioner in a lower income neighborhood wrote about his experiences with only 17 patients: "aside from the emolument, if there be any, and the gratitude of the parents, which is always abundant, and the increase of reputation, which surely results, there is another cause of gratification in the treatment of these cases; it gives a man a feeling of power over disease and consequently a sense of pride in his profession in a great degree."[22]

In retrospect, a fundamental limitation of the early studies was the very small doses of antitoxin. Holt's 1896 committee proposed that the dose for children ages two and above be increased to 1,500 to 2,000 units of antitoxin daily for up to three days. A 1902 New York City health department study of 166 fatal cases reported that two-thirds of the cases received a dose of 4,000 units or less, with only one dose being administered in two-thirds of the cases. In 1990 a single dose of 20,000 to 100,000 units was recommended.[23]

The controversies surrounding antitoxin treatment led many physicians to avoid it for years, as shown by mortality statistics compiled by the New York City health department. A 1904 study found a diphtheria case fatality rate in Manhattan of 10%, compared to 5.7% in over 3,700 Manhattan tenement cases treated by department physicians at the request of the attending physician. The department also reported that diphtheria mortality rates were declining more slowly in Brooklyn than in Manhattan and the Bronx, "the explanation of which is that diphtheria antitoxin has not been used to the same extent by the physicians of Brooklyn."[24]

In 1908 the department found it necessary to issue strict regulations to raise the standards of medical care in diphtheria: physicians were required to report all cases of diphtheria promptly; cultures were required for all diagnoses; patients with diphtheria were to be quarantined for at least ten days; and other children in the family were to be given immediate immunizing doses of antitoxin. Physicians were told that if they stopped taking cultures, they must notify the health department and department physicians would do so. If physicians desired, department physicians would administer antitoxin without cost to the poor. In 1908 and 1909, the municipal bacteriology laboratory analyzed about 70,000 specimens of throat cultures annually, with 62% having been taken by department physicians (including many follow-up cultures), compared to only 38% by the much larger number of private practitioners. Clearly the health department was leading and many community physicians were lagging in the use of bacteriological methods in diphtheria.[25]

Tuberculosis

Pulmonary tuberculosis was the most serious health problems of urban adults in the early twentieth century and a major concern of all municipal health departments. Tuberculosis has existed as a recognizable disease for at least several millennia, but it became the leading cause of death in Europe and North America with the rapid growth of cities after 1800. Tuberculosis of the lung, which accounted for more than nine-tenths of all tuberculosis deaths, was estimated to have caused 14% to 25% of all deaths in American cities in the mid-nineteenth century. Death rates began to decline spontaneously during the second half of the nineteenth century in many American and European cities.[26]

Statistical analyses of tuberculosis mortality rates were much more accurate than for many other diseases. Most of the victims were younger adults who had no other diseases that could have produced misdiagnoses. The terminal signs and symptoms were well known to physicians, so that the cause of death was usually obvious if the patient was under medical care. Most deaths were in cities, which maintained the best mortality statistics.

The most useful urban tuberculosis mortality statistics were compiled by the Metropolitan Life Insurance Company based on its industrial life insurance policyholders. According to Louis Dublin, the company statistician, in 1919 the 10 million Metropolitan industrial policyholders were predominantly urban and "more than any other group for whom data are available, typical of our industrial population" and representative of "all the important industries and occupations." The family breadwinners were mostly blue-collar or lower level white-collar workers and many lived in geographic areas that were not yet part of the death registration area. The policyholders were divided about equally between men and women. Reporting of death was essentially complete because claims were paid only after beneficiaries provided death certificates or other proof of death.[27]

The pulmonary tuberculosis mortality rates of industrial life insurance policyholders were much higher than the United States death registration area, which included rural as well as urban residents. In 1911–16 pulmonary tuberculosis accounted for 15% of the 635,449 deaths among Metropolitan Life Insurance Company industrial policyholders ages 15 and above. White men ages 15–19 had a pulmonary tuberculosis mortality rate per 1,000 policyholders of 1.0, which rose to 3.9 at ages 25–34, peaked at 5.4 at ages 35–44, and was still high at 3.7 at ages 55–64. White women ages 15–19 had a rate per 1,000 policyholders of 1.4, which peaked at ages 25–34 with a rate of 2.4 and declined to 1.5 for those aged 45–54 and 1.4 for those aged 55–64. For persons ages 25–54 the pulmonary tuberculosis death rate for male policyholders was almost twice that of the death registration area and the rate for female policyholders was about 25% higher.[28]

The modern epidemiology of tuberculosis began in 1882 when Robert Koch isolated the tuberculosis bacillus and demonstrated that it could produce tuberculosis in experimental animals. It was then discovered that infection in humans was produced primarily by the transmission of tubercle bacilli through the air from person to person, that tubercle bacilli were exceedingly slow growing, and that the tubercular process often ceased spontaneously and the patient returned to health.[29]

The presence of the tubercle bacillus in healthy persons was measured using the tuberculin test. In 1907 Clemens von Pirquet found that injections of tuberculin (a substance obtained from tuberculosis cultures) produced skin reactions in persons who had been infected with the tubercle bacillus even if they never developed clinical tuberculosis. Studies using the tuberculin test found that at least three-fourths of all adults in American cities in the early twentieth century had been infected by the tubercle bacillus at some time during their lives, with most never experiencing clinical disease. A 1917 study of 460 children ages 6–7 without clinical tuberculosis in Framingham, Massachusetts, found that 55% of the girls and 38% of the boys had reactions to the test. In the mid-1920s Chadwick and Zacks tested 42,071 Massachusetts school children without tuberculosis and found that the proportion who had reactions to the test increased from 21% at age 5 to 35% at age 15, a lower rate because of the inclusion of many rural children. The rates would have been higher in both studies had children with clinical tuberculosis been included.[30]

These rates were similar to those found in European studies. Clemens von Pirquet examined 693 children in Vienna with no symptoms of tuberculosis and found that the proportion with reactions to the tuberculin test increased from 2% of those aged 1–2 to 55% of those aged 11–14. A hospital study of 108 Viennese children ages 10–14 who were admitted with diseases other than tuberculosis found that 92% had reactions. Both studies excluded children with clinical tuberculosis. Similar rates were found in autopsy studies of persons who died from diseases other than tuberculosis. The ability of infected humans to resist clinical tuberculosis was most strikingly demonstrated by a tragic accident in Lubeck, Germany, in 1926 where 249 babies were inadvertently given massive doses of virulent tubercle bacilli. Although 31% died of acute tuberculosis, the remaining 69% developed only minor lesions and were free of tuberculosis twelve years later.[31]

Tuberculosis rates were highest in the lowest socio-economic groups. Louis Dublin compared tuberculosis mortality rates for three types of Metropolitan Life Insurance Company policyholders: low-income persons who paid small premiums weekly for industrial insurance; middle- and upper-income persons who paid much larger premiums quarterly or less often for ordinary insurance; and an in-between group that paid moderate premiums monthly for intermediate insurance. For white males ages 15–74 in 1925, industrial policyholders had a tuberculosis mortality rate of 1.4 per 1,000 policyholders, intermediate policyholders had a rate of 1.1 per 1,000 policyholders, and ordinary policyholders had a rate of 0.6 per 1,000 policyholders.[32]

Nationality groups with similar tuberculosis infection rates had strikingly different tuberculosis mortality rates. Chadwick and Zack's study in the early 1920s found that the reactions to the tuberculin test were about the same (from 25% to 30%) among Massachusetts schoolchildren whose mothers were born in the United States, Great Britain, Ireland, Germany

Table 7.1: Pulmonary Tuberculosis Mortality Rates By Place Of Birth: New York City, 1912–1193

| Place of Birth | Nationality of deceased | | | | Nationality of parents of deceased | |
| | 1912 | | 1913 | | 1912 | |
	deaths	rate	deaths	rate	deaths	rate
Austro-Hungary	347	1.3	330	1.2	380	1.0
England	165	2.1	147	1.9	160	1.4
Germany	503	1.8	479	1.7	1,152	1.9
Ireland	1,057	4.2	1,111	4.4	2,515	4.5
Italy	409	1.2	446	1.3	540	1.0
Russia	395	0.8	448	0.9	456	0.6
Scotland	58	2.5	69	3.0	71	2.0
Sweden	87	2.5	97	2.8	111	2.1
U.S.A.	5,021	1.8	4,939	1.7	1,595	1.6
Total	8,591	1.8	8,601	1.8	8,591	1.8

(rates per 1,000 persons)

Sources: New York City Department of Health, *Annual Report of the Board of Health for the Year Ending December 31, 1912* (New York: 1913), 166; New York City Department of Health, *Annual Report for the Calendar Year 1913* (New York: 1914), 178.

and Austria, the Scandinavian countries, Italy, and Russia and Poland. Yet tuberculosis mortality rates varied greatly by nationality in a manner similar to total mortality. In New York City in 1912 and 1913 tuberculosis mortality rates were lower for those born in Italy, Russia, and Austro-Hungary (the last two groups were mostly Jews) than for those born in the United States and Western Europe (see Table 7.1). Socio-economic factors were important within nationality groups, so that, for example, Jews in low-income neighborhoods in New York City had much higher tuberculosis rates than those in high-income neighborhoods.[33]

The downward secular trend in tuberculosis mortality that began in the second half of the nineteenth century continued unabated during the early twentieth century. Massachusetts, an urban state with the first reliable death registration statistics, showed a decline from 3.1 tuberculosis deaths per 1,000 population in 1880 to 1.9 in 1900 and 0.6 in 1930. This was much greater than the overall decline in the state's death rates, so that the proportion of all deaths that were caused by tuberculosis decreased from 16% to 5% over the period. Statistics from the U.S. death registration area showed a very similar trend, with tuberculosis mortality rates declining from 1.9 per 1,000 persons in 1900 to 0.7 in 1930 while total death rates declined from 17.2 to 11.3 per 1,000 persons.[34]

The decline in tuberculosis mortality rates benefited both low and high socio-economic groups, according to studies of Metropolitan Life Insurance Company policyholders. Between 1911 and 1943 white and nonwhite male and female industrial life insurance policyholders ages 16–24 and 26–45 experienced substantial declines in their tuberculosis mortality rates (see Table 7.2). The decline was greatest for white males age 26–45 and for nonwhite (primarily black) males and females in both age groups. Comparisons of the lower socio-economic status industrial policyholders with the higher socio-economic status ordinary policyholders showed that tuberculosis mortality rates declined by about two-thirds for both groups between 1911 and 1930. By 1936–39, female industrial policyholders had only slightly higher tuberculosis mortality rates than female ordinary policyholders, but male industrial policyholders continued to have much higher rates than male ordinary policyholders, mostly due to differences in occupations.[35]

Table 7.2: Tuberculosis Mortality Rates, by Age, Sex, and Race: Metropolitan Life Insurance Company Industrial and Ordinary Policyholders, 1911–43

| | (deaths per 1,000 policies) *Industrial Policyholders* | | | |
	white male	white female	colored male	colored female
Ages 16–25				
1911	2.2	2.2	5.5	7.1
1926	0.7	1.2	3.0	4.6
1943	0.2	0.2	1.3	1.8
Ages 26–45				
1911	5.1	2.8	5.2	4.4
1926	1.6	1.1	2.9	2.5
1943	0.6	0.3	1.5	1.1

1936–39
(deaths per 1,000 policies)

| | Male *Type of Life Insurance* | | Female *Type of Life Insurance* | |
Age	Industrial	Ordinary	Industrial	Ordinary
26–35	0.6	0.3	0.5	0.4
36–45	0.9	0.4	0.4	0.3
46–55	1.3	0.5	0.3	0.2
56–65	1.4	0.6	0.4	0.3

Source: Malvin E. Davis, *Industrial Life Insurance in the United States* (New York: McGraw-Hill, 1944), 302, 318–19.

Although most of the secular decline occurred during a period of rising standards of living, the decline did not result from that factor alone. Tuberculosis mortality rates continued to drop during the depression of the 1930s at a greater rate than the overall death rate despite steadily deteriorating economic conditions. The tuberculosis mortality rates per 1,000 population in the United States death registration area declined from 1.9 in 1901 to 1.1 in 1920, 0.7 in 1930, and 0.5 in 1940. The overall crude death rate declined from 16.4 in 1901 to 13.0 in 1920, 11.3 in 1930, and 10.8 in 1940. From 1930 to 1940, the proportion of all deaths from tuberculosis dropped from 6.2% to 4.6%. The pulmonary tuberculosis mortality crude death rates per 1,000 population in New York City dropped from 2.3 in 1901 to 1.1 in 1920, 0.6 in 1930, and 0.5 in 1937. The overall crude death rate in the city declined from 19.9 per 1,000 population in 1901 to 12.9 in 1920, 10.8 in 1930, and 10.4 in 1937. Between 1930 and 1937, the proportion of all deaths from tuberculosis dropped from 5.6% to 4.8%.[36]

Tuberculosis control was therefore an extremely complex problem. The secular downward trend began in the nineteenth century long before any tuberculosis control measures were in operation and declined steadily through good times and bad. Socio-economic status affected tuberculosis mortality, but different nationality groups with the same socio-economic status had widely varying mortality rates.

Louis Dublin distinguished two sets of factors involved in tuberculosis control. In the nineteenth century tuberculosis mortality rates declined because of the rising standard of living and sanitary measures. In the twentieth century the key factor was lifestyle changes resulting from a health education campaign that emphasized "personal hygiene"—"sufficient rest, adequacy of nourishing food, of recreation and of other influences."[37] The change from sanitary measures to health education is clearly seen in the programs of the New York City health department, which were unmatched by any other city in the world.

The New York City Health Department Tuberculosis Control Campaign

Tuberculosis mortality rates were higher in New York City than in most other cities. In 1913, the New York City pulmonary tuberculosis mortality rate per 1,000 population was 1.7, which was higher than Boston (1.5), Chicago (1.4), Cleveland (1.0), Detroit (1.0), Philadelphia (1.6), St. Louis

(1.3), and San Francisco (1.6), but lower than Los Angeles (2.2), Cincinnati (2.2), and New Orleans (2.3). These statistics must be considered in light of New York City's grim determination to track down every case of tuberculosis compared with the much more lax reporting in most other cities.[38]

The department's earliest attempts to control tuberculosis after the discovery of the tubercle bacillus began with anti-spitting ordinances and fumigation, disinfection, and repainting of tenement apartments of persons who died of tuberculosis. The programs were quickly found to be a waste of time and resources.[39]

The health department then adopted a new philosophy of control that focused on identifying all tuberculosis patients and preventing them from infecting others. In 1894 the department established a registry of all reported cases and in 1897 required all physicians and health care institutions to report tuberculosis cases within one week of treatment. Physicians objected to compulsory reporting, which they considered unnecessary for middle-income families and objectionable to families who believed that tuberculosis was a hereditary taint. Hermann Biggs insisted that reporting was essential in tenement districts and frustrated the medical profession's effort to have the state legislature repeal the ordinance. The department's conflicts with private physicians continued for many years. In 1922, the annual report complained that "an appreciable fraction of the physicians in New York do not fully co-operate in the prevention and control of tuberculosis. There are hundreds of cases [in which physicians and private tuberculosis clinics] certify to the Health Department that home conditions are eminently suitable and in compliance with the Health Department regulations, when, in fact, they know nothing of the home conditions." In response, the department had a department nurse visit every newly reported case to assure "herself that there is no menace to health."[40]

The program to maintain a registry of all active cases of tuberculosis was an expensive and labor-intensive failure. Many cases were never reported. In 1902, the department reported a 22% increase in registered cases from dispensaries and hospitals after insisting on better reporting from them. By 1904 it had lost track of so many cases that it reorganized the registration system and required private physicians and hospitals to report changes of address or discontinuance of treatment, with little success. In 1919, a typical year, 1,647 tuberculosis deaths occurred "in which no record of a previous report of the disease to the Health Department could be found." The status of most of the reported cases was unclear. For example, at the end of 1920 the department reported 27,919 registered cases. One-third were at home and not under professional care, constituting "one of the most important problems that the Department has to deal with." Another 19%, "all trace of whom has been lost," included homeless cases and were, "possibly, an even greater factor of danger to the community than the at home cases." The remainder were under the care of the city or private physicians or hospitals, but the department knew nothing about the quality of care or home environments of the patients receiving private care. Furthermore, twice as many cases were registered in Manhattan tuberculosis clinics as Brooklyn clinics, even though the two boroughs had similar populations. Last, nonpulmonary cases of tuberculosis were not required to be reported, so that the department had no information about them.[41]

The 1897 ordinance enabled the department to incarcerate pulmonary tuberculosis patients who were a danger to their families and others, but so few cases were confined that it was also a waste of effort and resources. For example, the number of cases involving "forcible removal to hospital" were 25 in 1909, 27 in 1910, and 68 in 1911. In 1919, when two cases were incarcerated, the annual report noted that "the use of the big stick and the exercise of summary police powers by the Health Department has in late years fallen into great disfavor," but added that "there are a certain group of individuals with whom persuasion even though it comes from the tongues of angels is not effective in securing compliance with the regulations of the Health Department." In 1926 six cases "considered a menace to others" were incarcerated in a city hospital, with the annual report commenting that "the procedure would be more often employed were it possible to obtain evidence sufficient to warrant such action." In 1930 the department conceded that some cases were being detained "indefinitely" for "questionable" reasons and began periodic evaluations of the cases to expedite their return to the community.[42]

Compulsion was used regularly by New York City and other cities to deal with disease carriers or potential carriers. Josephine Baker reported about vaccinating the homeless at lodging houses in the Bowery district: "Few of them were nature's noblemen, so I always had a Health Department policeman by my side when I marched in . . . . The policeman would wake a man up and tell him to put out his arm. Then I would vaccinate him and pass on to the next. They were usually too far gone from bad whiskey to know very much about what was going on." The most famous forcibly incarcerated disease carrier, known as Typhoid Mary, lived for over twenty years until her death in a cottage set aside for her use on the grounds of a New York City municipal hospital. When she died in 1938 the department annual report referred to her as the "famous typhoid disease carrier" and noted: "Her death brings to mind the successful struggle of the Department to protect the public by detention of those individuals unwilling or unable to abide by the regulations set up for proper control of communicable disease. Typhoid Mary persistently refused to cease working as a cook and to her activities were ascribed at least 50 cases of typhoid fever."[43]

Another method of preventing patients from spreading tuberculosis was to institutionalize them in hospitals or tuberculosis sanatoriums. The 1902 annual report stated: "the chances for recovery of a tuberculosis patient confined to a city tenement are so small as to be negligible, whereas each of these patients becomes, with the progress of the disease, more and more a menace to the health of every person with whom he comes in contact." In 1906 the city opened a free municipal sanatorium in Otisville, New York. In January 1910 the sanatorium had 320 beds and in that year treated 1,051 patients for an average length of stay of about three months. The size of the sanitorium was increased regularly, and in December 1913, it had 583 beds. The department also maintained records of all cases in private sanitariums in the city or elsewhere. Department standards for hospitalization about 1915 were based exclusively on sputum tests, even though they were often inaccurate: patients were hospitalized when they had positive sputum tests and discharged when their sputum tests were negative three times in succession. Children with active tuberculosis who were excluded from school were treated at sanitoriums, day camps, and fresh air schools.[44]

The institutionalization program failed to prevent the spread of tuberculosis because many active cases were released from the sanitoria. The Metropolitan Life Insurance Company operated a tuberculosis sanitorium for its employees and found that the tuberculosis mortality rate of the discharged patients from 1919 to 1937 was five times the rate for all company employees. This ratio was similar to that found in a study of patients hospitalized only once for at least 90 days in ten Minnesota sanitoria between 1925 and 1935. Evidence from other sanitoria was even more discouraging: of 547 patients discharged from one New York sanitorium between 1902 and 1905, more than 60% died before 1912. The deceased included 17% of the released patients who were considered cured, 51% of those in whom tuberculosis was arrested, and 72% of those considered improved. A study of patients discharged in 1909 from the Pennsylvania State Sanitorium found that 44% died by 1913 and 14% were in unsatisfactory health.[45]

The New York City health department bacteriological laboratory tried to improve diagnosis by testing sputum cultures supplied by department and private physicians, but the program was only marginally effective. The number of sputum cultures tested annually increased from 5,000 in 1900 to almost 65,000 in 1916, with tubercle bacilli found in one-fifth to one-half of them. In general, the more cultures tested in a year, the lower the proportion with tuberculosis bacilli, which suggested that the periodic drives to induce private physicians to submit sputum cultures produced more cultures but few additional cases. In 1907, private physicians provided 56% of 27,277 tuberculosis cultures, whereas they also provided 41% of 64,282 diphtheria cultures and 76% of 10,212 typhoid cultures. Thus the small number of health department physicians, not the private physicians, were the most active users of the bacteriological laboratory to diagnose tuberculosis and diphtheria.[46]

The health department operated tuberculosis clinics, but these identified few new cases of the disease and duplicated the work of the sixteen other clinics in 1908, most in municipal and private hospitals. In 1910, the department maintained eleven tuberculosis clinics that employed 55 physicians and 31 laboratory assistants. Most of their patients were previously identified cases who were referred by private physicians, dispensaries, and hospitals. In 1908, of the almost 8,000 new patients examined at the health department clinics, the large majority had been diagnosed with tuberculosis previously and most of them were later transferred to a public or private clinic near their homes.[47]

Clearly, the health department's efforts to control tuberculosis by separating patients from the community were failures. The department formulated and implemented a wide variety of programs that approached the problem from different perspectives, but none of them achieved the stated objectives of identifying tuberculosis patients and preventing them from infecting others.

The most productive and cost-effective department strategy involved making the public an active rather than a passive participant in tuberculosis control. It sent visiting nurses to educate patients and their families in their homes. Tuberculosis patients, unlike those with other infectious diseases, were continuing sources of infection because they were sick for months or years. Hermann Biggs called home visitation a "simple but very powerful means of attacking disease."

> Home visitation aims to bring to light other cases of the disease in the same family; it strives, if possible, to trace the cause or source of the infection; it aims to learn what influence the patient's environment has on his disease and on the health of others in the home; it attempts to devise means of curing

the infections which have already occurred and of preventing further infections. It tries, by an intensive study of many cases, to gather experience to guide in the care of all. In short, home visitation constitutes the absolutely necessary and only means of learning the conditions surrounding, and the causes of, the infection.[48]

The department first employed a few nurses to visit tuberculosis patients in their homes in 1902 and the 23 who were employed for this purpose in 1910 were increased to 159 during the year. Each nurse was assigned a number of cases not being treated by private physicians. She made frequent visits to cases who had a high risk of transmitting the disease because of their failure to follow hygienic rules and less frequent visits to other cases. In 1909 the nurses made 26,109 visits, in 1910 the enlarged nursing staff made 241,181 visits, and in 1911 226,859 visits, which enabled the department to reduce the number of physician visits from 23,583 to 4,324 and the number of patients who were removed to hospitals from 452 to 68.[49]

The home visitation program reflected a new philosophy of tuberculosis control based on the personal education of as many patients as possible. In the 1923 annual report, the department claimed that it had direct responsibility not only for the tuberculosis patients who made 76,000 visits to department clinics, but also for those not under the care of private physicians and clinics and the "refractory" cases. The report continued: "our nearly 200 field nurses . . . are valuable agents who disseminate education, and who, by personal oversight of the homes of many thousands of patients do yeoman service in preventing or confining the spread of disease."[50]

The educational role of nurses was part of a growing awareness of the importance of education in tuberculosis control. The public had to be educated to recognize the early symptoms of tuberculosis and seek medical care. Patients had to be educated to maintain high levels of personal hygiene in such matters as using separate towels, bed linens, and a sputum cup for expectoration. The family needed to learn how to prevent the patient from infecting other family members. As early as 1893 the New York City health department distributed a pamphlet about tuberculosis in four languages, a method of education that was used by many cities, states, and private groups, including the National Tuberculosis Association. Another popular educational tool was motion pictures, which were shown by the department in theaters, parks, and other locations. They described the housing and factory breeding grounds of the disease and its treatment and curability.[51]

The health department also tried unsuccessfully to enlist private physicians in identifying and reporting early cases of tuberculosis to improve their chances of recovery. It viewed the local medical profession as the "first line of defense" and wanted it to be "an active friend and ally of the Health Department," according to the 1919 annual report. Yet the report also referred to "the many difficulties preventing closer affiliation which have been responsible for breeding misunderstandings that have not infrequently bordered on open hostility." It blamed these on "the system of individual-istic practice of medicine."[52]

In 1929, due to declining tuberculosis rates, the health department converted its control program to one of prevention and diagnosis by establishing tuberculosis diagnostic clinics. In 1934 twenty of thirty-two tuberculosis clinics were diagnostic facilities for the department's patients and ten were "for patients of private physicians who are unable to pay the standard fee for consultation and x-ray." In 1939 the clinics examined 53,771 cases, including 10,600 for patients of private physicians. By this time, the rates of positive diagnoses had declined to 7.4% of the cases examined. Low rates were also found in mass X-ray screenings. Only 2.2% of the 232,475 persons X-rayed in New York City from 1933 to 1939 had active cases of tuberculosis.[53]

Even though the number of new cases of tuberculosis was declining steadily, virulent tuberculosis bacilli were still prevalent and infected susceptible newcomers. This was most evident in New York's small black community, which grew from 61,000 to 328,000 inhabitants between 1900 and 1930 due to immigration from the rural south. In 1940, blacks, who comprised only 6% of the population, produced 27% of the tuberculosis deaths and had a tuberculosis mortality rate of 2.1 per 1,000 compared to 0.4 per 1,000 for the combined native-born and foreign-born white populations. The health department's interest in tuberculosis control among blacks dated to 1905, when it offered its tuberculosis clinic on three evenings each week to a group of black physicians for the care of black patients. According to the annual report, "it was hoped that this would stimulate the interests of the colored people of this city, physicians, clergymen and laymen, in the subject of the control of tuberculosis, which disease is so prevalent among their people." However, black patients preferred the regular clinics and black physicians lacked expertise in tuberculosis, so the experiment was stopped after six months. In the 1920s the health department operated two clinics in Harlem that served the black population, which had 25% of all visits for tuberculosis in the city.[54]

The Framingham Tuberculosis Study

The most plausible explanation for the lack of success of the New York City health department tuberculosis control programs was its focus on changing individual behavior. An alternative approach was to consider tuberculosis a social problem and involve the entire community in tuberculosis control.

To test the social approach, in 1917 the National Tuberculosis Association carried out a six-year tuberculosis control program that transformed an entire community. The program was undertaken at the initiative of the Metropolitan Life Insurance Company, which contributed $200,000 and considerable technical, clerical, and other support. The site was Framingham, Massachusetts, a township of 17,000 inhabitants near Boston, which comprised an industrial city and a surrounding rural area. It had average mortality rates and a large proportion (27%) of foreign-born residents, most from Italy, Canada, and Ireland. It also had well-trained physicians, good hospitals, proximity to Boston medical schools, and support from an excellent state health department. The study was originally designed to terminate after three years, but additional Metropolitan funding extended it to six years.[55]

The Framingham study was part of the community social survey movement, which originated in the late 1880s in England. Charles Booth (1840–1916), a wealthy industrialist, financed and directed an extensive study of the population of London published as *Life and Labour of the People in London*. The report, which concluded that one-third of the population of London lived in poverty, attracted world-wide attention, but the methods consisted mostly of personal observations and interviews with people who worked with the poor. Community social surveys became extremely popular and hundreds of them were conducted in the United States by private and public agencies from 1900 to 1930 to evaluate social problems such as housing, schools, sanitation, nutrition, wages, unemployment, and crime. The studies were supposed to include statistical data, interviews, government records, and other information, but many of them lacked methodological rigor. The surveys stressed the involvement of local residents, partly to improve information gathering and partly to persuade politicians, government officials, and business leaders to implement the findings.[56]

Health was the focus of only a few studies. The 1914 Locust Point demonstration project used health education to improve the health of 900 public school pupils in a "highly underprivileged section of Baltimore," according to Means. Students were given information on diet, rest, sleep, outdoor exercise, and other activities conducive to good health. The goal was to design a program that would interest teachers and stimulate children to share the information with their families. It attracted national attention and influenced similar programs elsewhere.[57]

The Framingham tuberculosis study was as much a field experiment as a social survey. The investigators devised and implemented a wide range of community-level interventions and measured their impact on mortality and morbidity rates. The original objective was to lower the tuberculosis rate, but it was soon expanded to include the overall health of the city. Many of the interventions, such as school and industrial health programs, had multiple consequences and others, such as hospital improvement, could be better justified in that way.[58]

In evaluating tuberculosis mortality trends, the investigators could not use before-and-after comparisons because of the secular trend of declining tuberculosis mortality rates. Instead they compared the tuberculosis rates in Framingham to seven similar Massachusetts towns selected as controls. The researchers also foresaw that the number of tuberculosis cases would increase during the first years of the study due to more accurate diagnosis and comprehensive screening. They reviewed all deaths in Framingham from 1912 to 1916 and recoded the number caused by tuberculosis from 58 to 71 of a total of 808 deaths from all causes. As predicted, the number of tuberculosis cases under observation increased from 40 in the year preceding the study to 185 in the first year of the study (39–40, 51, 68).

The study was launched with an elaborate community education campaign. The investigators obtained the cooperation of political, business, community, and neighborhood leaders, health professionals, and the press. Local Metropolitan Life Insurance Company agents informed their policyholders about the study and the Metropolitan conducted a sickness survey of more than one-third of the population similar to others it had carried out. Agents, nurses, and home visitors interviewed families and recorded the amount and types of disease. The interviewers, aided by widespread publicity, recruited 4,473 individuals to undergo medical examinations in the program health center or their homes in order "to measure actual illness as contrasted with admitted or recognized illness. . . as a device for measuring new cases of tuberculosis, [and] as a measure for giving publicity to the idea of health examinations in general," according to the study final report (49–50).

A key feature of the study was a far-reaching health education campaign, which was described by the final report as including "popular leaflets, street care placards, [store] window displays, health exhibits, literature for distribution in the schools, the factories, the baby clinics, etc." The local newspaper provided free space for a weekly "Health Letter," which discussed tuberculosis, "child welfare, fresh air, the danger of common [shared] utensils, personal hygiene, pasteurized milk, the importance of birth registration, first aid in summer, influenza, rural hygiene, cancer, mental hygiene, health examinations, etc." The articles stressed methods of transmission of tuberculosis, including direct contact with infected adults, sputum, and "infected utensils, such as common cups, common towels, carelessly washed eating utensils, etc." (53–56).

Children received special attention, with hundreds given the von Pirquet tuberculin test. Although 54% of those ages 6–7 had positive reactions, no active cases were uncovered. The program operated a summer camp for five years for several hundred children with poor overall health (62–63, 65–66). Local physicians were given clinical lectures on tuberculosis by members of the study staff. The physicians were encouraged to refer questionable cases to a consultation service of tuberculosis specialists on the staff, who examined the patients in their homes and elsewhere (51, 81–83).

The city was scoured for sanitary problems, according to the final report, including surveys of "commercial establishments, industries, schools, housing and home congestion, food handling, privies and wells, sewage disposal, stables and fly breeding nuisances, etc." A thorough investigation was made of the schools, which led to the elimination of common drinking cups and recommendations for better toilets, washing facilities, heating, illumination, and seating. Factories were examined for dust ventilation, safety, and other problems. An estimated 11,000 persons—almost two-thirds of the total population—received complete medical examinations at schools, factories, and other sites from twenty-five physicians and seventy-five nurses. To eliminate bovine tuberculosis, the researchers tracked down every cow in the region and found that one-fifth of them had evidence of the disease. Sale of pasteurized milk increased from 15% to almost 80% of all milk sold (74–79).[59]

Louis Dublin observed that "the most important over-all achievement of the Demonstration was the development of a series of rounded health activities in the community and the stimulation of public sentiment in favor of them." According to the study report, the city of Framingham raised its budget for "infant welfare, tuberculosis, general sanitation, and other fields" from $8,000 to $20,000. The school health budget increased from $1,500 to $6,000. Industrial health expenditures rose from $2,800 to $11,000. Private organizations and hospitals increased their health promotion activities. Most of the programs initiated by the study were later taken over by public or private agencies.[60]

The achievements of the program were measurable and impressive: tuberculosis mortality rates per 1,000 population in Framingham declined from an average of 1.2 in 1907–16 to 0.4 in 1923. In the seven control towns, the decline was from 1.3 in 1907–16 to 0.8 in 1923. Framingham continued to have a considerably lower tuberculosis mortality rate than the control towns for more than two decades. The benefits extended to infant mortality, with Framingham infant mortality rates declining from 81 per 1,000 births in 1916 to 49 per 1,000 births in 1922–23, a decline of 40%.[61]

The Framingham study contributed to growing national recognition that community-wide public health programs could have an impressive impact on health.[62] The study was at the forefront in applying the principle that a wide range of community-level changes was required for effective control of tuberculosis or any widespread disease. It demonstrated the importance of public education and participation. By the end of the study, Framingham residents understood that they were collectively responsible for and could improve the health of their community.

The Framingham study confirmed three conclusions that many public health officials had reached. Effective public health programs required the active participation of the public. Active participation occurred only when the public was systematically educated about the nature of the programs and the role of the public. Last, the programs could be evaluated only by statistical analyses. Statistics had became the final arbiter of all public health programs, and it would play an equally significant role in the campaign to reduce infant mortality.

8

HEALTH EDUCATION AND INFANT MORTALITY IN NEW YORK CITY

There is a very great amount of poverty and overcrowding in [New York City]. . . . In many parts housing is still most unsanitary; . . . furthermore, there was up to the time of [World War I] an unending stream of immigrants arriving, so that the task of educating them was never done, those who were educated to our health standards being continually replaced by others who were not. Again, the climate is most trying.

(New York City Health Department, 1917 annual report)[1]

In all large communities, the poorer element of the foreign-born population presents the greatest problem encountered in municipal health work. Diversified in their habits, often superstitious and resentful of any interference with their mode of life, oppressed by poverty, frequently ignorant or neglectful of the simplest sanitary requirements, their assimilation as citizens of their adopted country comes only as result of education—persistent, inclusive, and never-ending. . . . Lectures, printed instructions, and publicity in all its forms are used, but the most valuable and effective form is found in individual instruction in the home. . . . We have found the employment of trained nurses for this purpose of inestimable value.

(Thomas Darlington, New York City Health Commissioner)[2]

119

> Health education is the method through which the [New York City]
> Health Department . . . enlightens people and induces them to act in
> a manner that will conserve their health. . . . The idea of promoting
> public health by education . . . goes back to the nineties when the New
> York City Department of Health first applied it to tuberculosis. Sub-
> sequently it was successfully used to combat infant mortality, diphthe-
> ria and other communicable diseases. Today the entire Health De-
> partment is an educational undertaking.
>
> (New York City Health Department, 1939 annual report)[3]

Programs to reduce infant mortality provided the strongest evidence that
public education was the keystone of all effective public health programs.
Health departments learned that the education of the mother was essential
to a healthy baby. In order to focus on mothers and families, the New York
City health department provided integrated care in neighborhood health
centers throughout the city.

Infant Mortality

Few aspects of urban life in 1900 were more dispiriting than the seemingly
ceaseless numbers of deaths of infants in the first year of life in the overcrowded, congested, and unsanitary tenement districts populated by new
immigrants from Europe. In an era when life was becoming more pleasing
and satisfying even among the poor, so many little lives entered the world
and passed out of it in the flicker of a few moments, so many "lean, miser-
able, wailing little souls carried off wholesale by dysentery," according to
Josephine Baker, who worked in the New York City health department and
headed its Bureau of Child Hygiene for many years after its organization in
1908. "One could hardly walk a block in any tenement district in the city"
in the summer, she wrote, "without meeting a 'Little White Funeral'" with
"a cheap white coffin and a few wilted flowers."[4]

    Programs to improve infant health had the unwavering allegiance of
public health administrators. The commissioner of health of New York
City observed in 1923, a year when the city had the lowest infant mortality
rate of the ten largest cities in the United States:

> Reduction of infant mortality is looked upon by public health workers all
> over the world as "a consummation devoutly to be wished." The Depart-
> ment of Health is especially proud of the results obtained, because it feels

that they are a practical demonstration of the efficiency and efforts of the field forces—the conscientious, hard-working staff of doctors and nurses who have kept at their tasks through most trying circumstances, day in and day out.[5]

Reductions in infant mortality rates were of less interest to the native-born middle and upper classes. They had little sympathy for the unwashed, ignorant, and impoverished immigrants who overwhelmed the cities and seemed to procreate at a staggering rate. No voluntary association for the health of infants and children ever compared to the National Tuberculosis Association or the March of Dimes (for poliomyelitis) in the number of local chapters or financial resources. Infants in immigrant families usually died of gastro-intestinal disorders or respiratory infections that posed no risk to the middle classes. Their deaths only confirmed the middle-class belief that immigrants were unable or unwilling to adopt American values and follow the rules of elementary hygiene.

Infant and child health programs were more popular with the urban political machines, such as Tammany in New York City, that appealed to immigrants for votes. Baker wrote: "I must confess that I would rather work with a Tammany administration than with a reform administration [despite its] graft and wholesale corruption," because Tammany bosses were much more sympathetic to her infant and child health programs. Reform administrations, after taking months to consider her proposals, found them useful but financially impractical. The Tammany bosses, on the other hand, always included some leader "who could be approached and told what was on my mind and how great the need was" and would arrange for funding. The Tammany bosses were particularly sympathetic to a woman administrator: "Being a woman was an enlightening asset in dealing with the old-time Tammany crew of chieftains and hangers-on. . . . I liked them and I liked to work with them. That is heresy, I know, but I couldn't help it."[6]

Health departments in New York City and elsewhere secured public backing for their infant and child health programs by stressing different benefits to different groups. When they sought support from the middle and upper classes, they emphasized the need to protect the general public from diphtheria, scarlet fever, and other contagious diseases that were prevalent among poor immigrant infants and children. To satisfy the political machines that depended on immigrant voters, the departments put most of their resources and efforts into reducing gastro-intestinal and other noncontagious conditions that were the primary causes of infant mortality, even though the conditions posed no risk to the middle classes. When the interests of the middle classes and the immigrants coalesced, the results were impressive. The total budget of the New York City Health Department increased from $1 million in 1900 to $3.9 million in 1913, much greater than the increase in the city's population from 3.4 million to 4.9 million. Equally important, department leadership during most of this period was in capable hands.[7]

Infant mortality rates declined steadily in New York City in the early twentieth century, as they did in cities throughout the country. In 1902 New York City's rate was 181 deaths in the first year of life per 1,000 reported live births. In 1912 the rate was 105 deaths per 1,000 live births, in 1927 it was 56, and in 1937, 44. The decline in infant mortality rates was due primarily to improvements in urban living conditions, as indicated by the growing proportion of infant deaths resulting from congenital disorders, which are least affected by these factors. From 1901 to 1937, the infant mortality rate per 1,000 live births from congenital causes remained fairly level at about 30, while the rates from diarrhea and enteritis declined from about 40 to about 5 and from all other causes from about 70 to about 15. As a result, the proportion of deaths from congenital causes increased from 21% to about 60%. Because many deaths due to congenital conditions occur early in infancy, the proportion of deaths in the first year of life that occurred in the first month of life increased from 36% in 1910–15 to 61% in 1937.[8]

Milk

The public health campaign to lower infant mortality rates began with important bacteriological discoveries about milk. Most milk contained bacterial pathogens responsible for infectious diseases and nonpathogenic bacteria that could overwhelm the infant's gastro-intestinal tract and produce fatal cases of diarrhea and dysentery. The bacteria had many opportunities to enter and multiply in milk because the New York City milk supply came from thousands of dairy farms within a radius of hundreds of miles. At the farms the milk was often exposed to rodent infestation and contamination with dirt and cow dung and hair. It was transported in unrefrigerated railroad cars to city dairies that processed and delivered unrefrigerated and unbottled "loose" or "dipped" milk to thousands of retailers 24 to 36 hours later. Grocers stored the milk in unrefrigerated large cans, from which they poured the milk into unsanitary and often bacteria-laden containers provided by customers. Other dealers drove horse-drawn carts through city streets and ladled out unrefrigerated milk exposed to dust and dirt into similarly unsanitary containers. Bottled milk had much lower bacterial counts, but it was too expensive for the poor.[9]

The difficulties for the urban consumer were described in a Metropolitan Life Insurance Company pamphlet written by Milton Rosenau, the noted public health authority. Rosenau noted that "milk is the most difficult of all our foodstuffs to collect, handle, and transport. . . . it spoils quicker than any other food." He recommended that consumers inspect their milk because "frequently milk contains so much dirt that the specks may be seen as sediment in the bottom of the bottle or glass." Milk should be tested by pouring it through several layers of white cloth and looking for a "brownish or blackish stain." He warned that filtering would remove the dirt but not the germs and listed the diseases that were transmitted through germs in milk.[10]

The great dilemma for public health officials was that milk was one of the few economical sources of many essential nutrients needed by children. Immigrant children often had bread and coffee or tea for breakfast or a pickle for lunch. Rosenau warned that children raised on tea and coffee "are apt to be pale and sickly." "Milk is the best food we have" and "one of the cheapest foods," he insisted, "there is no substitute. Save on other things if you must, but not on milk. You cannot afford to do without it—growing children especially need plenty."[11]

Milk inspection and production were revolutionized by bacteriology. The old methods of inspection relied on taste and appearance, which were disguised after dairies began to use chemical additives. Bacteriology made it possible to establish objective quantitative standards, such as the total bacterial count, that could be used to test milk samples at the farm, the dairy, and the dealer and were accepted as evidence in court. Bacteriological studies showed that raw milk sold at retail in hot weather could contain millions of bacteria per cubic centimeter, compared with hundreds of bacteria in milk fresh from the cow's udder. Pasteurization, the most important innovation in milk processing, retarded the multiplication of the bacteria and was quickly accepted by health departments and many commercial dairies, because it also lengthened the shelf life of the milk. Pasteurization was required by major cities after 1910 and in 1916 88% of New York City's milk was pasteurized.[12]

New York City regulated every step in the milk distribution process. Inspection of city dairies began in 1895 and was extended to dairies and farms elsewhere after 1905, when the U.S. Supreme Court ruled that the city could require permits for the sale of milk. In 1912 the city began to inspect retail stores and enacted measures that practically banned the sale of loose milk. The health department periodically sent its inspectors throughout the milk-producing region and employed local inspectors to examine up to 590 creameries in five states located up to four hundred miles from the city. By 1927 the department was inspecting 60,000 dairy farms in seven states and two Canadian provinces that produced and shipped 3.1 million quarts of milk daily to New York City.[13]

This approach was based on the belief that milk safety could be achieved by delivering it to the consumer in a sanitary condition. Yet the department soon learned that many consumers in tenement districts could not afford to purchase quality bottled milk, had no effective method of refrigerating milk, or diluted it with bacteria-laden water. Milk safety was as much a problem of the home as of the farm, the dairy, and the grocer.

In order to provide low-income mothers of infants with inexpensive pure milk, beginning in 1889 some European cities established milk stations or milk depots that distributed pure milk to the mothers. In the same year, Henry Koplik, a New York City physician, brought the idea to America. At first Koplik prepared sterilized milk in small bottles for sick infants and instructed the mothers to dilute it with barley gruel, but "they could not be trusted to dilute it correctly. The milk became contaminated or spoiled in the handling of it." Ultimately, he reported, "I went into the open market and bought the best bottled milk, [and] sterilized it in separate portions. . . . I felt the patients who came to be treated were so troubled and often so ignorant that the milk must be placed in their hands ready for the infant, and all they would have to do was to give it at proper intervals."[14]

In 1893 Nathan Straus, a New York philanthropist, opened several milk stations in New York City and later in other cities that sold bottles of pasteurized milk modified to the age of the baby. The milk was provided gratis to the very poor and at low cost to others. Within two years his New York City stations distributed 500,000 bottles of milk a year, and by 1910 the 18 seasonal or year-round stations distributed more than 4 million bottles of pasteurized milk a year. Other private groups also organized milk stations, and the New York Milk Committee operated 31 milk stations in 1911 either year round or during the summer. The movement spread elsewhere and by 1913, 297 milk stations were in operation in thirty-eight cities.[15]

The popularity of private milk stations in New York City led the health department to participate in the program and rationalize their operations. In 1904, the department contracted with a private charity operating five milk stations to provide free milk to poor tuberculosis patients to improve their nutrition. By 1908 48 private milk stations were in operation. In 1911 the city established 15 milk stations in neighborhoods not being served by the then 64 private stations. In 1912, after 48 private stations closed, the department opened 40 more so that there were now 55 public milk stations and 24 private ones. In 1920 the health department assumed responsibility for 8 stations operated by Strauss, raising its total to 68. Once the health department gained control, it instituted uniform record keeping and eliminated the "former duplication of work, overlapping of territory, and waste of effort," according to the 1912 annual report. Its stations sold quart bottles of pasteurized whole milk, dispensing 1.6 million quarts in 1912, which increased to 4.6 million in 1923. The mothers who visited the stations were given instructions on modifying the milk for their infants, and the annual report noted that "few mothers are found too ignorant or negligent to follow the instructions." The locations of the stations were widely publicized using newspapers, school teachers, visiting nurses, private charities, and letters mailed to new mothers.[16]

The milk depot movement had a limited impact on the quality of milk used by poor mothers. Many mothers were unable to go to the stations daily and others supplemented depot milk with milk from unsafe sources.[17] More basically, the concept was based on the belief that the best programs treated the mothers as passive recipients. Yet even the purest milk quickly became contaminated if the mother diluted it with tap or river water or let it sit uncovered at room temperature. Such programs were doomed to failure unless the mother also received education in handling milk.

The most widely advocated alternative to bottled milk was breast feeding, another method that did not require educating the mothers. In 1901 William Park and L. Emmett Holt undertook a study of 632 infants for the New York City health department and concluded that "most of the bottle-feeding is at present very badly done, so that as a rule the immense superiority of breast-feeding obtains. This should, therefore, be encouraged by every means. . . . The time and money required for artificial feeding, if expended by the tenement mother to secure better food and more rest for herself, would often enable her to continue nursing with advantage to her child." The health department sought to induce mothers to breast feed their infants using pamphlets and the personal recommendations of city physicians and visiting nurses. The 1923 annual report observed that "every effort is made to encourage breast feeding and in many instances even the husbands of foreign-born mothers are appealed to on the subject, as they seem to understand the situation more readily and can always be depended upon to instruct their wives as to what should be done."[18]

The advantages of breast feeding were subjected to research, most notably Robert Woodbury's brilliant statistical study of infant deaths in the early 1920s. He found that 87% of mothers used only breast feeding for infants in their first month, which declined to 71% in the third month, 57% in the fifth month, and 13% in the twelfth month. The mortality rate per 1,000 births in the first month for the breast-fed-only group was 17, compared to 55 for those who were artificially fed and 36 for those with mixed feeding. In the sixth month the mortality rates per 1,000 infants were 2 for the breast-fed group, 18 for the artificially fed group, and 6 for those with mixed feeding. The study also found that breast feeding produced a much greater reduction in infant mortality rates in families with the lowest earnings than those with the highest earnings.[19]

Research studies of tenement districts by the New York City health department discovered that breast feeding was far from a panacea. A 1912 study found that mothers who worked outside the home could not breast-feed their babies exclusively and that some mothers were so poorly nourished that they were not able to breast-feed. A 1907 study found that many breast-fed infants were also fed bottled milk and other foods, with the accompanying risk of exposure to bacterial pathogens. The problem was exacerbated by the "bad hygiene prevailing in many tenements during the summer months, owing to poverty and ignorance," according to Park and Holt. They found that the "depressing effects of great atmospheric heat [over 90 degrees] were very marked in all infants no matter what their food. Those who were ill were almost invariably made worse, and many who were previously well became ill."[20]

Park and Holt concluded that the knowledge and skills of the mother were the key to successful infant care:

> It was practically the unanimous opinion of the physicians who made the observations that intelligent care had more to do with the results of feeding than any other factor. Many individual instances were reported of infants living under the worst surroundings and whose food was of a very inferior kind of milk, and yet if the mother was intelligent and the infant well cared for, it throve in spite of the unfavorable conditions. On the other hand, if the infant had no proper care it made little difference how good the milk furnished might be, the results were usually bad.[21]

They stressed the importance of educating mothers in methods of intelligent care, including "clean bottles and nipples; the willingness and ability to carry out directions as to methods of feeding, quantities, frequency, the stopping of milk at the first signs of serious diarrhea, etc.; proper care of the milk itself while in the house, and methods of sterilizing; suitable clothing and cleanliness of the children, and as much fresh air as possible."[22]

For those tenement children who survived infancy, malnutrition was the great health problem, especially during the frequent periods of inflation or depression. A 1918 study of 184,374 school children in public and parochial schools found that 19% in each type of school were "definitely undernourished." In 1919 nurses of the New York City health department found undernourishment in 19% and "definite malnutrition" in 7% of 19,037 children ages 1–7 in 11,007 low-income families in the "congested" districts throughout the city.[23]

Recommendations for improving the diets of malnourished children were increasingly based on scientific discoveries in nutrition. In 1917 the federal government issued a food guide that recommended five food groups: flesh foods for protein, starchy foods for carbohydrates, fat foods, watery fruits and vegetables, and sweets. In the 1920s the food guide emphasized foods containing vitamins, which had been discovered about a decade earlier as agents that retarded growth when removed from the food of young rats.[24] Vitamins were thus considered primarily growth-promoting factors that were of greatest importance to children. Vitamins also prevented childhood diseases like rickets and scurvy and were essential to nursing mothers, whose diets influenced the vitamin content of their milk.

The nutrition of children could be improved only by educating the immigrant mothers, whose food choices were influenced by both economic constraints and cultural preferences. Michael M. Davis, a leader in the immigrant health movement, observed in 1921 that immigrants could neither afford nor obtain all of the foods that they ate in Europe, so they "limit themselves to the few familiar foods easily obtainable, thereby eliminating various essential elements and completely upsetting the balance of the traditional diet, which is not restored by the gradual addition of American products chosen without regard to food values." Italians considered milk a beverage rather than a nutritious food and favored but could not afford fresh vegetables, so they and their children subsisted on a diet of pasta with a few vegetables, sausages, bread, and coffee. Jewish children consumed "too many pickles, too few vegetables, and too little milk." Davis's solution was straightforward: "It is much easier for the dietitian to learn the foods of the foreign born than for these people to adjust their finances to a new dietary."[25]

Thus studies from a variety of perspectives all pointed to the same conclusion: the health of infants and children depended on the education of their mothers. Science had provided the knowledge and mothers needed to be taught it so that their children could live healthy lives, achieve normal growth, and resist infection.

Visiting Nurses

The need to educate mothers and families was greatest in tenement districts inhabited by low income immigrants with little understanding of urban life and limited knowledge of English. Tenement programs would also reach the great majority of infants in New York, because about 75% of the approximately 130,000 births in 1920 occurred in tenement districts.[26]

The most popular early method of education was "printed slips of directions," according to Park and Holt. They were highly critical of this approach and urged personal instruction in their 1901 study of infant feeding in immigrant families:

> Mothers are often anxious and willing, but ignorant and stupid. Many cannot read and many more have not the wit to apply in practice what they read. When, however, such printed advice was preceded or accompanied by personal explanation, it was found of great assistance. Personal contact is the only way to influence these people, and this must be frequently repeated to influence them permanently; as an aid to this, printed slips are useful.[27]

Convincing statistical evidence that personal instruction could reduce infant mortality rates was provided in a 1921–24 demonstration project in Thetford Mines, Quebec. The project was funded and carried out by the Metropolitan Life Insurance Company, which had many policyholders in Quebec, and endorsed by the provincial and local governments and the Roman Catholic Church. The French-speaking asbestos mining town of 9,000 persons was selected because it had an infant mortality rate of 276 deaths per 1,000 live births from 1917 to 1920. The rate was almost twice the Quebec rate of 145 and three times the overall Canadian and American rates. Only 10% of the mothers received prenatal care and most children lived on boiled potatoes, milk, and cornstarch for their first two years. Three Metropolitan nurses visited all pregnant women weekly during the third trimester and visited the mothers and infants frequently for the first month and thereafter saw them in a clinic. The nurses made 14,731 visits in 1922. The pregnant women and new mothers were also invited to the clinics for classes in infant care. Infant mortality rates per 1,000 live births plunged to 96 in 1923 and then rose to 117 in 1924, practically identical to the 1924 Quebec rate of 119. After 1924, the local government and the mining companies continued the programs, Quebec established similar clinics throughout the province, and in 1925 the University of Montreal founded the first training school for French-speaking nurses, with financial support from the Metropolitan.[28]

More complex problems confronted a major city like New York. Physicians and midwives were the most suitable providers of health information to mothers, but the health department's relationships with both groups were strained. Both groups often failed to report many home births, despite a legal requirement that they report all births promptly. In 1905 the city obtained state legislation that made physicians personally responsible for filing birth certificates with the department for all births that they attended. In 1910–11 more than two hundred physicians and twelve midwives were prosecuted and fined for failing to report births or deaths.[29]

Midwives posed the greater problem because they served so many immigrants. The department observed in the 1920 annual report that "every expectant mother has the right to ask, if she so desires, that she be delivered at home. The cornerstone of American society is the home, the family unit, and effort should be made to maintain rather than disrupt it. [T]he midwife . . . acts as accoucheur, attendant nurse, and confidant, [and] occupies a unique position in cosmopolitan cities." Equally important, New York did not have enough physicians and hospital beds to perform all of the deliveries. Nonetheless, according to the 1912 annual report, "many [midwives] are unfitted for their profession and do not maintain either the ethical or technical standards that are essential. The habitual delinquents are, generally speaking, the older midwives who have practiced many years, unsupervised and unrestrained." The department's solution was to improve and strengthen midwifery by developing a corps of well-trained midwives of the "superior character and ability of the graduates of foreign schools." European schools were under government supervision and usually required completion of a course of study of twelve to eighteen months.[30]

In 1907, after the city obtained state authority to regulate midwives, the health department established compulsory midwife registration based on certain standards and provided education for midwives in their own languages. In 1914 it required all future midwives to be graduates of an approved school, such as the School for Midwives in the city's Bellevue Hospital, a free six-month program organized in 1911, or a comparable European program. Midwives who were already practicing were allowed to continue to do so. The program became less important with the increase in hospital births. In 1909, 3,131 registered midwives delivered 40% of the 123,000 births; in 1924, 1,309 midwives delivered 20% of the 130,000 births; and in 1931, 863 midwives delivered only 9% of the 116,000 births, when two-thirds of all births occurred in hospitals. By 1940, 89% of all births occurred in hospitals and midwives delivered only 3% of them.[31]

In 1915 the department reported that "practically complete registration of the births occurring in the City has been attained, only those at which neither a physician nor a midwife was present remaining unreported." The major problem remaining was the failure to report births within the ten-day limit.[32]

In order to educate mothers, the health department turned to a new and growing profession, visiting nursing. Visiting nursing originated in Liverpool, England, about 1859 when a philanthropist organized a nursing school and employed its graduates to provide free care for the sick poor in their homes. The system soon spread to other English cities and a national organization was founded in 1875. Visiting nurses did not dispense material relief, thereby making them professional nurses rather than representatives of charitable organizations. The first visiting nurse associations in America were organized in 1885, and American private charities organized twenty-one visiting nursing agencies by 1890, including a few that provided material relief. Some agencies stressed education as well as patient care. The charter of the Instructive District Nursing Association of Boston, incorporated in 1888, stated that nurses had a responsibility "by precept and example to give such instruction to the families which they are called upon to visit as shall enable them henceforth to take better care of themselves and their neighbors by observing the rules of wholesome living and by practicing the simple arts of domestic nursing."[33]

Visiting nurses soon specialized in fields such as tuberculosis nursing. In 1903 in Baltimore, Maryland, tuberculosis visiting nurses replaced the Johns Hopkins University medical students who had been sent since 1899 to the homes of dispensary patients with tuberculosis to educate them in hygienic precautions. According to a 1922 account, the students found patients "in the last stages of consumption, . . . living with half a dozen other people, crowded into one or two rooms. . . . [O]ften they slept in the same bed with one, two, and sometimes three others: always they ate with the family, sharing the same cups, spoons and other dishes, and often giving the baby a sip of coffee from their own cup, or a bite of food from their fork. Was there any wonder that when one case was found, others were almost sure to follow?" In 1910 the Baltimore public health department assumed responsibility for the program. The New York City health department and several public and private dispensaries employed tuberculosis visiting nurses about 1903 and greatly expanded the program thereafter.[34]

Visiting nursing in New York City began in 1893 with the establishment of the privately funded Nurses' Settlement (later called the Henry Street Settlement) by Lillian Wald and others. Nurses who lived in the settlement provided nursing care to poor sick immigrants on the city's lower east side. When the health department began medical inspections of schoolchildren about 1900 and sent home large numbers with contagious conditions like head lice and trachoma, Wald offered in 1902 to send nurses to the homes of children in four schools with high exclusion rates to teach their families how to destroy the head lice. The results of what Baker called "home missionary work" were so successful that the department employed additional nurses in the tenement districts of Manhattan in the same year to expand the work. In 1903 visiting nurses made 16,000 visits to homes and an equal number to schools and treated 400,000 cases of head lice and eye and skin diseases. By 1905, when fifty nurses were employed (although many more were needed), the annual report emphasized the educational functions of nursing visits: parents "are instructed in keeping the children clean, carrying out treatment begun in school by the nurses, obtaining glasses for the children with defective sight, taking children to their physicians or to dispensaries for treatment."[35]

In the summer of 1903, a small experiment completely transformed visiting nursing. The thirty-three school visiting nurses of the health department, who had no summer responsibilities, became a "summer corps" who visited the mothers of newborn children recorded at the Bureau of Vital Statistics to dampen the annual summer epidemic of diarrhea and dysentery that killed 1,500 infants each week. Initially the nurses followed up the visits of department physicians to sick infants. The great innovation occurred when the nurses were instructed to visit only healthy newborns and educate their mothers. When they encountered sick infants, they informed department physicians, who visited the homes and treated the infants. The neighborhood selected for the experiment, according to Baker, was a "complicated, filthy, sunless and stifling nest of tenements on the lower east side of the city . . . largely populated by recently landed Italians, willing to learn new things in a new country." The experiences of the nurses were similar to those of Baker when she started working in the health department as a physician five years earlier and visited homes daily from 7 to 11 A.M. and 4 to 6 P.M.

> I climbed stair after stair, knocked on door after door, met drunk after drunk, filthy mother after filthy mother and dying baby after dying baby. It was the

hardest physical labor I ever did in my life: just backache and perspiration and disgust and discouragement and aching feet day in and day out. . . . The babies' mothers could not afford doctors and seemed too lackadaisical to carry their babies to the nearby clinics and too lazy or indifferent to carry out the instructions you might give them. I do not mean they were callous when their babies died. Then they cried like mothers, for a change. They were just horribly fatalistic about it while it was going on. Babies always died in summer and there was no point in trying to do anything about it. It depressed me so that I branched out and went looking for healthy babies too and tried to tell their mothers how to care for them. But they were not interested. I might as well have been telling them how to keep it from raining.[36]

Each nurse obtained the addresses of newborn infants from the birth certificates received the previous day. She visited each home and urged, according to Baker,

breast-feeding, efficient ventilation, frequent bathing, the right kind of thin summer clothes, out-of-door airing in the little strip of park around the corner—. . . all of it completely new to Mrs. Capozzi and all of it new in public health. Many of these mothers were a little flattered to have an American lady take all that trouble about little Giovanni, and were likely to go out of their way to learn and to co-operate. If the mothers were sulky or apprehensive, the nurses went again and again, wearing down their resistance, establishing friendly contact, until they were ready and willing to cooperate. . . . As soon as they saw their babies were flourishing, despite the cruelly hot weather, they became our most efficient aides.[37]

In 1908 the New York City Department of Health established the Division (later Bureau) of Child Hygiene with Baker as its first chief. Under her leadership, it achieved world-wide influence and renown. In 1908 the summer corps of the division employed 106 visiting nurses and 28 physicians in the tenement districts with the highest infant mortality rates in the city. The 41,000 infants in the districts constituted 37% of the approximately 106,000 infants in the city who were under one year of age. The program was so successful that 1,200 fewer deaths occurred in the districts than in the previous summer. The nurses visited 41,510 infants and made 9,905 revisits, while the physicians visited 1,688 sick infants. Nurses and physicians also delivered lectures in local recreations centers and distributed a pamphlet that urged breast-feeding, light clothing, daily bathing, and fresh air. The pamphlet advised mothers not to wean their babies in hot weather and warned them: "If the baby vomits or has diarrhea, stop all feeding, and give cool, boiled, water. Send for your doctor at once, or notify the Department of Health." Mothers who used artificial feeding were advised to "give the baby only good milk, prepared exactly as the doctor directs. Keep the milk always cold and covered. Do not ask your neighbor's advice about feeding, ask your doctor."[38] Few of these mothers could afford any doctor other than the free health department physician, but the phrasing was intended to mollify local physicians.

The visiting nursing program expanded steadily each summer for years. From 1911 to 1920 between 10,000 and 22,000 infants up to one year old participated in the program each year, with the nurses concentrating their efforts in districts with the highest infant mortality rates. In 1922, the 16,377 babies received 72,733 visits from nurses. Every nurse was assigned 150 infants, with the number of infants reduced in districts with higher infant mortality rates. The nurses gave only emergency care to sick babies and referred them to hospitals, dispensaries, or to the 20 part-time physicians employed by the department. The nurses' educational activities were supplemented by lectures given at milk stations, school playgrounds, recreation piers, and offices of charity organizations.[39]

From the beginning the summer visiting nurse service was coordinated with financial assistance for the family and health care for infants who were not making normal progress. The 1909 annual report stated that nurses were told to refer "cases of sickness or destitution" to other public agencies and private organizations. Visiting nurses met daily with department physicians in the milk stations to have them visit delicate and sick infants, and in 1913 the physicians made 1,211 such visits, compared with 119,645 for the nurses. In 1912, at the urging of the health department, a number of private and public agencies organized the Babies Welfare Association (later renamed the Children's Welfare Federation) to coordinate their activities. Even some private businesses provided material relief. In the summer of 1912 a newspaper fund-raising campaign and a large ice company joined to donate 317,700 pounds of ice to indigent families, a program that was continued by charities and businesses for many years.[40]

By 1915, the death rates of older infants were declining so much that a new emphasis was inaugurated on prenatal care and education. According to the annual report: "renewed efforts were made to reach the mother as early in pregnancy as possible and to have her place herself under medical care at the earliest opportunity." Nurses visited healthy pregnant women every several weeks and educated the mother in personal hygiene and child care and urged breast feeding. Pregnant women who visited the Baby Health Stations with previous children were given similar advice. Newborns were visited frequently in the first week and every ten days thereafter, and "sick, delicate or weak ones as frequently as required." The number of home visits each July and August varied from 15,000 to 20,000 annually in the 1910s. The health department program was limited by financial constraints, but private charities provided material and other assistance to the mothers.[41]

When the summer visiting program was discontinued at the end of each summer, the nurses returned to their duties in the schools. The mothers were referred to the neighborhood baby health stations "for a continuation course of advice," according to the 1918 report, but only 3% of the mothers took advantage of the centers. The 1912 annual report observed that "the mothers are generally fully aware of the need of additional care of their babies during the summer, but in winter it is difficult to convince them that special attention is necessary, and there is a well-rooted aversion to bringing infants to the stations in cold weather." The 1918 report observed: "it is sadly true that very often babies who need care most never reach the stations because of ignorance or carelessness of their mothers." In 1919, the department began to visit those infants at their homes, which it called "a definite step forward in infant mortality control."[42]

During the 1920s the health department was joined by many private agencies in providing visiting nursing. In 1929, the health department provided 793,000 home visits and 27 private agencies 728,000 home visits (most patients received multiple visits). The private agencies made 90% of the 305,000 maternity visits, while the health department made 96% of the 493,000 child health visits and 99% of the 150,000 tuberculosis visits.[43]

An especially successful innovation that began in 1909 was education in infant hygiene for older daughters. According to the annual report:

> Realizing that many babies were often left entirely in the care of the older children of the family, it was judged proper to formulate a method by which these so-called "Little Mothers" might receive adequate and practical instruction in this subject. All girls over 12 years of age in the schools were required to attend the lectures [in] elementary infant hygiene and feeding [in the spring]. The interest and eagerness for information aroused in the girls who attended the lectures was one of the most encouraging features of the year's campaign.[44]

The program was expanded to include younger girls and had 18,000 girls enrolled in 1912. In 1920 the annual report stated that the department instructed 15,000 girls "in poorer sections of the City where [foreign-born] mothers, by reason of poor financial status and ignorance of rules for healthful living, need assistance and co-operation of the older girls." Baker, who was responsible for this and many other innovations, described the typical participant as a "scrawny child of eight or nine, dirty and dishevelled, lugging a dirtier and more dishevelled baby which alternated between peevish wailing and sucking at something anonymous, crying all the louder when the little mother slapped it in understandable childish impatience with the nagging noise." Baker said that the girls received:

> practical instruction from nurses in baby feeding, baby exercising, baby dressing and the other parts of baby care. . . . These youngsters were among our most efficient missionaries, canvassing tenements for us, cajoling mothers of their acquaintance into giving baby health stations a trial, checking up on mothers who had backslid in attendance at the stations, telling every mother they met all about what they were learning. They organized fresh-air outings for their own mothers and babies.[45]

The little mothers' program became so popular nationally that at one time 50,000 girls were enrolled in 44 American cities. Baker's system was to have each group of girls elect their own officers and operate their league with a nurse as a advisor. They heard talks by nurses and physicians, learned how to use equipment to bathe, change, and care for babies, practiced on dolls or occasionally live babies, read materials on health, and performed health plays that they wrote. A key aspect of the program was teaching the girls personal hygiene and preparing them for motherhood.[46]

The department also expanded its health programs for schoolchildren. In 1897, following the lead of Boston and Philadelphia, New York City began inspecting children for contagious diseases and in 1905 it instituted inspections for other types of diseases and physical defects such as hearing and eyesight. In 1914, about the same time as other cities, it established a policy of examining all children upon entrance to school and, when financially feasible, in their third and sixth school years. In response to complaints by local physicians, the department advised students to have private physicians perform the medical examinations. Unfortunately, many families failed to bring their children to a physician or clinic after the school physician had diagnosed dental, hearing, or vision problems. In order to educate the parents, the health department urged them to attend their child's school health examinations. According to the 1922 annual report, "parents are also encouraged to come to school to discuss their children's health and hygiene problems with the nurse. In this way, the [nurse] can conserve her own energy, especially in the elimination of stair-climbing, and at the same time reach a larger number of parents than she could if she had to go into the district to see them individually." Given the ratios in 1926 of about 11,300 schoolchildren per physician and 5,040 per nurse, as well as the lack of facilities in many schools, little time was available for such consultations.[47]

The health of schoolchildren could not be improved unless parents were educated about children's health needs. For years, according to Baker, visiting nurses were often unable to get impoverished families to "pay some doctor to treat an ailment that seemingly did not cripple the child." The nurse would make repeated visits and "offer to take the children to a free clinic. But either fear or plain neglect offered a sufficient rebuff" in the majority of the cases. In order to remove economic barriers to the treatment of the most common problems, the department established eye clinics to provide refractions and treat contagious eye diseases in 1912 and dental clinics in 1913. These grew to treat tens of thousands of schoolchildren annually in the 1920s and 1930s, but the demand always exceeded the capacity of the clinics. Their success provided the strongest evidence of the department's achievements in educating parents. The 1923 report observed that "after years of instruction, parents of today seem to realize that a child with physical defects is handicapped in its school work, and are therefore willing to do what they can to have the condition removed."[48]

The health department also recognized the need for health education in the schools. The 1920 annual report observed: "teaching health habits to children, and [a] determination to make children the most interested persons in their own health, is the most important type of work that the community can carry on." The goal was a child "who knows how to keep well." To implement this policy, health instruction increased from ten minutes a week in 1916 to four hours a week in 1929, and after 1920 school health week became a major annual event.[49]

Neighborhood Health Centers

Health education encompassed many different aspects of the lifestyles of the families. When visiting and school nurses educated immigrant parents about the health of infants and children, they discussed topics such as feeding, diet, growth, immunizations, physical defects, mental deficiencies, childhood diseases, and regular checkups. Yet the public and private agencies that provided these services were geographically dispersed and often inaccessible to immigrant mothers and their children. Each agency also had its own bureaucratic requirements that constituted an additional obstacle for the mothers. Consequently, mothers often did nothing until the child's health problems became severe. If health education was to be an effective method of improving health, the health department had to organize health services to mesh with the education of parents. The optimum structure for immigrant families was a conveniently located facility that housed educational, preventive, and therapeutic health services, expedited referrals among them, and minimized paperwork by the family.

The health facility used by immigrant families that anticipated this model was the milk station. By 1912, according to the annual report, the 55 city milk stations provided "places where a mother may obtain pure milk for infant feeding at the lowest market price and in addition may receive such instruction as may be necessary from a physician and nurse to teach her how to keep her baby well and the exact method by which it should be fed." The stations registered all mothers and infants who visited them, and 38,000 mothers were registered in 1912. Many mothers visited the milk stations only for infant medical care, with 60% of the babies in 1912 brought to the stations for the first time being ill. In order to focus the stations' efforts on prevention rather than treatment, the department charged them with all deaths of babies in their districts. The visiting nurses were assigned to milk stations in the summer of 1912 and given the added responsibility of making home visits to mothers who stopped attending. The nurses made 114,000 visits to registered mothers in that summer.[50]

In 1916 the health department acknowledged the expanding functions of the milk stations by renaming them "baby health stations." In 1917 the annual report explained that the change was designed "to emphasize educational and prophylactic objects of service rather than value of milk, as the primary factor in control of infant and child welfare." Five major functions were proposed for the stations in the 1919 annual report: pre-natal care; care and feeding of babies under two years of age; home visiting during the year and especially the summer; physical examinations of pre-school children ages 2 to 6 with advice to the family on correcting physical defects; and provision of space for public and private social service agencies. Implementation suffered because of inadequate resources and insufficient staffing, which consisted of one nurse and one assistant daily at each station and one physician for every three stations.[51]

The 1918 annual report observed that the baby health stations "have come to be recognized as community or neighborhood centers to which most inhabitants of the vicinity come for advice and instruction which relates to the family." Station physicians made emergency visits to homes day and night. The nurses secured the prompt admission of sick infants to hospitals and of women to maternity institutions, and found temporary shelters for infants and day nurseries for children of working mothers. They conducted classes in subjects such as personal hygiene in the home, disease prevention, and corrective exercises for those with orthopedic problems. Trained dietitians held cooking classes that emphasized nutrition and cost. Weekly sewing classes and educational programs were held for pregnant women. The annual report noted that the "gatherings afforded them a certain amount of social intercourse which relieved the monotony of their daily life, and gave them a healthier mental attitude, which is so essential during pregnancy." Meetings were also held for high school girls and Little Mothers' Leagues (which were now year-round programs that included cooking classes). The centers furnished desks for private "child-caring, social service, philanthropic, and other agencies, as well as maternity centres." Health education was provided at the centers to nurses, physicians, midwives, social workers, and public health students.[52]

One of the most successful devices for attracting residents to the centers continued to be the sale of milk, which the department characterized as "the poor man's food." The milk was originally intended for infants, but was later consumed by nursing mothers, pregnant women, older children suffering from malnutrition and other disorders, adults suffering or convalescing from tuberculosis and other diseases, and others in need and unable to pay regular prices. Approximately 5.8 million quarts were sold annually from 1917 to 1920 at a price per quart varying from eight cents in 1916 to eighteen cents in 1920 (after a period of war-time inflation), a savings of three-to five cents compared to the market price.[53]

A basic deficiency of the stations was their failure to serve certain groups of children, including many of the sickest and neediest infants. In 1919, 43% of all deaths during the first year of life occurred in the first month of life, yet from 1915 to 1920 only 11% to 14% of the approximately 40,000 infants under one year of age who attended the stations annually were brought there in their first month. The infants brought to the stations were increasingly in good health and the mothers regular in attendance and receptive to the advice of the nurses. This suggested that the poorest and least educated mothers were not using the centers. To reach these women, the 1920 annual report stated that the stations lengthened the intervals between visits for healthy infants and sent visiting nurses to the homes of infants who were "weak, delicate, sick, or suffering from malnutrition." It observed, "these babies should not be made to suffer for the sins of omission or commission of their parents."[54]

The largest group not receiving systematic care was pre-school children, who were brought to the attention of the department only if their mothers brought them to the baby health stations. Infants and schoolchildren, on the other hand, were the responsibility of visiting and school nurses respectively. Most of the 500,000 children ages two through six were not registered at the stations and never received physical examinations, vaccinations, or follow-up health advice. The 1920 annual report observed: "The Bureau of Child Hygiene has preached for a great many years the importance and necessity of directing attention to the pre-school age period. We have had neither the appropriations nor the personnel to conduct this work on the large scale that it merits." It urged private child-care agencies to assume responsibility for these children, but a 1929 survey of public and private health agencies estimated that only 3% of the 500,000 pre-school children received "any definitely planned health service."[55]

In order to address these deficiencies, according to the 1915 and 1917 annual reports, in 1914 the health department inaugurated "a new departure in public health administration" by opening an experimental Health District to serve 30,000 Russian and Austrian Jewish immigrants in an area of twenty-one square blocks on the lower east side of Manhattan. The objectives were to locate many health department functions in the district and use health education to "cultivate among the people of the district a co-operative spirit for the improvement of their health and sanitary conditions." The "family became the basic unit of Health Department service," with a "Family Record Card" describing the family and its residence and providing a "continuous history" of health department services rendered to all family members. Each family was cared for by a single nurse, which reduced home visits and combined the functions of the school nurse, the tuberculosis nurse, and the visiting nurse. The district administered visiting nursing, tuberculosis and venereal disease clinics, school medical inspection and nursing, employment certificates, contagious diseases, health education, and sanitary inspections. The program's success was indicated by the increase in the number of infants enrolled at the district from 100 to 651. Four more districts were opened in the next few years, but the First World War forced the department to terminate the program.[56]

The health department suffered a major setback from 1918 to 1925 when a new mayor tried to politicize it and replace existing workers with political appointees. The baby health stations survived because of their strong community support. In 1922, mothers made 740,000 visits to the clinics, 5.7 million quarts of milk were sold, visiting nurses assigned to the stations made 206,000 home visits, and 15,000 children were vaccinated. However, the new political and financial exigencies forced the department to depend more on private health organizations. According to the 1919 annual report:

> child care is no longer to be considered an individual problem nor the problem of a municipal health department alone. It is now a community problem. . . . Such results as are being attained in this City can come about only through a well-organized, co-ordinated and correlated effort on the part of all [public and private] agencies interested in infants and children, with the health department acting as a clearing- house. The control of infant and child morbidity and mortality is more of a socio-economic than a medical problem.[57]

Most changes in the health stations during the early 1920s were byproducts of the rising standard of living, such as the decline in the sale of milk from 5.7 million quarts in 1922 to 4.1 million in 1924. More important, according to the 1927 annual report, was that "the number of babies suffering from diarrhea, dietary disorders, malnutrition, has become so greatly reduced that it is now rare indeed for the nurse or [physician] to be called upon for actual nursing care of the babies." The staff could now focus on babies who needed special care. According to the 1923 report: "All sick, delicate and malnourished babies are kept on the rolls of the stations and are visited repeatedly by the nurse and nurse's assistant, if the mother refuses or cannot come to the station clinic. The doctor also makes a home visit, if the nurse believes the baby is not making the progress it should."[58]

An unanticipated consequence of the health stations was their impact on the values and beliefs of immigrant mothers. Many immigrant mothers lived traditional lives that emphasized the home, the family, and the dominance of the husband. The visiting nurses were often the first American women with whom they had a personal relationship. The nurses urged the mothers to make their own decisions about infant care and to visit the health stations, where they participated in classes and clubs for the first times in their lives. The nurses advised mothers to limit the number of their children to their economic ability to raise them properly, in contrast to traditional values favoring large families. The outcome was a breakdown of many aspects of traditional cultures as they concerned the roles of women.[59]

By the mid-1920s, the health department, by collaborating with other public and private agencies, had a greater impact on the lives of tenement families than any other organization in the city. The 1926 annual report observed:

The Health Department is the largest social service agency in the city. With its several thousand field employees, it reaches and sees more families than any similar organization possibly can. The nurses in our clinics, baby health stations and schools are constantly being called upon for advice and even material help. . . . [T]hey call upon the various [public and private] social service agencies for co-operation and help. At the holiday season, hundreds of dinners and food baskets are obtained by them for needy families. . . . Hundreds of bundles of clothing and pairs of shoes are regularly distributed. The nurses arrange for free operation for adenoids and hypertrophied tonsils for children at different clinics, dispensaries and hospitals and get hundreds of pairs of glasses for children, either entirely free, or, better still at a reduced price on the installment plan. Large numbers of children have been sent to the country in the summertime.[60]

As the health department retrenched in the early 1920s, private organizations assumed responsibility for innovations, such as two neighborhood health center demonstrations on the east side of Manhattan. A small one was established in 1921 in East Harlem, a neighborhood of Italian immigrants, and a much larger and more influential demonstration opened in 1926 in Bellevue-Yorkville, an area of Italian and Irish immigrants with exceptionally high infant and total mortality rates. A major objective of the Bellevue-Yorkville experiment was to improve cooperation among the 65 public and private agencies operating there. It was originally funded with $1 million from the Milbank Memorial Fund, but the health department assumed leadership in 1929 and financial responsibility subsequently.[61]

The success of the experiments and a new supportive mayor led a commission to recommend in 1929 that 30 health department neighborhood centers be constructed in all five boroughs of the city to serve those "too poor to engage private doctors." Each center would bring together in one location a number of public and private agencies providing different types of health and social services. Health services would be provided to children and adults and the family would be made the basic unit of service.

The commission recommended that the first neighborhood center be constructed in North Harlem to serve the city's most recent immigrant group "because the need there is most pressing. . . . In this community of 174,000 is the largest urban colored population in the world. The numbers are increasing at an accelerated rate due . . . especially [to] the exodus of colored labor from the south. The change from rural to urban life creates health hazards, noticeably the spread of tuberculosis." The small Harlem community also lacked the private charitable and religious organizations of the much larger and older immigrant groups. The center was opened in

1930 with enhanced resources and received more attention in succeeding years than any other center.[62]

The recommendations became public policy and in 1937 Mayor Fiorello LaGuardia stated that "the health center has become the basis of our health program." In that year 20 centers were in operation, due largely to funding by federal government agencies, including the Public Works Administration, Public Health Service, Children's Bureau, Works Projects Administration, and later the Social Security Administration. Between 1934 and 1940, federal funds assisted in the construction of 15 new health centers, a laboratory building, and nine child-health stations. Federal agencies paid the salaries of physicians, dentists, nurses, technicians, and social workers who provided school, maternal, and child health services, maintained health department records, conducted diagnostic and laboratory work (including chest X rays of 210,000 persons), and carried out other projects such as social surveys and mosquito control. Federal government funds contributed $1.3 million to a total cost of $5.2 million for the construction of fourteen health centers and a laboratory building between 1936 and 1940.[63]

In 1939, 30 health districts were in operation, 11 with new buildings. Each health center was designed to be a largely self-contained health department serving a district of about 250,000 population. According to the 1939 annual report, most buildings provided "space for maternity and child health services; tuberculosis, dental, and venereal disease stations; nursing services; space for local offices of visiting nurse and welfare agencies; and an auditorium and exhibit room for health education." Some of the districts had separate substations that provided maternity and child health services. Health statistics were compiled on a district level to identify local problems. In districts housing one of the city's five medical schools, the centers were located near the schools and "extra space is provided in the five centers to accommodate laboratories and teaching rooms for the schools' professors of preventive medicine." The professors trained both medical students and department staff members.[64]

Community groups were involved at both city-wide and district levels, reflecting the position in the 1937 annual report that the district health program "must be a vital, integrated part of the community which it serves." At the health department level, committees composed of health department staff and representatives of medical societies and health and social service organizations assisted with planning and coordination with the private health sector. At the district level, some districts had committees of representatives of local community and medical, nursing, health, and welfare organizations.[65]

Conflict between the health centers and private physicians was a continuing problem. Local physicians were quite willing to let the centers undertake health education programs but objected to their provision of medical care. To appease local physicians, the health commissioner often urged, as in a 1937 statement, "all who can possibly afford it to use the services of private physicians. For those unable to go to a private doctor the centers provide such clinic services as are needed for the particular district."[66]

Although the health department was integrating services in the neighborhood health centers, specialization was disconnecting specific health services from each other. The process is shown by the twelve prenatal care clinics opened in Baby Health Centers in 1924 using federal grants from the Sheppard-Towner Act and funded by the city and other sources when the act expired. The clinics used visiting nurses to encourage more pregnant women to obtain prenatal care, provided continuing medical care of the women throughout pregnancy, and educated the women by furnishing the clinics with "layettes, model beds, trays and other supplies necessary for the expectant and nursing mother, and [demonstrating] these articles to groups when they call at the station for instruction and advice," according to the 1924 annual report. In 1925, the clinics served 5,186 pregnant women who made 15,049 visits and another 2,896 who received care in their homes, during a year when about 125,000 births occurred. More than 55% of the women were supervised for three or more months. By 1930, the eighteen prenatal clinics had 25,000 visits and provided the following services: "complete history, physical examination, pelvimetry, blood pressure, Wasserman and urine tests, special care of abnormal cases, careful follow-up, arrangements for confinement, post-partum supervision, and instructions as to the care of the child."[67]

In 1938, this integrated approach was replaced by one based on specialization. By this time 90% of the approximately 100,000 yearly births occurred in hospitals and only about 7% of pregnant women registered at the twenty-three prenatal stations. The department expressed "increasing recognition of the desirability of continuous medical supervision of the pregnant woman by the hospital where the delivery takes place." The department therefore eliminated prenatal care clinics in areas with "adequate hospital facilities." The hospitals made every effort to ensure that the woman had a safe pregnancy and delivery and a healthy baby but did not provide the same outreach or educational programs.[68]

A similar development occurred when the health department organized bureaus based on professional specialty. In earlier years, major bureaus were organized on the basis of constituency served, such as the Bureau of Child Hygiene, the Bureau of Industrial Hygiene, the Bureau of Infectious Diseases, and the Bureau of Food and Drugs, all organized in 1913–15.[69] The achievements of these bureaus were measured in terms of socially desired outcomes: infant mortality rates and number of childhood immunizations; number of industrial accidents and diseases; number of cases of infectious diseases; and food and milk safety. The bureaus achieve these goals by bringing together workers with different skills.

Each of the new bureaus grouped the workers in a particular professional specialty. For example, the 608 visiting, school, and baby health center nurses, and the 72 nurses' assistants were organized into a separate Bureau of Nursing in 1928. The bureau measured its achievements in terms of professional training, standardization, supervision, and productivity. It deemphasized home care and devoted more time to schools and clinics, where nurses could see more patients per day, had better resources, and could be supervised more easily. In 1931, 45% of the department's total of 1.1 million nursing hours were spent on home visiting. In 1937, only 27% of the 1.3 million nursing hours went for home visits.[70]

The specialty bureaus were centralized in the health department's headquarters, while the health districts were decentralized and located throughout the city. The specialists serving at the health districts were supposed to report to their central bureaus on technical matters and to their district health officers on administrative matters, but the distinction was never clear in practice. A series of department reorganizations from the 1940s through the 1970s expanded the authority of the central bureaus and diminished the power of the districts. By the 1970s, the health districts had to compete with approximately 25 bureaus and other central units for funding, personnel, and authority. In addition, some health functions became the responsibility of new city agencies. A fiscal crisis in the 1970s produced the closing of seven of the twenty remaining health centers and reduced the functions of the others.[71]

The advantages of integrated health care for a community were shown in another demonstration project of the Metropolitan Life Insurance Company in Kingsport, Tennessee. Kingsport grew rapidly to 7,000 inhabitants in 1916 after a railroad employed city planners to design a model town to attract industrial firms. The firms constructed plants that drew rural job seekers and their families, but the town lacked suitable housing, plumbing, a safe water supply, and sewers. The newcomers had little understanding of urban life, and infectious disease rates quickly escalated. In 1919 the Metropolitan Life Insurance Company convinced the local firms to purchase group life and sickness/accident insurance for their employees and brought in visiting nurses, provided loans for housing purchases, and established a health unit with baby, prenatal, general, and school clinics. The total mortality rate dropped from 26 per 1,000 population in 1917 to 12 in 1921 and the infant mortality rate declined from 231 in 1914 to 75 in 1921. After a few years, the Metropolitan, which was incurring substantial deficits, asked for more local financial support. New firms had not purchased insurance, older ones did not renew their policies, the town government refused to provide additional funding, and some local physicians opposed the program. When additional local funding was not provided, the Metropolitan discontinued its support in 1931 and the city's health problems returned.[72]

Thus health programs were most effective when they were integrated to serve the needs of the family and community. The keystone was health education, which taught families to live healthy lives, to know when to seek professional help, and to follow regimens to restore health or reduce the effects of illness. The 1938 annual report of the New York City health department aptly summarized this new philosophy:

> School children owe their favorable health status not merely to medical examinations, corrective work and health instruction given in the schools today. They owe this in a large measure to a more intelligent attitude and care within their own family circle. The prenatal instruction of mothers, better professional attention at birth, training in baby feeding and care, immunization against diphtheria, all have played their part in the well-being of today's children. . . . There are family responsibilities for children which no Department of Education and no Health Department can assume. Public agencies can only help people to help themselves. They cannot possibly take over normal family responsibilities. This is a problem of adult health education.[73]

9

THE METROPOLITAN LIFE INSURANCE COMPANY HEALTH EDUCATION PROGRAMS

> It seems to us that the best thought of the age has fixed upon insurance as the solvent for most of the economic ills of society. One can in imagination picture the time when instead of but one-third of the population, practically all living in the cities and towns shall be insured in Industrial mutual companies; and in the development of these companies along Welfare lines one may look to the time when the people shall take care of themselves through life insurance in a service covering health in life, care in sickness, indemnity in death, sanitation in community life, the financing of home-owning, of public utilities and civic conveniences—a mutual service of cooperation among such a large proportion of the population that it may be called The New Socialism!
>
> (Haley Fiske, President Metropolitan Life Insurance Company, 1924)[1]

After urban public health departments adopted health education to improve the health of their residents, the Metropolitan Life Insurance Company undertook a vast nationwide health education campaign as a distinctive advertising and public relations program. The multifaceted campaign included free nursing care for sick policyholders and materials to educate the general public about personal behaviors that contributed to infectious and chronic diseases. It reached more persons than any other public or

146

private health campaign and made the Metropolitan the private counterpart of a national health department during the first half of the twentieth century.

Health education for the general public was considered the newest dimension of public health in the early twentieth century. According to a New York City study in 1929, it had three components: "(1) the spread of knowledge of the facts of disease and health, (2) the increase of the individual interest in healthy living, and (3) the development of the social interest in healthful conditions in the community." These objectives were to be achieved by "teaching hygiene and training in health habits for individuals."[2]

Health education was provided to varying degrees by a number of public and private organizations. The health departments of large cities had active programs, but little was done in the towns and villages where most of the population resided. Most states deferred to local jurisdictions on matters concerning health. Federal government agencies like the Children's Bureau, the Census Bureau, and the Bureau of Labor Statistics conducted outstanding research and provided excellent publications on selected topics, but their roles were narrowly defined. Voluntary health associations, especially the National Tuberculosis Association, and some private corporations developed and published educational materials for the public. Public schools provided health education. A survey of 341 school superintendents in the 1920s found that 73% of the school systems taught courses entitled health or hygiene. The subjects included nutrition, exercise, fresh air, personal and mental hygiene, care of eyes and teeth, and disease transmission. Few teachers were properly trained and the textbooks were often outdated. Classroom materials were also prepared by corporations, trade associations, and nonprofit organizations such as the Child Health Organization, some of whose materials were published by the federal government.[3]

Health-related products were advertised in the growing number of publications being read by a more educated population. Between 1900 and 1929, daily newspaper circulation increased from 15 to 42 million copies and magazine circulation increased from an estimated 65 million copies to 202 million. Newspapers and magazines enabled advertisers to inform consumers about many new products, including automobiles, refrigerators, cigarettes, and prepared foods. Some of the most popular new products were for personal hygiene in response to social and technical changes such as indoor plumbing, more clerical and white collar jobs in offices and stores, greater employment of women, and more leisure time. By the 1920s, millions of Americans were brushing their teeth, bathing frequently with soap, and using deodorants, mouthwash, and toiletries. A 1938 survey of 53,000 homes in sixteen cities found that 94% had soap for personal use, 89% had toothpaste or tooth powder, and 69% had toothbrushes.[4]

Advertisements for personal hygiene products sometimes urged users to support public health programs concerning their products. A 1912 toothpaste advertisement in a woman's magazine stated: "It is for you as a parent to urge the teaching of dental hygiene in the schools and to practice it in your home." The need for such education was considerable, given the statement in the 1909 annual report of the New York City health department that "most of the children showed a more or less complete lack of dental hygiene." The city undertook to remedy the problem and by the early 1920s dental hygienists provided classroom instruction in brushing teeth to all New York City schoolchildren and in the 1930s the department set up dental clinics (largely funded by the federal government) that had 518,000 visits from schoolchildren to 136 clinics in 1939.[5]

The soap industry conducted a major advertising campaign about the health benefits of its products. Before the mid-nineteenth century soaps were manufactured locally because the animal fats spoiled quickly. All soaps, except expensive glycerine soaps, were designed for laundry use and were extremely harsh to the skin and of poor quality and consistency. New soap formulations with vegetable oils retarded spoilage and permitted the manufacture of individually wrapped small bars of mild soap intended for personal use. Soap manufacturers advertised extensively to inform the public about the new soap and its ability to destroy invisible microbes that could spread disease. The Association of American Soap and Glycerine Producers funded the Cleanliness Institute between 1927 and 1932 to encourage schools to teach cleanliness and the benefits of soap. Certainly the schools needed improvement in this regard. A survey of 145 schools with 124,000 students in fifteen states found that only 57% had soap and 31% had soap, hot and cold water, and towels. The Institute distributed hundreds of thousands of copies of pamphlets, storybooks, posters, and teachers' guides, and its *Cleanliness Journal* was distributed free to educators, social workers, and health officials. It also provided lecturers to schools and civic and professional organizations.[6]

Food advertisements made health-related claims. They emphasized pure ingredients, sanitary methods of production, and their ability to maintain health and prevent disease. Food producers contrasted the cleanliness of their new sealed packages with the often rodent- or insect-infested bulk containers in grocery stores. Health themes were especially prevalent in advertisements for commercial breakfast cereals and other products designed to replace inexpensive home-made foods.[7]

Advertising in the early twentieth century was almost entirely for products rather than services. The fifty-eight corporations that spent $100,000 or more annually advertising in national magazines during at least one year from 1913 to 1915 included only one service organization, the American Telephone and Telegraph Company. Other service industries that advertised nationally were involved in travel, such as railroads, hotels, and steamships. With few exceptions, notably the Prudential Insurance Company, life insurance companies did not advertise because they believed that life insurance was sold by the personal influence of a salesman.[8]

During the 1920s many corporations inaugurated public relations programs to explain corporate goals and activities to the public and receive information from the public. Previously, according to Tedlow, "leading capitalists seemed to accept the criticism and even hatred their activities provoked as occupational hazards." Their efforts to blunt the attacks, if any, consisted largely of philanthropy. When the entrepreneurial capitalists retired or died, they were replaced by a new generation of professional managers who recognized the social and economic impact of their corporations. They adopted public relations, a term first used for that purpose in 1916, to improve their corporate images among the public, politicians, and community leaders. Corporations employed individual public relations experts early in the century and some experts formed public relations agencies in the 1920s.[9]

Public relations was used most extensively by the American Telephone and Telegraph Company, a government regulated monopoly. Theodore Vail, who became president in 1907, created an information department to convince the public that a government regulated private monopoly was superior to either government ownership or open competition. The department published advertisements in newspapers and magazines, provided motion pictures free to theaters and organizations, maintained a speakers bureau, and distributed editorial materials for newspapers and magazines that could be reprinted without attribution. It was widely credited with improving service to customers and informing the company about customers' opinions. At the same time, AT&T withheld advertising from uncooperative newspapers and kept secret its successful efforts to harass and undermine other telephone companies.[10]

By the 1920s advertising and public relations had become so pervasive that many thought that they had reached the point of saturation.[11] Any corporation that sought a distinctive place in the crowded advertising marketplace needed a novel approach. The health and welfare programs of the Metropolitan Life Insurance Company were probably the most innovative and successful advertising and public relations campaigns of all time.

The Health Programs of The Metropolitan Life Insurance Company

At the turn of the twentieth century, the life insurance industry was under unrelenting attack. The most damaging disclosures occurred at the nationally publicized hearings on industry practices of the Armstrong commission in New York State in 1905–7. The commission uncovered so many unethical and illegal practices that nationwide life insurance sales dropped below the 1905 level for the next five years. The investigations in New York and elsewhere produced a number of state statutes, including a 1911 Wisconsin law that created a public life insurance company. To regain public confidence, some life insurance companies advertised that they were regulated by the stringent New York State statutes that resulted from the Armstrong hearings. Industrial life insurance companies were particularly vulnerable because government life insurance programs using tax revenues, which existed in Europe, could provide similar death benefits at much lower cost than private insurance companies. Government programs eliminated the expenses of selling and underwriting policies, collecting premiums, investing income, and maintaining reserves.[12]

The three largest industrial life insurance companies—Metropolitan, Prudential, and John Hancock—made concerted efforts to show urban working-class Americans an honorable side of the industry. They dominated industrial life insurance, selling 95% of the industrial life insurance policies that were purchased by more than one-fifth of all Americans in 1909. They provided badly needed burial insurance to millions of urban tenement dwellers for a few cents a week and paid death benefits promptly and unhesitatingly, unlike some ordinary life insurance companies. They were financially secure, as opposed to the many banks that took the family's money and failed to return it when they went bankrupt during the next depression. They employed thousands of immigrants and their children as agents, managers, and clerical staff, which not only demonstrated the companies' commitment to the immigrant communities, but also provided upward mobility for immigrants and enabled them to influence the practices of the companies. Although early policy provisions were disadvantageous and high agent turnover provided poor service, the companies steadily improved the quality of their products, services, and agents and made industrial life insurance a superior investment for many lower-income Americans.[13]

The Metropolitan and some other leading life insurance companies also engaged in a form of industry self-policing. Between 1893 and 1918, the Metropolitan assumed responsibility for some or all of the policies of thirty-one life insurance companies that failed or were otherwise unable to meet their obligations. The companies included twenty-two industrial life insurance companies with 770,000 policyholders.[14]

From 1909 until well after mid-century, the Metropolitan was the largest life insurance company in America. Its assets of $1.6 billion in 1925 were $500 million greater than those of any other company. In 1927 the Metropolitan had $13.5 billion of individual policies in force, compared to $10 billion for the Prudential Insurance Company and less than $6 billion for every other company. The Metropolitan also led the industry in group life insurance beginning in the 1920s. In 1934 the company insured 20.6 million industrial policyholders, 5.3 million ordinary policyholders, and 1.4 million group policyholders, covering about 20% of the population of the United States and Canada. In 1935, a typical year, 20% of all individual life insurance policies sold in the United States were sold by the Metropolitan Life Insurance Company.[15]

The Metropolitan had become one of America's greatest and most powerful corporations, but such prominence had its dangers. The many critics of the life insurance industry could easily direct their attacks at the largest and most recognizable company. The Sherman Anti-trust Act of 1890 had led to the divestiture of great corporations like the American Tobacco Company and Standard Oil in 1911 and the Metropolitan might experience a similar fate. The muckrakers' incessant and widely publicized attacks on great corporations would sooner or later produce an attempt to sully the Metropolitan's reputation. According to Haley Fiske, then Metropolitan vice president, in 1909 one New York State Senator denounced "industrial insurance as back-door insurance and servant-girl insurance, and there was a strong intimation that the business was one which robbed the poor." A much more serious condemnation occurred in the 1890s when life insurance companies, especially those selling industrial insurance, were charged with encouraging infanticide by insuring children. It was alleged that some parents neglected or even murdered their children to obtain the death benefits. Legislation was enacted in some states to ban life insurance on children below a certain age.[16]

To justify its dominant position and industrial life insurance generally, between 1909 and mid-century the Metropolitan Life Insurance Company adopted a far-reaching program to improve the health and welfare of its policyholders and the American people. Its objectives were consonant with the historical support of the life insurance industry for public health and sanitation programs and universal birth and death registration. They also paralleled the activities of other kinds of insurance companies, as the Metropolitan observed in 1924: "With fire insurance companies striving after fire prevention and casualty companies spending large sums for the prevention of accidents, it logically follows that life insurance companies may just as properly devote a very considerable part of their energies to the conservation of that most precious possession, human life."[17]

The Metropolitan's health programs were distinctive because they reached more Americans than the health programs of any federal, state, or local government agency or any single private organization before 1965, when the federal government enacted Medicare and Medicaid. The programs made the Metropolitan the nation's health department in the eyes of millions of Americans. In his history of early corporate public relations activities, Roland Marchand has concluded, "The clear public service provided by [the Metropolitan] ads and programs, particularly the many that promoted preventive health care, won Metropolitan Life a reputation as the most philanthropic advertiser of the era."[18]

The contributions of the Metropolitan were acknowledged by prominent public figures of the period. William H. Welch, then Dean of the Johns Hopkins University medical school and a leader of American medicine, observed that the Metropolitan was "probably the most powerful agency for stimulating interest in public health in this country." Herbert Hoover, as U.S. Secretary of Commerce, called the Metropolitan in 1923 "the greatest single institution dedicated to public welfare in America." Similar sentiments were expressed by governors, senators, mayors, religious leaders, Canadian prime ministers, and even the presidents of other life insurance companies. The president of one of the leading ordinary companies, the New York Life Insurance Company, praised the "welfare work of that amazing institution, the Metropolitan Life." The president of the Pacific Mutual Life Insurance Company called the Metropolitan "the best and the greatest life insurance company in the world . . . , a company of which all insurance men are proud. It is a credit to our business."[19]

The Metropolitan was not a philanthropic organization and its health and welfare programs were designed not only to improve the health of policyholders, but also to enhance public relations, increase sales, and deflect criticisms of the company and the industry. The programs were not expensive. In 1933, the health and welfare programs cost the Metropolitan

$5.4 million, 0.6% of the company's total expenses of $889 million. The bulk of company expenditures, $565 million, were spent on claims, cash value returns of surrendered policies, and dividends. The health and welfare programs were carefully targeted to the company's main source of policyholders, urban working and lower middle class families. They were designed to gain the respect of physicians, nurses, and public health and other government officials in order to enhance the company's image. They also had an extraordinary impact on sales. For example, although the Metropolitan was not a pioneer in group life insurance, its unrivaled reputation among factory and office workers enabled it to dominate the rapidly growing market for group life insurance until well after mid-century. Metropolitan thus became the largest seller of both individual and group life insurance in America, a remarkable achievement. The group life insurance contracts alone repaid the cost of the company's health and welfare programs many times over.

The health and welfare programs were initiated and strengthened by Haley Fiske (1852–1929), who served as the Metropolitan's vice president from 1891 and president from 1919 until his death at age 77 in 1929. Fiske was born in New Jersey of working-class parents and attended Rutgers University. He completed a legal apprenticeship and entered a New York City law firm, where he advanced rapidly and was assigned to handle the legal affairs of the Metropolitan. He joined the Metropolitan in 1891 at the request of its incoming president and soon assumed full responsibility for most of its operations. Fiske's early actions reflected his experiences as a lawyer who served the interests of corporations and the wealthy. He revived the company's ordinary life insurance operations, increasing the amount in force from $5 million in 1892 to $700 million in 1909, thereby attracting more middle-class clients. He developed an intermediate policy for policyholders who could pay premiums quarterly but could not afford ordinary policies. During the early 1890s, because of his experience as a trial lawyer, he represented the company and the industry in responding to the allegations that industrial life insurance on infants and children lured parents into committing infanticide. To defeat legislation introduced in some states to ban sales of life insurance to children, Fiske traveled widely, spoke to many state legislators and community leaders, and defended industrial insurance while acknowledging its many limitations.[20]

The experience of justifying industrial life insurance before critical legislators and public leaders transformed Fiske from an aggressive business executive into a devout churchgoer with a deep personal sense of social responsibility. According to Louis Dublin, the company statistician during much of Fiske's term as president, "those who knew him during his tempestuous career as a successful trial lawyer could hardly recognize the new personality of the insurance executive." During the economic depression of 1893 the company voluntarily paid death claims on some policies that had been in force for years but had lapsed due to unemployment. After the depression Metropolitan reinstated the policies of hundreds of thousands of policyholders on favorable terms. Both practices were repeated in the next three decades during ordeals such as earthquakes, floods, fires, and strikes, which Fiske compared to natural disasters to justify his actions. In 1896 the company paid cash bonuses in the form of lower premiums on nonparticipating policies that could not legally receive dividends and Fiske called the bonuses profit-sharing to evade the legal barrier. In 1897 the company resolved a major criticism of the industry by providing paid-up policies when policies lapsed after five years. In 1915 he converted Metropolitan from a stock company into a mutual company owned by the policyholders to eliminate the possibility of stockholder misappropriation of company surpluses (the Prudential also mutualized and John Hancock was always a mutual company). During the 1920s he endeavored unsuccessfully to convince the New York State insurance commissioner and the state legislature to permit life insurance companies to offer unemployment insurance, a type of policy that could never have been more than marginally profitable.[21]

Every year as president Fiske traveled thousands of miles to meet with agents, community leaders, and politicians to describe his vision of the Metropolitan. Every third year he completed a 12,000-mile tour to attend conventions of the company's field force in the United States and Canada. He justified the trips by saying that he had "no right to try to govern a company" composed of "different nationalities, different traditions, in different parts of the country, different local feelings, from a swivel chair" in New York City. He also believed that the field force "has got a right to have me and the other officers appear before them and size them up" and a receive "an account of their stewardship." Fiske took great pride in his relationships with his employees and proudly referred to the company's employee benefits, especially the free tuberculosis sanitorium and convalescent home, as a model for all of industry.[22]

The views he expressed to Metropolitan employees were highly atypical of a business executive. At one convention in 1922 Fiske stated: "The Metropolitan desires that it shall not be considered by the public a money-making institution, which is doing work for profit, whose business is to get in as much money and pay out as little as possible. . . . what we are trying to do is to use that business as a public institution for the purpose of serv-

ing the American people, and especially the working people of America."
He replied to critics of the Metropolitan free visiting-nursing program by
saying: "There has been the temptation on the part of some to say it is
illegal, and to that charge I have been able to make one answer and that is
that we save lives so that they can continue to pay for their insurance. That
was not the real original motive, but it furnished the legal basis." He used a
similar justification for Metropolitan health research and public health programs in 1921: "Will it be said that this management is taking money from
some working people [policyholders] and spending it broadcast for the
public welfare? Let it be said. The answer is the reduction in mortality; the
last year shows the lowest mortality [rate that the company has] ever experienced . . . a reduction 6 per cent greater than that in the [death registra-
tion] area. . . . This relative saving in mortality means over three and one-
half million dollars a year to this Company, a sum much greater than what
we are spending in this health and welfare work. . . . There is a lesson for
the states, that they can spend money scientifically and wisely, for building
healthy people, and make money by it."[23]

His death in 1929 was prominently reported on the front page of the
New York Times. The newspaper's long obituary called him "one of America's
most conspicuous advocates of popular education in matters of health, and
credited with having done much to increase the longevity of the average
man and woman." An editorial noted the many achievements of the company and concluded: "To have conceived and carried out a plan for helping
millions of policy holders to lead more healthful and longer lives is one of
the great triumphs of this new century."[24]

Fiske was one of a new generation of professional managers who
claimed that their role was to serve the best interests of the community and
their employees as well as the stockholders or policyholders. Yet few corporate executives actually served as stewards of the public interest. No other
insurance company executive displayed Metropolitan's commitment to social welfare. Theodore Vail of AT&T and Alfred P. Sloan of General Motors, two of Fiske's most famous counterparts, were best known for their
strategies of corporate cartelization in order to dictate to the public the
terms on which they conducted business. Vail was uninterested in extending telephone service to the kinds of families who purchased industrial
insurance (the proportion of all households with telephone service did not
reach 50% until 1946[25]) and General Motors under Sloan never produced
an inexpensive automobile comparable to the Ford Model T. Haley Fiske
was unique among the nation's major business executives in his commitment to improving the lives of the great mass of urban Americans.

The Metropolitan Visiting Nurse Service

Fiske's first programs were motivated by the disparity between the mortality rates of the lower-income industrial and the higher-income ordinary policyholders. In 1923, when the situation had improved considerably, a 30–year-old white male Metropolitan ordinary policyholder could expect to live 6.6 years longer than a comparable industrial policyholder, and a 50–year-old ordinary policyholder could expect to live 4.2 years longer than a comparable industrial policyholder. Between the ages of 25 and 54, white male industrial policyholders had mortality rates more than twice those of ordinary policyholders. These were the ages when the costs of death were greatest to life insurance companies.[26]

In 1909 Fiske invited Lee K. Frankel (1867–1931) to establish a social welfare program for the company's industrial life insurance policyholders. The objective was to reduce policyholder mortality rates and maintain the health of wage earners so that they would not lose their jobs and lapse their policies by not paying the premiums. Frankel had obtained a Ph.D. and worked as a chemist in Philadelphia for some years. He then headed the United Hebrew Charities in New York City where, according to an announcement of his appointment in the policyholder magazine, *The Metropolitan,* "his work brought him into close and constant contact with the industrial classes." The article stated that Frankel's appointment signified a new "progressive policy of attempting to reduce the cost of industrial insurance, so as to give the workman and his family a larger measure of benefit than has been possible heretofore."[27]

Frankel established a free visiting nursing service for sick Metropolitan policyholders, published hundreds of millions of health education pamphlets, conducted sickness and unemployment surveys throughout the country, used Metropolitan agents to prod governments at all levels to sponsor health programs, and funded enough health research to make the Metropolitan the precursor of the National Institutes of Health. His obituary in the company's *Statistical Bulletin* stressed another of his skills. It noted that life insurance agents were

> a body of business men engaged in tasks usually so different from that of the social worker. Yet he succeeded in making of the managers and agents first-class social service workers. It was no small achievement to build up, in a relatively short time, a cooperating group of 25,000 people, widely distributed over the United States and Canada, who were ready at his behest to take on one task after another, if he only would say that it was socially desirable.

. . . They were often rallying points in their own States for the passage of social and health legislation. They collected numberless schedules for various research purposes, whether it be on the cost of medical care, on unemployment, or the prevalence of disease.[28]

The agents did not participate solely because of altruism or their respect for Frankel and Fiske. They recognized that collecting premiums weekly at the homes of policyholders did not by itself establish a personal relationship conducive to the sale of additional life insurance. Frankel's programs enabled agents to rise above their role of bill collectors to demonstrate their personal interest in the health and welfare of the families. The resulting friendships laid valuable groundwork for future insurance sales.

Frankel's first innovation in 1909 was the Metropolitan visiting nursing service, which became Metropolitan's most acclaimed health program in the minds of policyholders, political leaders, public health officials, physicians, and the public. By 1909 nursing was well established as a profession and nurses were employed in many schools, factories, businesses, and hospitals. Visiting nurses were employed by municipal health departments, settlements, and charities to care for the sick poor at their homes, at dispensaries, and at milk stations. The Metropolitan program was distinctive, according to the superintendent of nurses of the Visiting Nurses Association in Kansas City, Missouri, because it reached a "class of people that had long been neglected and overlooked. . . . [T]he extremes, the rich and the very poor, have always been able to secure attention, the rich because they were able to pay for it, and the very poor because it was provided for by various charitable institutions, but the great industrial class had been left to get on as best it could." From the company's perspective, visiting nursing could induce persons to buy policies, return working policyholders to their jobs promptly and prevent lapses, and might reduce mortality rates.[29]

The visiting nursing program was proposed by Lillian Wald of the Henry Street Settlement in New York City, who worked with Frankel at the United Hebrew Charities. She pointed out to him soon after his employment that Metropolitan agents who visited homes to collect premiums often found sick policyholders who were receiving inadequate medical care. Wald suggested that the agents inform the visiting nurses in her Henry Street Settlement who would then visit the patients, with the nurses' fees being paid by the Metropolitan. Even though the nursing fees could hardly be justified by the few cents paid weekly by many policyholders, Fiske approved a three-month experiment. The program proved to be immensely popular with policyholders and agents, who recognized its extraordinary appeal in selling life insurance. A Metropolitan industrial life insurance policy now included a health insurance policy at no extra cost (the Metropolitan never included the visiting nurse service in its policy contracts, however). The visiting nursing service became company policy and by the end of 1909 it was in operation in thirteen cities and the nurses made 4,700 patient visits. By 1924 the service was in operation in four thousand cities and towns and the nurses made 2.5 million visits in that year and a total of 20.8 million visits since the program began. Coverage was extended to group policyholders in 1918 and intermediate policyholders in 1926, though it was never available to ordinary policyholders. The John Hancock Mutual Life Insurance Company introduced its own visiting nursing service in 1925, but Hancock was much smaller than the Metropolitan.[30]

The Metropolitan emphasized to policyholders that its nursing service differed from the charity nursing visits dreaded by so many of the poor as visible evidence to their neighbors of their personal failings. It also stressed that the nurse's function was as much education as medical care. It explained to policyholders in the *Metropolitan* magazine in 1916:

> Prompt medical attention and good nursing care will, in very many instances, cut short what might otherwise be a long and serious illness. This is the reason the Company is extending to you the privilege of Nursing Service. . . .
>
> The Nursing Service is in no sense a charity. Every visit made by our Nurses to Industrial policy-holders *is paid for by the Company.* This is so, not only where we employ an Independent Nurse of our own, but it is also true in localities where our work is done by nurses connected with organizations carrying on visiting nursing. . . .
>
> This personal care of the sick in their homes affords our Nurses opportunities while carrying out their nursing duties to teach policy-holders how they may best keep well and prevent sickness by carrying out the simple but necessary rules of health. . . . [W]e want you to feel that we are sending you, not only a Nurse to nurse you or yours in sickness, but also a *friend* who can and will help you by her advice and guidance.[31]

The Metropolitan repeatedly stressed the educational role of the nurse. A company history observed in 1924:

> Her practiced eye is quick to detect unhygienic conditions in the home, and through kindly advice she endeavors to remedy those conditions. She teaches the value of fresh air, sunshine and cleanliness, and makes helpful suggestions for the selection and preparation of food. In maternity cases she gives advice as to the proper clothing for the child and as to its care after her visits are no longer needed. Through her teaching of hygienic living, her visits

have a permanently beneficial influence on the welfare of the households she visits.[32]

Once the company embarked on this extraordinary program, many operational policies needed to be established. The most fundamental was the decision to establish affiliations with local visiting nursing associations wherever possible and to employ its own nurses only where no associations existed. This was an immense undertaking because many visiting nursing associations were poorly managed, gave no training and little supervision to the nurses, and did not establish standards designed to achieve and maintain high-quality service and control costs. The Metropolitan, with decades of experience in organizing a very similar kind of agency force, employed a professional nurse as superintendent in the home office and a number of field supervisors who visited the existing local associations and helped organize new associations in communities where none existed. By 1916, nearly 500 of the 843 Metropolitan local nursing services were under the auspices of nursing associations and the Metropolitan insisted that such associations maintain the standards specified by the National Organization of Public Health Nursing. Elsewhere, the company employed its own visiting nurses either on salary or a per-visit basis; in some small communities the Metropolitan visiting nurse was the only professional health care provider.[33]

The Metropolitan published training materials beginning in 1914 and later *A Manual of Instructions for Visiting Nurses* prepared and revised periodically jointly with the National Organization for Public Health Nursing. The company held regular training sessions in the field and prepared a required correspondence course for the nurses. It created a system of record keeping, later adopted by the National Organization for Public Health Nursing, that made quantitative analyses of the illnesses of the patients and the activities of the nurses. It published a number of pamphlets on patient care for the nurses to give to families after explaining procedures to them.[34]

The scope of the visiting nurse service operation was comparable to the company's agency force. In 1916, the service was available in 1,862 communities and provided 1.2 million visits to 221,566 cases at a cost of $613,000. By the early 1940s, the Metropolitan provided nursing service in 7,728 communities in the United States and Canada through affiliations with 819 public health nursing agencies, as they were then called. At that time it employed 571 nurses in communities with no agencies. Between 1909 and 1949 the service cost the company $106 million.[35]

The nursing program emphasized the care of infectious rather than chronic diseases. According to Frankel and Dublin in 1918, the Metropolitan "endeavored to limit its public health nursing to diseases and conditions that have been demonstrated to yield the largest practical returns. . . cases of acute illness, of accidents, and of after care of childbirth." All patients were required to be under the care of physicians after the initial nursing visit and nurses were instructed to make no revisits to patients not under such care. In 1915 and 1916 the average case that received nursing care under physician management was treated for thirteen days and was given eight visits by the nurse. Seventy-five percent of the patients were female, and a large proportion of the visits to them involved pregnancy and/or post-natal care. The most common medical problems of the male patients were accidents and injuries.[36]

A study of the outcomes of all patients treated in 1915 and 1916 revealed that infectious diseases involved both fewer nursing visits and much better outcomes. The 18,111 cases of influenza and the 19,663 cases of pneumonia each accounted for 7% of all visits. On average, the influenza cases were treated for nine days and received an average of five visits, at the end of which 95% of the patients recovered or were improved and only 1% deceased. The pneumonia cases were treated for an average of twelve days with nine visits, after which 84% recovered or were improved and 8% deceased. The 7,368 cases of communicable diseases of childhood (measles, scarlet fever, whooping cough, and diphtheria) accounted for 3% of all visits. On average, they were treated for eleven days and received six visits, after which 83% recovered or were improved and only 4% deceased. Patients with chronic diseases were often in the terminal stages; their care, according to Frankel and Dublin, involved the "humanitarian services" of the "promotion of their comfort and the easing of the burden of suffering." The 6,020 cases of pulmonary tuberculosis accounted for 2% of the cases. On average, they were under care for 32 days and received 11 visits, after which 31% were deceased and 36% were unimproved, with 34% transferred to institutional care. The 3,252 cases of cancer, on average, were under care for 27 days and received 14 visits, after which 36% were deceased and 40% unimproved, with 30% transferred to institutional care.[37]

The guidelines and rules for nursing visits demonstrated the range of this free service. A 1937 manual listed three major functions for the nurse: "to give skilled nursing care, under the physician's direction, to eligible policyholders who require this service in their homes; to teach the care of the sick and the control and prevention of communicable disease; and to give instruction in the prolongation of life and the promotion of health." Nurses could not diagnose, prescribe, assist at operations, or visit patients in the hospital, but they could administer hypodermic injections, although not intravenous ones. Only two visits could be made unless the patient was under the care of a physician, an increase from one visit in 1924. Visits could be continued for six weeks in acute illnesses, and six visits within six months were permitted in chronic illnesses, although exceptions were allowed. Up to six visits were permitted to teach patients or family members to administer insulin intravenously. Two visits daily were permitted for the critically ill. In order to prevent families from purchasing policies solely for prenatal and postnatal care (in 1929 36% of all visits were for maternity or newborn care), prenatal visits were denied unless the policy had been in force for one year, later reduced to six months, except for those covered by group policies. One visit monthly was permitted for the first seven months of pregnancy, two in the last two months, and eight in the three weeks after uncomplicated home delivery, with fewer visits for hospital deliveries.[38]

The visiting nurse service was described in detail to policyholders, who were then told: "Remember: The Nurse can do the most good early in illness; so be sure to call her promptly." They could obtain nursing service by contacting the nurse directly, their Metropolitan agents, the local Metropolitan office, the visiting nurse association, their physician, or their employer in group policies. Before the widespread availability of telephones, policyholders were given postcards to mail to the local Metropolitan office. They were informed that "this service is for nursing care and health instruction. The nurse does not diagnose illness or prescribe medicine." The importance of patient education was always stressed: "She will teach someone in your home how to give care between her visits and how to prevent the spread of sickness."[39]

Company agents played a key role in the nursing program. In 1933 the Metropolitan employed 26,000 agents who made about 240 million home calls a year. The typical agent serviced 250–300 families and made 177 calls weekly. The company observed: "He is known and trusted by the family. Often he is of the same nationality as the policyholders. He speaks their language. He is one of them." He was often asked by the family to send a nurse or recommended to the family that a nurse visit the home. Agents received instruction about the nursing service from nursing supervisors and were kept informed about health problems in their communities. When diphtheria immunization became available in the 1920s, the company offered to immunize the children of its 25,000 agents and staff members in the field force at no cost and urged the agents to have their children immunized as models for their policyholders. Agents were asked to participate in local health campaigns and to cooperate with local health departments.[40]

The nursing service had an extraordinary impact on sales and policy-holder relations. Thankful families purchased life insurance on other family members, directed agents to new neighbors, and recommended Metropolitan policies to acquaintances. Workmen urged their employers to purchase Metropolitan group life insurance policies. Heartfelt letters of appreciation poured into the home office, as Fiske observed: "I could bring tears to your eyes by letting you see the ill-spelled, scratchy letters from grateful fathers, happy mothers, contented husbands for lives saved."[41]

The impact of the visiting nursing service on Metropolitan life insurance sales can be shown in several ways. The Metropolitan lapse ratio (net terminations divided by number of policies in force) about 1916 was 5.63, compared to 8.12 for Prudential, the most comparable industrial company, and from 6.28 to 8.34 for three leading ordinary companies (which should have had much lower lapse rates because of their higher-income policyholders and less frequent payment of premiums). Another indicator was the recurring problem of sales of life insurance on children and infants. Visiting nurses could provide maternity care to insured mothers beginning in 1914 but could not care for the newborn in the many states where life insurance policies could be sold on infants only after they reached one year of age. The key to eliminating this limitation was New York State, which was the home of Metropolitan and many other large life insurance companies and had insurance regulations that were a model for many other states. The Metropolitan persuaded the New York State legislature to changes its laws in 1923 by pointing out that denying life insurance policies to infants prevented them from receiving free nursing care. The same tactic had been employed successfully two years earlier when the company convinced the Colorado state legislature to repeal its law banning the sale of life insurance to children under age 15.[42]

Because the Metropolitan was by far the largest employer of nurses in the country, it recognized the need to attract capable women to nursing and used its publications for that purpose. As part of its school health education program, the company published pamphlets in the 1920s with biographies of "health heroes." Women were prominently included, and their biographies were written to make nursing and health careers particularly appealing to women, in contrast to the more descriptive and historical accounts of the men. The biography of Florence Nightingale informed readers: "The visiting nurse, or public health nurse, as she is generally called, is a graduate nurse employed by a community to safeguard the health of everybody within reach of her care [including] Big and Little, Old and Young, Rich and Poor. . . . She is the doctor's colleague in the labor and hope of conquering disease. She goes into the home as a friend. She helps the loved ones at the patient's bedside. She does what they would do had they her knowledge, skill and training. . . . She teaches the family how to care for the sick—how to keep well—so that her visit not only brings immediate relief but lasting benefit." The nurse educates the mother of the new infant "not by books—for the foreign mother cannot read English and many American mothers do not read. [She] teaches by demonstration." The pamphlet described school and industrial nursing as well as the Metropolitan visiting nurse service and informed readers that "young women interested in becoming nurses will be advised as to the selection of a school by the Metropolitan Life Insurance Company," giving Frankel's name, title, and address.[43]

The Metropolitan's financial support enabled visiting nursing to became more economically secure, existing visiting nursing associations to expand, and new ones to be organized. According to a superintendent of a visiting nurses association in 1920, prior to the Metropolitan program visiting nurses "went into the homes that were very, very poor. We were charity nurses." Now "there is a large body of the middle class of people, self-respecting, who do not want charity to-day, and who feel absolutely free to call upon the [Metropolitan visiting] nurse. They know that when they do, her services are paid for, and that she is coming to them in . . . an absolutely business way." The very poor, who were not policyholders, benefited because no one knew that their nursing visits were charity visits. In the 1930s and 1940s the Metropolitan provided between one-fourth and one-third of the total budgets of its affiliated visiting nursing associations, with the nurses making 4 million visits to 700,000 policyholders annually in 1933. A nursing historian wrote in 1922 that the Metropolitan advertised visiting nursing "as perhaps it could not be advertised by any other association. It has brought the public health nurse into homes where she would not otherwise have been; it has been largely instrumental in removing from visiting nurse the stigma of charity and placing it on a pay basis. In fact we might almost say that the Metropolitan Life Insurance Company has *popularized* public health nursing."[44]

The visiting nurse service was terminated on January 1, 1953, having made 107 million visits to more than 20 million policyholders since 1909. Many policyholders now had Blue Cross hospital insurance and in 1952 Metropolitan introduced its own hospital and surgical insurance, which it wanted policyholders to purchase. Most important, the number of nursing visits had declined steadily since the 1930s. Patients preferred to be treated by physicians, who offered them revolutionary new methods of diagnosis and treatment not available from nurses, including antibiotics, sulfa drugs, insulin, and vitamins. The nursing service was now providing maternity and newborn care and nursing care for the chronically ill rather than returning patients to health and preventing disability and death. Between 1929 and 1949 the proportion of nursing visits for acute and contagious diseases fell from 49% to 16%, those for chronic conditions rose from 5% to 18%, and those for newborn and maternity care rose from 36% to 53%. The company, which was then paying nurses $1.5 million to make 750,000 visits annually, considerately made the announcement in 1951, thirty months before the termination date, to enable the local nursing services to adjust to the change.[45]

Metropolitan ordinary policyholders were provided with a different health program. In 1914 a group of private individuals opened the nonprofit Life Extension Institute (later Life Extension Examiners) to administer periodic physical examinations to life insurance policyholders to facilitate the early identification of disease. To encourage policyholders to obtain the examinations, the insurance companies paid for them but did not receive reports about the policyholders. The Metropolitan was the first company to subscribe to the service in 1914. In 1924, the Metropolitan provided free examinations to intermediate and ordinary policyholders with policies exceeding $500 at intervals graded by the size of the policy. The Institute provided over two million physical examinations to Metropolitan policyholders before it was discontinued in 1947.[46]

The Metropolitan Health Education Campaign

The Metropolitan also created a wide variety of materials to educate the public about ways to improve their health. The company published dozens of different pamphlets providing guidance for healthy living, the care of the sick, and the prevention of illness. Health pamphlets were a popular form of health education used by municipal and state health departments, the federal government, and private organizations. The Metropolitan health pamphlet program greatly exceeded that of any other public or private organization. For example, in 1921 the federal government distributed 1.2 million scientific and popular health pamphlets, while the Metropolitan distributed 25 million popular health pamphlets in that year and 33 million in the next. Although the earliest Metropolitan pamphlets stated that they were "for the use of its policyholders," hundreds of millions were distributed to the general public and students by company agents, visiting nurses, state and municipal public health departments, schools, physicians, hospitals, and private businesses. Many health departments and schools relied on Metropolitan health pamphlets. By 1929, 535 million copies had been distributed, by 1934, 800 million, and by 1959 1.7 billion. Every pamphlet displayed the name and address of the Metropolitan Life Insurance Company but contained no advertising material.[47]

The Metropolitan health education campaign began in 1909 with the change in the editorial content of *The Metropolitan,* a policyholder magazine established in 1871, from general to health topics. The *Metropolitan* was distributed by the agents four times a year for many years in English and French, with occasional issues in Italian, Polish, Yiddish, German, Hungarian, and Bohemian. The overall philosophy was described in 1909: "In the study of disease today, medicine plays but a small part. It is the policy of prevention that is now the focus of the world's attention." Education about sanitation was the aspect of prevention most needed by the tenement dwellers who comprised the magazine's readers. A 1910 article cautioned: "Flies are disease carriers. They live and breed in all kinds of filth. Flies infect food and liquids by germ-laden feet . . . . The great secret of how to get rid of flies is cleanliness. Screen all food. Keep receptacles for garbage carefully covered. . . . Screen all windows and doors." Another article warned: "Don't let drinking water stand uncovered. . . . Keep your cooking utensils clean and off the floor. Vermin and mice carry infection; they never stay in clean places. . . . Select a milkman who has clean hands, clean clothes, clean wagon, clean cans, clean bottles. Do not select a milkman because he sells cheap milk. Refuse milk that shows a deposit of dirt in the bottom of the bottle. DO NOT FORGET THAT DIRTY MILK MAY KILL THE BABY."[48]

In 1912 the Metropolitan began to publish pamphlets on specific health topics using the most recent scientific knowledge. They were written in simple and concise language and attractively designed using colors and illustrations. Some of the authors were leading public health and medical authorities and all were revised periodically. The more popular ones were published in as many as ten different languages for the immigrant groups that were the core of Metropolitan's market. Most were four-to-eight pages in length, but some were longer and the cookbook, first issued in 1918, was sixty-four pages.[49]

Many pamphlets concerned the health of infants and children. Between 1909 and 1945 the Metropolitan distributed 33 million copies of a pamphlet entitled in various editions *The Child, The Baby,* and *Your Baby,* in half a dozen or more languages. The pamphlet provided detailed descriptions of every period from pregnancy through early childhood. The 900,000 copies distributed annually by the Metropolitan may be compared to the 200,000 copies of *Infant Care* distributed annually by the U.S. Children's Bureau between 1914 and 1921 and the 600,000 copies of a pamphlet on infant care and feeding distributed by the Prudential Insurance Company in 1917. The Metropolitan also distributed many millions of copies of pamphlets on infantile paralysis, diphtheria, pneumonia, influenza, scarlet fever, tonsils and adenoids, whooping cough, dental care, milk, first aid, goiter, colds, foot health, eyesight, posture, child psychology, and the transition from infancy to childhood.[50]

The child-care pamphlets urged families to seek professional medical care and avoid advice from neighbors. An early handbill on infant care urged: "Do not feed it on coffee, beer, syrups, or solid food. Buy the best and cleanest milk you can. . . . If the baby is sick, stop feeding it altogether. Give it water instead, and SEE THE DOCTOR AT ONCE. Do not let the neighbors tell you what to do. More babies are lost through delay in seeing the doctor and from continuing to feed them after they are sick than from any other reason." A later pamphlet urged pregnant women to consult a physician as soon as they suspected that they were pregnant. Women who did not have personal physicians were told to obtain advice from the Metropolitan nurse. They were warned: "Do not consult your neighbor about your condition. Even if she has had children, her experience may be wholly unlike your own."[51]

The pamphlets also corrected common misconceptions about childhood diseases. The pamphlet, *Scarlet Fever,* said: "Scarlet fever is a very contagious disease. It is easy to catch but not so easy to cure. No child has to have it. Because one child has it, is no reason why other children should have it. Do not let the well children be near the sick child." Pamphlets stressed the serious health problems that could result from infections. The scarlet fever pamphlet observed that the "heart, kidneys, and ears, are often seriously affected by scarlet fever." Another pamphlet, *Measles: Protect Your Children,* advised: "Unless you give him good care, your child may develop pneumonia and other diseases. The kidneys may . . . develop chronic disease in later life. The eyes and ears often become inflamed, which sometimes results in loss of sight or hearing. Your child's future health will depend largely upon the care that you give him at this time." The pamphlet *Whooping Cough* stated: "Whooping cough is very dangerous to children and sometimes fatal to grown-ups. More people die from whooping-cough than from scarlet fever. The mother whose children have had whooping-cough . . . can remember her child running to her gasping for breath, catching hold of her skirt for support and finally breaking into that painful rasping cough."

Early pamphlets recognized the severe economic constraints of most Metropolitan policyholders. The child care pamphlet urged mothers to sew their own inexpensive and practical clothing for their infants. It suggested a large clothes basket as a cradle and clean rags as diapers. A 1922 edition of the *Metropolitan Cook Book* began: "a great many families are not well nourished, not because they do not spend enough money for food, but because they do not get enough food value for the money spent." The book provided recipes for a variety of cereal grains for breakfast and other meals, suggested inexpensive sources of protein, and urged the use of fruits and vegetables in season because they were less expensive. It advised: "a variety of food from day to day, rather than a great variety at one meal, will not only keep the cost of food down, but also lessen labor, to say nothing of its good effect on the body."[52]

Pamphlets directed at adults emphasized healthy living as the best method of preventing disease. The very first pamphlet, *A War on Consumption*, observed: "strong, healthy people possess the power of resisting [tuberculosis] germs, otherwise it is likely that the disease would kill off whole communities. NEARLY EVERYBODY at some period of life BREATHES IN the living GERMS of the disease, but owing to the power of resistance of a HEALTHY body, the germs are not able to multiply." Later editions expanded on this point: "The first requirement is to live the sort of life that will keep the body at its best. You may have the germs of tuberculosis in your body and yet not develop the disease if you have good bodily resistance." Techniques for leading a healthy life were described in many pamphlets. *Health, Happiness, and Long Life* presented a straightforward "prescription" similar to the tuberculosis pamphlet: sleep and rest, fresh air, exercise, sunlight, cleanliness, proper diet, comfortable clothing, work and play, good posture, and "good mental habits." *Overweight and Underweight* included Metropolitan height and weight tables, menus for dieting and gaining weight, calorie counts, and exercises.

Later Metropolitan pamphlets discussed chronic and degenerative diseases. One on diabetes stressed the importance of avoiding obesity, especially in those with a family history of the disease. Another, *Give Your Heart a Chance*, urged annual physical examinations and gave advice on daily activities for those with high blood pressure or a "weak or disordered heart." Pamphlets on hearing loss and cancer discussed strategies for living with the diseases.

For a number of decades beginning in 1922 the company published monthly advertising messages in leading national magazines (the total magazine circulation began at 17 million and reached 38 million in 1950). The messages were concerned primarily with health problems of adults and their writing style and vocabulary were directed more toward a middle-class than the working-class audience of the early pamphlets. Each advertisement listed the name and address of the company but contained no commercial message. Readers were offered free copies of relevant pamphlets if they wrote the home office and the company received as many as 50,000 requests each month. According to Dublin, three themes were stressed: "the importance of keeping fit; the danger of neglecting even minor illnesses and injuries; and the need for periodic medical examination for the early detection of chronic disease." The advertisements described commonly overlooked symptoms of serious diseases, such as acute or chronic indigestion and persistent headaches. The topics included cancer, heart disease, diabetes, appendicitis, anemia, tuberculosis, diphtheria, and syphilis; health behaviors such as dental care, mental hygiene, exercise, recreation, and automobile safety; and medical problems like eyesight, hearing, and overweight. New treatments were prominently described, including insulin for diabetes, serum therapy for pneumonia, surgery and radiation for cancers, and diphtheria immunization. According to Marchand, "the ads were both informative and socially beneficial. Metropolitan . . . boldly explored diseases such as cancer and syphilis in a straightforward way virtually unknown in articles in family magazines of the day." The messages won numerous awards and were widely acclaimed by the public, health professionals, community leaders, and the advertising profession.[53]

Some of the Metropolitan disease campaigns combined several types of media. To educate the public about rheumatic fever, the Metropolitan sponsored at least one national magazine advertisement on the subject each year in the 1930s and 1940s, published a popular pamphlet, and issued a clinical booklet that was distributed to 40,000 physicians. Agents sponsored speakers who discussed the subject at their service clubs. The publications were prepared with the cooperation of the American Heart Association, the Academy of Pediatrics, the U.S. Children's Bureau, and the U.S. Public Health Service.[54]

The Metropolitan was among the first organizations to use the newly popular radio for health education. In 1925 it set up a studio in its home office and broadcast an early morning program that emphasized "diet and exercise as a secret of health," according to a company executive. The programs guided the listeners through physical exercises and offered health advice on diet and other topics. The broadcasts were aired on stations in Boston, New York City, and Washington. In the first few months the radio stations received 39,000 approving letters from listeners (about two-thirds of them women), many of whom were sent Metropolitan pamphlets. According to an article in the *New York Times,* "Overweight, old age, blood pressure, heart trouble and nervousness are prominent among the conditions broadcast listeners want to overcome by exercises." The radio programs continued until 1935, without ever including a commercial message.[55]

The Metropolitan also provided health exhibits at state and county fairs, sometimes with a nurse in attendance to treat sick visitors. It produced several motion pictures, similar to those of other organizations, on topics such as diphtheria immunization, smallpox vaccination, overweight, and annual physical examinations. To reduce the widespread use of common drinking cups, the company distributed millions of paper drinking cups in railroad passenger cars and schools with warnings against the use of shared cups.[56]

Other Metropolitan Programs

In 1925 the Metropolitan, which had millions of schoolchildren among its industrial policyholders, established a School Health Bureau. In 1929 it began publication of a periodical, *Health Bulletin for Teachers,* that was distributed regularly to 35,000 teachers in 1959. The company prepared pedagogical materials for teachers and recommended individual Metropolitan health pamphlets for use in specific grade levels and courses. Other life insurance companies followed the example of the Metropolitan in providing school health materials.[57]

Biographies of "health heroes" were among the most popular of the Metropolitan publications for schoolchildren, with 3.7 million copies of at least one of them distributed by 1951. Each biography had a specific theme, often involving the use of scientific medical knowledge in daily life. The biographies of Edward Jenner, Edward Trudeau, and Frederick Banting emphasized the benefits of vaccination, the sanitorium movement, and insulin respectively. Careers in medical research were encouraged in the biographies of Robert Koch, Louis Pasteur, William Welch, and Florence Sabin. The biography of Ellen Richards stressed the importance of a knowledge of nutrition by mothers, that of William Sedgwick the need for public health officials to educate the public about health and disease, and Josephine Baker was quoted as saying in her biography: "The way to keep people from dying of disease . . . is to keep them from falling ill. Healthy people don't die."[58]

As the Metropolitan group insurance division grew to insure one-fourth of all workers covered by group life insurance in 1942, the company sought to improve the health of its group policyholders beyond the provision of visiting nursing service and Metropolitan health pamphlets. The Metropolitan organized the Policyholders Service Bureau in 1919, which employed a staff of technical specialists who visited the firms and provided assistance on turnover, absenteeism, personnel policies, safety, production, and profit sharing. The Industrial Health and Hygiene Service was concerned with health issues associated with working conditions and company medical departments. It undertook studies in several dangerous industries to reduce industrial hazards and improve ventilation, lighting, and sanitation, and published numerous manuals for businesses based on the research. In 1923 Fiske stressed an ethical justification for his decision to offer group insurance:

> In some way or other, we might through Group Insurance, ameliorate that class antagonism which for so many years has existed between these so-called capitalists and labor. In the last few years we have seen much of this antagonism. Strikes; lockouts; incendiarism; bombs; murder; and we have been shocked. Ah, perhaps we would not have been so shocked if we had read the history of capitalism for the last hundred years. Labor exploited and underpaid; poorly housed; children uncared for; put out to work too early; women living like animals; all ground down for the profits that were to be made in keeping down labor. . . . Human beings were treated not as human beings but as machines, to be scrapped like old iron, and the cry comes up — . . . "We are entitled to be treated as human beings, with a fair wage and with a right to the comforts of life." . . .
>
> You and I have some sympathy after all, with these poor people who are uniting in a protest against wrong methods of living and carrying on business. We thought we could see through Group Insurance some opportunity of carrying home to employers some sense of responsibility.[59]

The Metropolitan used its home office employees as a testing ground for new group insurance programs. These included free lunches, an employees' dispensary, free physical, dental, and eye examinations, a medical rest room for sick employees, and special nutrition supplements. The Metropolitan owned and operated its own tuberculosis sanitorium with an adjoining Rest House for employees who suffered from other conditions. The facility was located in the Adirondack Mountains in New York State. It opened in 1913 and closed in 1945 when only 26 of its 350 beds were occupied. In order to construct the sanitorium, the company obtained a

New York State court decision that permitted business organizations to develop programs for the health of their employees.[60]

The Metropolitan expended millions of dollars on health research and health demonstration projects. Fiske justified them by saying: "We are teaching the State its duty. . . . sooner or later it will be brought home to the legislators and to the municipalities that we have shown what can be done by them and what must be done. And thus indirectly, as well as directly, we are teaching the laws of health to large bodies of people, bringing the means of improving health to them." The Framingham, Thetford Mines, and Kingsport demonstration projects were described in previous chapters. The company helped fund diphtheria immunization and tuberculosis control campaigns in a number of cities and states. It provided funding for an Influenza-Pneumonia Commission in 1919 after the great influenza pandemic and supported it for more than two decades. It funded research on diabetes by Elliott Joslin at the New England Deaconness Hospital in Boston, on rheumatic fever by the American Heart Association, on tuberculosis at the Henry Phipps Institute and the Saranac Laboratory for the Study of Tuberculosis, on the B.C.G. tuberculosis vaccine, and on the use of mass X rays as diagnostic techniques (contributing almost $60,000 for the last two projects). It published important research reports and provided funding for health pamphlets published by governments and voluntary health organizations.[61]

The Metropolitan used its agents as interviewers for numerous social surveys of industrial policyholders. At the request of the federal government, in 1915 its agents conducted the country's first national unemployment survey and in 1930 they surveyed 200,000 families to obtain estimates of nationwide unemployment levels. The company undertook several studies of the cost of medical care during the 1920s and 1930s, some of which were published by the federal government. One was a 1930 replication of a major study carried by the Committee on the Costs of Medical Care. The company carried out sickness surveys in a number of major cities in order to encourage greater municipal spending on health care. It encouraged communities to draw on its agency force for smaller projects. An advertisement addressed to community leaders in *Adventure* magazine in 1923 noted that in 1922 the company conducted 440 Community Clean-Up Campaigns and published literature to assist such campaigns. The advertisement warned about refuse and stables in alleys and back lots and stated that "unless all of a community is clean, no part of it can be entirely safe" from the germs that cause disease. It continued: "Have a great Spring Cleaning in Your Town, too! Let the Metropolitan agents in their daily round of visits to the homes of policyholders, help you to enlist your house-holders in the Campaign."[62]

Among the most striking of the Metropolitan's activities were those involving direct political action. Fiske observed that "the only people I know who have a right to walk into the domestic circles of [working class families] once a week are industrial agents." From 1909 on, these agents often brought with them militantly political circulars. Some urged the poli-cyholders to support and vote for public tuberculosis sanitoria in Chicago, Cleveland, Cincinnati, St. Louis, and other cities and states. Others advo-cated Workmen's Compensation laws, adequate appropriations and orga-nizational structures for state health departments, full time county health officers, birth and death registration, and funding for playgrounds. Some opposed proposed antivaccination and antivivisection legislation. Policy-holders in several cities were informed of their rights and responsibilities under tenement house laws. Agents also assisted individual health depart-ments, informing local policyholders of health programs such as free vacci-nations or baby clinics. On a more scholarly but no less polemical level, the Metropolitan published research monographs on European national pen-sion, unemployment, and health insurance programs.[63]

The Metropolitan developed programs to assist its many immigrant policyholders. It published two colorful pamphlets that described the ad-vantages of citizenship, provided elementary information on American his-tory, and spelled out the steps to obtain first and second (citizenship) pa-pers. An Immigrant Service and Citizenship Bureau was organized in 1921 to help policyholders obtain citizenship papers and provide personal assis-tance to those with families members coming from abroad or detained at American ports. It handled 7,100 cases from forty-two countries through 1924.[64]

As the company became more knowledgeable about its industrial policyholders, it recognized the profitability of investments in working-class urban housing. The Metropolitan decided to construct large, self-contained communities of low-rent apartments, which retained their value much longer than isolated individual buildings. In 1922, at the urging of the Metropolitan, New York State enacted legislation permitting life insur-ance companies to construct housing with a specified maximum rent per room. The company then constructed fifty-four apartment buildings in Queens in New York City for 2,125 families to help relieve a major hous-ing shortage. Preferences were given to low-income families and those with children. The company's Welfare Bureau operated a model apartment in one of the buildings and employed an instructor who provided classes on child care and homemaking and took housewives on tours of local food stores to explain the nutritional value of foods and give advice on food purchases. The apartment complex, which was the largest housing construction project in the history of New York City, proved extremely popular with residents, provided an attractive return on Metropolitan's investment, and led other insurance companies to invest in housing. The public relations benefits were clearly indicated by an editorial in the *New York Times*:

> It does not detract from the credit due to the Metropolitan Life Insurance Company for its interest in promoting modern, low-priced housing to point out that it is an enlightened self-interest. . . . Many [Metropolitan] polices are taken out on children's lives, and it is a sad fact that too many of these claims went to pay for the funeral expenses of the infant "beneficiaries." . . . Our great insurance companies might go in still more emphatically for housing reform as affecting the poor. Civilized living conditions hold a place beside diphtheria antitoxin as a preserver of child life.[65]

In the late 1930s when it had considerable capital to invest and few attractive prospects during the Depression, the Metropolitan constructed Parkchester, a self-sufficient community of fifty-eight buildings with twelve thousand low-to-moderate rental apartments on 129 acres in the Bronx in New York City. Parkchester was the largest private or public housing project ever built in the United States and housed families with incomes between $2,000 and $4,500 a year. The project was enormously popular and provided a higher rate of return for the company than other available investments. After the Second World War, the Metropolitan invested $100 million in moderate-income housing for thousands of residents in four projects in New York City and others in Washington, D.C., San Francisco, and Los Angeles. Although the housing was criticized for insufficient open space, a *New York Times* editorial noted in 1947 that the Metropolitan has been "one of the greatest builders of all time, clearing slums and providing apartments that the great mass of families in the middle income group could afford and enjoy."[66]

The 1940s housing projects in New York City brought to public attention a long-standing inequity in the practices of the Metropolitan and most other life insurance companies: discrimination against blacks. Richard Plunz writes in his history of New York City housing that three of the four projects "were clearly intended for white middle-income occupancy, and only [one] in Harlem, admitted black tenants. Apparently, it was planned partially as a response to the accusations of racism which had surrounded [one of the other projects] from its inception." A much more serious problem was that the Metropolitan and other companies had historically sold blacks policies with smaller death benefits because of their higher mortality rates, but did not engage in similar practices for nationality groups with higher mortality rates. In states that essentially banned this form of racial discrimination, such as New York after 1935, the Metropolitan apparently refused to sell life insurance to blacks, although the evidence is conflicting. Its policy was less regressive than that of other companies, including some of the largest ones, that refused to sell policies to blacks under any conditions. In the 1940s 8% of Metropolitan policyholders were black, similar to the proportion of blacks in most cities.[67]

Frankel had recognized from the beginning the need for evidence to demonstrate the benefits of the health programs. In 1911 the Metropolitan organized a Statistical Bureau, which was headed for many years by the statistician-epidemiologist, Louis Dublin, assisted by a demographer, Alfred Lotka, both eminent scholars in their fields. The bureau undertook hundreds of research studies, many of which were published in scholarly journals, popular articles, monographs, books, and, beginning in 1920, in the company's own monthly scholarly journal, *Statistical Bulletin of the Metropolitan Life Insurance Company.* The Statistical Bureau was the Metropolitan's most successful public relations program per dollar expended. At that time federal government vital statistics were rudimentary, published belatedly and infrequently, and omitted major areas of the country excluded from the death registration area. Consequently newspapers and magazines cited Metropolitan statistics on the mortality rates of its industrial policyholders as evidence of national trends. The science columnist of the *New York Times* observed in 1937: "Though the Metropolitan Life Insurance Company is a commercial institution, its reports on the state of its policyholders' health have the value and the authority of a governmental publication. . . . [Its Statistical Bureau] is the finest statistical department of its kind to be found anywhere."[68]

The Statistical Bureau also contributed to public awareness of specific medical problems. In 1926 the *New York Times* reported: "The latest attack on the problem of cancer comes not from a research worker's laboratory but from the statistical bureau of a life insurance company—the Metropolitan of New York. For fifteen years the Metropolitan has been analyzing the cancer deaths . . . among its industrial policyholders. The result is probably the most careful statistical inquiry into this most dreaded of diseases that has ever been made." In the late 1940s the statistical bureau was among the first to point out the growing importance of childhood accidents as a national health problem, which provided an impetus for a national campaign by government and private organizations.[69]

The Metropolitan Life Insurance Company thus behaved for more than a third of a century as though the nation's health were its corporate responsibility. Its nursing service was America's alternative to socialized medicine and enhanced the economic viability and social prestige of nursing. Its pamphlets and advertisements were the single most widely used source of information about health and disease for adults and schoolchildren. It sponsored more research on primary and preventive health care than any other private or government organization. It compiled national health statistics that were more widely cited than those of the federal government. It sponsored school health education programs that helped make the health of schoolchildren a national concern. It was the largest builder of low-cost apartment housing in the nation. The company spurred state and local governments to strengthen their public health and health care programs. In return, the Metropolitan secured a level of trust and goodwill from the public, health professionals, and governments that enabled it to maintain its dominant position in the industry with little criticism.

After mid-century, the Metropolitan programs were no longer sufficiently distinctive to warrant their continuation on the same scale. The demand for visiting nursing was reduced by health insurance and patient preferences for physicians. Metropolitan's health publications became less significant with expanded media coverage of health topics, greater health knowledge of the public, and improved school health materials. The reports of the Statistical Bureau became less comprehensive than federal government vital statistics. As the programs lost their benefits for public and policyholder relations, they were scaled back or eliminated.

The Metropolitan's programs thus introduced millions of Americans to the idea that individual health was affected by personal behaviors and that lifestyle changes could reduce the risk of death and disease. The programs also went beyond the customary infectious diseases to familiarize the public with public health's newest challenge: preventing chronic diseases.

PART III

The Coronary Heart Disease Epidemic

10

EARLY TWENTIETH-CENTURY MORTALITY TRENDS AND RHEUMATIC HEART DISEASE

> Far from being the sole property of the aged and infirm, various forms of heart disease impair and kill more people in all walks of life and all ages groups than do any other four diseases combined. The grim harvest of child lives exacted by such spectacular terrors as infantile paralysis is as nothing compared with the hundreds of thousands of little children who suffer and die from [rheumatic] heart disease today. (Senator George Smathers, 1948)[1]

During the early twentieth century the declining mortality rates from infectious diseases brought chronic diseases to greater public attention. The history of rheumatic heart disease, then a major chronic disease, demonstrated the many difficulties involved in their management and control.

Mortality Trends in the Early Twentieth Century

Between 1900 and 1940 overall mortality rates declined more than in any comparable period in American history, but the amounts varied widely among age and sex groups. This is indicated by vital statistics from 1900 to 1940 for those states that were included in the death registration area since its inception in 1900 (see Table 10.1). These states, primarily in the North-

Table 10.1: Mortality Rates for 1900 Death Registration Area by Age and Sex
1900–1940

	(deaths per 1,000 population)									
Age	*White Males*					*White Females*				
	1900	1910	1920	1930	1940	1900	1910	1920	1930	1940
1–4	20.2	15.4	11.0	5.0	2.2	18.7	13.9	10.1	4.3	1.9
5–14	3.8	3.1	2.9	1.8	1.0	3.8	2.9	2.5	1.4	0.7
15–24	5.8	4.6	4.3	2.8	1.7	5.6	4.1	4.3	2.4	1.2
25–34	8.1	6.7	5.9	3.8	2.5	8.1	6.1	6.5	3.5	1.9
35–44	10.6	10.2	7.9	6.6	4.9	9.6	8.1	7.3	5.1	3.6
45–54	15.5	15.8	12.9	13.4	11.8	14.0	12.7	11.8	10.1	8.0
55–64	28.5	30.3	26.3	28.0	27.1	25.5	25.3	23.7	22.0	19.0
65–74	59.1	61.7	58.5	57.9	57.9	53.4	55.3	54.8	49.5	45.4

Source: Forrest E. Linder and Robert D. Grove, *Vital Statistics Rates in the United States: 1900–1940* (Washington, DC: U.S. Government Printing Office, 1943), 177–78.

east and Midwest, had the most trustworthy reporting and comprised about one-fourth of the total United States population.[2] Their mortality rates declined by about 90% for children ages 1–4 and by more than 50% for males and females through ages 35–44. The oldest age groups had much smaller reductions. Women ages 54–65 experienced a 25% decline in their mortality rates and those 65–74 experienced a 15% decline. Men ages 55–64 and 65–74 experienced a 10% decline over the four decades, but practically no decline after 1920. For all practical purposes, the great mortality decline excluded men ages 55 and older.

The best statistics on mortality trends in urban areas are those of the industrial policyholders of the Metropolitan Life Insurance Company. The number of policyholders was enormous: between 1879 and 1929 the Metropolitan sold 100 million industrial policies and in 1929 it had 19 million industrial policyholders. The policyholders were overwhelmingly urban, with only 5% of deceased male industrial policyholders ages 15 and over employed in agriculture compared to 25% of all deceased occupied males in the death registration area.[3]

The decline in urban mortality rates from about 1910 to the early 1930s, as shown by white[4] Metropolitan industrial policyholders, generally paralleled the trends of white urban and rural residents of the states in the original death registration area (see Tables 10.1 and 10.2). The greatest declines occurred among urban adult males: about 1910, male policyholders ages 25 and older had much higher mortality rates than the general male population, but by the early 1930s they had only slightly higher rates. The convergence was probably

Table 10.2: Mortality Rates by Age and Sex: Metropolitan Life Insurance Company Industrial Policyholders, 1911–1935

| | (deaths per 1,000 policies) | | | | | | | |
| | White males | | | | White females | | | |
Age	1911–1913	1920–1922	1927–1929	1933–1935	1911–1913	1920–1922	1927–1929	1933–1935
1–4	11.9	8.8	5.9	3.8	11.0	7.8	5.2	3.3
5–9	3.8	3.1	2.4	1.7	3.5	2.6	2.0	1.4
10–14	2.4	2.3	1.3	1.3	2.2	2.0	1.4	1.0
15–19	4.1	3.3	2.8	2.0	3.7	3.4	2.5	1.5
20–24	6.4	4.4	3.6	2.8	5.7	4.9	3.7	2.6
25–34	10.2	5.6	4.9	4.0	7.3	5.7	4.3	3.3
35–44	17.0	9.1	9.0	7.6	9.9	7.1	6.2	5.0
45–54	25.0	15.4	17.5	15.8	15.4	11.6	11.3	10.0
55–64	42.9	30.4	34.6	33.0	31.4	24.5	24.8	22.6
65–74	84.4	66.8	70.6	67.5	70.1	59.0	56.3	53.5

Source: Louis I. Dublin and Alfred J. Lotka, *Twenty-Five Years of Health Progress* (New York: 1937), 541–42.

due to employment in new industries and occupations with much safer working conditions. The mortality rates of urban female policyholders ages 25 and over were slightly higher than the general female population throughout the period. Among younger males and females, ages 5–24, policyholders and the general population had similar rates and similar declines throughout the period. Comparisons of children ages 1–4 are rendered problematic by the inability of seriously ill children to qualify for life insurance.

Most of the reduction in urban mortality rates was due to the decline in death rates from infectious diseases, as shown by the causes of death of Metropolitan industrial policyholders. Mortality rates per 1,000 insured children ages 1–14 declined from about 0.5 to about 0.2 annually between 1911–15 and 1931–35, more than half of which was due to lower mortality rates from influenza, pneumonia, measles, scarlet fever, whooping cough, and diphtheria. Among those ages 25–34, mortality rates per 1,000 policyholders dropped from 1.0 to 0.4 annually for men and from 0.7 to 0.3 for women, with about one-half of the declines resulting from fewer deaths from tuberculosis. Among those ages 35–44, death rates per 1,000 policyholders dropped from 1.6 to 0.7 for men and from 1.0 to 0.5 for women, with tuberculosis accounting for about half of the decline among men and somewhat less among women. Infectious disease mortality rates also declined among policyholders in older age groups, but other causes of death were more important.[5]

Within urban areas, the greatest beneficiaries of the decline were lower rather than higher income groups and young and middle-aged men rather than women. According to Metropolitan statistics, in 1923 the lower income industrial policyholders had mortality rates that were from 65% to 107% higher than the higher income ordinary policyholders for age groups up to age 65, and 21% higher for those ages 65 and older (see Table 10.3). In 1940–41 mortality rates for industrial policyholders were 12% to 55% higher for age groups from 25–34 to 55–64 and 11% higher for those ages 65 and over. Considering sex differences in mortality rates per 1,000 Metropolitan industrial policyholders, among those ages 25–34 men had 2.9 more deaths than women in 1911–15 but only 0.7 more deaths in 1931–35 (Table 10.2). Over the same time period, the sex differences narrowed from 7.1 to 2.6 for those ages 35–44 and from 9.6 to 5.8 for those ages 45–54. Among older age groups, the sex differences remained large primarily because men had higher death rates from cardiovascular/renal diseases and experienced increasing death rates from cancer while the rates for women declined.[6]

The trends in mortality rates were often misinterpreted because of simultaneous changes in the age distribution of the population. With regard to children, between 1900 and 1940 the total population increased by 74%, but declining birth rates limited the increase in the number of children under age 5 to 15% and those ages 5–14 to 32%. The combination of lower birth rates and lower death rates from infectious diseases exaggerated the decline in childhood diseases. With regard to older persons, the number of persons ages 45 and older tripled, which greatly increased the number of cases of chronic diseases and incorrectly suggested that the rates were

Table 10.3: Mortality Ratios by Age: Metropolitan Life Insurance Company Industrial and Ordinary Policyholders, 1923–1941

	Industrial Policyholder Mortality Rates as Proportion of Ordinary Policyholder Mortality Rates		
Age	1923	1930–34	1940–41
25–34	187	155	147
35–44	207	157	155
45–54	192	146	129
55–64	165	134	112
65+	121	131	111

Sources: Louis I. Dublin and Robert J. Vane, "Occupational Mortality Experience of Insured Wage Earners," *Monthly Labor Review* 64 (1947): 1009; Malvin Davis, *Industrial Life Insurance in the United States* (New York: McGraw–Hill, 1944), 120.

rising. The actual situation is indicated by comparing trends in crude death rates, which do not consider changes in the age distribution of the population, and standardized death rates, which give the population in each time period the same age, sex, and race distribution. The crude death rate per 1,000 Metropolitan industrial policyholders for cancer increased from 0.66 deaths in 1911 to 0.96 deaths in 1935, while the standardized rates increased much less, from 0.76 to 0.87, and that was due largely to improved diagnosis. The crude death rates per 1,000 policyholders from all forms of heart disease rose from 1.34 in 1911 to 1.49 in 1935, but the standardized rates actually declined from 1.58 in 1911 to 1.39 in 1935. The crude rates for stroke dropped from 0.69 in 1911 to 0.55 in 1935, while the standardized rates declined even more, from 0.83 to 0.48.[7]

Rheumatic Heart Disease

The most common form of heart disease early in the twentieth century was rheumatic heart disease, a chronic, disabling, and often fatal disease of children and younger adults. Although it was declining steadily as a cause of mortality and morbidity, it became conspicuous because of greater declines in other serious diseases. By 1929, rheumatic heart disease rates were surpassed by other types of heart disease. A New York City study at that time estimated that 25% of all cases of heart disease were rheumatic, 40% were arteriosclerotic, and the remainder due to syphilis and other diseases.[8]

Rheumatic heart disease was always preceded by rheumatic fever, a non-infectious childhood disease. Its multiple symptoms include fever, joint pains that migrate from joint to joint, and involuntary jerky movements known as chorea or St. Vitus's dance. About 75% of the patients who contracted rheumatic fever early in the century experienced one or more subsequent attacks of several months duration, most often within five or six years. The term "rheumatic" was adopted in the eighteenth century because the disease was considered a form of rheumatism, a group of afflictions associated with joint pain and fever. The association between rheumatic fever and rheumatic heart disease was first discovered in pathological studies at the turn of the nineteenth century and by 1850 the condition was established as a clinical entity.[9]

The great danger of rheumatic fever is endocarditis, an inflammation of the inner lining of the heart muscle that produces scarring of the heart valves. The scarred valves do not close properly, which permits blood to leak through them and produces a murmur that was used for diagnosis.

Each succeeding acute episode of rheumatic fever further scars and thickens the valves, especially the mitral valve (called mitral stenosis). This narrows the valve opening and reduces blood flow through it. Severe rheumatic heart disease ultimately produces congestive heart failure and a premature death. In 1949, Charles K. Friedberg estimated that between 65% to 75% of children who suffered from rheumatic fever developed clinical heart disease sooner or later, excluding those with minimal heart damage.[10]

Rheumatic fever was accepted as a specific disease entity very slowly. The epidemiologist John Paul noted in 1930 that rheumatic fever "has been, and is as yet, poorly defined. It certainly is not recognized as a clinical entity by most of the physicians in the United States. . . . Everything from the clinical viewpoint speaks for non-specificity." Symptoms of rheumatic fever occurred in different combinations among patients, were sometimes so mild as to go unnoticed by families and physicians, and the joint pains were often considered "growing pains." Frequently the disease revealed itself only after multiple attacks.[11]

Most victims of rheumatic heart disease were young children. A statistical study of 413 patients in New York City in the 1920s found that the average age of the initial attack was seven years and that 98% of the patients had their first attack before age 15. The most poignant aspect of this terrible disease was that children would recover from one attack, gradually improve to the great satisfaction of themselves and their families, and then undergo another attack that further damaged their hearts and left them more disabled than before. In severe cases their range of activities gradually deteriorated until they became completely bedridden and died in their 30s or 40s.[12]

The prevalence of rheumatic heart disease was difficult to determine because many deaths were attributed to rheumatic fever or chronic heart disease. Paul estimated about 1930 that rheumatic heart disease occurred in about 1% of all age groups up to age 44. The disease comprised an estimated 80% of all cases of heart disease in the 5–to–14–year-old group and declined gradually to 50% in the 35–to–44–year-old group. Especially useful statistics were provided by medical examinations for military service. In the First World War, 2.6% of 2.5 million draftees were excluded from military service because of organic heart disease, the largest number with rheumatic heart disease. Between 1940 and 1944, 1.8% of 1.5 million men ages 18–25 examined by Second World War selective service boards had evidence of rheumatic heart disease. A similar survey of 1.6 million draftees ages 19–25 in 1950–51 found 1.2% who were disqualified for military service because of rheumatic heart disease. The 1917–19 and 1950–

51 statistics underestimated the prevalence of the disease because they included only those with heart damage sufficient to cause disqualification.[13]

The etiology of rheumatic fever remained a matter of controversy for decades. Laboratory investigations were impossible because the disease occurs only in human beings. As a result, clinical observations served as the basis of medical knowledge. The first etiological agent recognized as being associated with rheumatic fever was the patient's standard of living. In 1862, an English physician stated that the victims of rheumatic fever were "weak, ill-nourished, overworked and often underfed and insufficiently clad, unhealthy . . . children, students, and young people." In 1940 an American physician, Ernst Boas, noted: "rheumatic infection is closely related to poverty, to poor housing, overcrowding, and inadequate diet. As in the case of tuberculosis, prevention is in large measure a matter of providing decent living conditions."[14]

During the early decades of the century, clinical evidence accumulated that rheumatic fever was always preceded by streptococcal infections. Many physicians rejected the idea of a causal relationship because a very small proportion of cases of streptococcal infection developed rheumatic fever. In 1930 Paul observed that "the mere bringing together of a patient and a streptococcus of one of the types thought to be of etiological significance is not sufficient to give rise to this peculiar and insidious disease. It would seem as if there were some other unknown factor or factors operating either directly or indirectly which are of great importance."[15]

The turning point occurred when statistical studies demonstrated that antibiotics could prevent patients with streptococcal infections from contracting rheumatic fever. The first studies in 1939 used the sulfa drugs and subsequent studies the more effective penicillin. Statistical studies also found that penicillin administered prophylactically to rheumatic fever patients prevented the recurrence of rheumatic fever attacks. One study of 434 children with rheumatic fever who were treated with penicillin for five years found a recurrence rate of only 2.9% per patient-year.[16]

Even though multiple etiological factors are necessary for the occurrence of rheumatic heart disease, subsequent research has focused almost exclusively on the streptococcus. As a result, according to a 1989 review, "a lot is known about the streptococcus, and a lot is known about the rheumatic fever, but little is known about what connects the two." It is accepted that rheumatic fever is a "post-streptococcal rather than a streptococcal disease."[17]

Another barrier to the effective management of rheumatic heart disease was diagnosis. Rheumatic heart disease has no distinctive electrocardiographic pattern that always provides an accurate diagnosis. No convenient mass screening tests could be administered routinely to schoolchildren comparable to mass X rays for tuberculosis. In 1960 a report of the American Public Health Association concluded: "The mechanism of the disease is unknown, its boundaries are indefinite, and its differentiation from other diseases is sometimes impossible. There is no specific laboratory diagnostic test. The diagnosis must therefore be arbitrary and empirical."[18]

Before antibiotics, the cardinal principles in the treatment of the "subacute phases" of rheumatic fever were, according to Paul, "rest, sunlight, carefully regulated life, adequate diet and medical supervision." These recommendations were seldom satisfactory. Active children with subacute symptoms could never be induced to remain bedridden continuously for weeks or months, and low income families did not have the funds for regular medical care or the physical space to isolate the child. Furthermore, no evidence existed that the regimen prevented future attacks.[19]

The long-term care of rheumatic heart disease patients before antibiotics was the responsibility of public health, education, and social service departments. New York City established the nation's first cardiac disease clinic in 1911 in Bellevue Hospital to provide treatment in the evenings for workmen discharged from the hospital. Later the city opened trade schools to provide care and vocational training for cardiac cases, almost all with rheumatic heart disease. In 1921 New York City had 31 public and private clinics, including 14 for children and 17 for adults, with a total patient population of more than 4,500. By 1925, the number of clinics had increased to 44. The clinics provided diagnosis, medical advice, and employed social service workers who assisted patients in finding employment and visiting nurses who visited them in their homes. By that time 28 other cities also had clinics. The 1939 annual report of the New York City health department stated that "until more is known of the etiology of rheumatic fever, weapons of attack are: early discovery, regular medical supervision, and the educational and vocational guidance of children with rheumatic heart disease." Schoolchildren suspected of having the disease were referred to cardiac clinics or private physicians and those applying for working papers were sent to a vocational consultation service.[20]

Sanitoria and convalescent homes were established in some cities and states to care for children seriously ill with rheumatic heart disease; in 1920 New York City had five such facilities. Unfortunately, the sanitorium movement was too limited to make a significant contribution. In 1920 more than 20,000 of New York City's public school children and thousands more in the parochial schools were "handicapped by permanent heart damage," according the *New York Times,* but the available sanitoria could house only a very small proportion of them. Paul observed that "rheumatic children cannot be moved en masse from the slums and kept for the rest of their childhood in sanitoria." According to Friedberg, "the results have not always been impressive" and outbreaks of streptococcal infections have occurred in them.[21]

After antibiotic prophylaxis was discovered in the 1940s, the responsibility for the control of rheumatic fever devolved on the patients' physicians. Yet most physicians did not accept the streptococcus as an etiological factor. As late as 1965, a presidential commission complained that only an estimated 100,000 of the 1.3 million cases of rheumatic heart disease were "receiving rheumatic fever prophylaxis. These figures underscore a shameful failure to control a potentially preventable disease." It added that "although the medical profession for 20 years has known of the effectiveness of chemical [sulfa drug] and antibiotic prophylaxis against the development and recurrence of rheumatic heart disease, the use of prophylaxis against this disease has been quite limited and disappointingly low."[22]

Physicians did adopt one misguided prophylactic surgical procedure for rheumatic fever enthusiastically: the tonsillectomy, millions of which were performed after 1920 with the idea of preventing rheumatic fever. Belief in the tonsils as an etiological factor began with the recognition that sore throats often preceded rheumatic fever. It was strengthened by occasional findings of streptococci on tonsils and the "focal infection" theory that certain organs served as the foci of infection and should be removed if possible. This led to the further recommendation that all children should have prophylactic tonsillectomies. An article on heart disease in the *New York Times* in 1920 stated that "acute inflammatory rheumatism" was a "germ disease" that entered the body through "the diseased tonsils or adenoids or decayed teeth. The removal of such tonsils and adenoids and the proper care of the teeth seem to be the most direct and effective measure against rheumatism." In the 1930s some physicians questioned the benefits of tonsillectomies and in 1957 Paul commented: "It is all the more extraordinary when one considers that during the half century in which the operation has been used, its value as an important therapeutic or prophylactic measure in this disease has never been proven." Subsequent statistical studies found no evidence that tonsillectomies reduced the incidence of streptococcal or other respiratory infections.[23]

Given the confusion surrounding so many aspects of rheumatic heart disease, professional leadership was essential to carry out research, educate physicians, and develop and evaluate preventive and treatment programs.

The American Heart Association (AHA) was organized in 1924, according to Howard Rusk, the noted specialist in rehabilitation medicine, "to develop a national public health program directed against heart disease and rheumatic fever." However, Senator Claude Pepper observed at the 1948 Senate hearings concerning the establishment of the National Heart Institute that the AHA "was doing the best it could, but it had not been able to arouse public opinion to the extent of any large number of donations being made. The public conscience and the Congressional conscience had not been sufficiently moved to appropriate any appreciable public funds, and very little was being done in the field where the greatest amount of damage was being done." Arlie R. Barnes, the AHA president, replied that before 1946 the AHA was "primarily concerned with the publication of scientific data for postgraduate education of physicians and the establishment of standards. . . . We have never had a national organization whose object was to bring this to the attention of the public so that funds could be collected. It is a difficult thing to collect funds. . . . because the people were not receptive to the idea; they didn't know the magnitude of the problem."[24]

In fact, the public was very receptive to solicitations from organizations concerned with health problems. In 1945, when the American Heart Association raised $39,000, the National Foundation for Infantile Paralysis raised $16 million, the National Tuberculosis Association $15.5 million, and the American Cancer Society $4 million. The AHA, which was then dominated by physicians and medical researchers, was unwilling to undertake a fund raising campaign even though rheumatic fever and heart disease caused almost five times as many deaths as infantile paralysis, whooping cough, diphtheria, and scarlet fever combined. In 1944, the AHA organized the American Council on Rheumatic Fever for public education, research, and control programs. In 1947, the AHA was reorganized to admit lay members and began large-scale fund raising, but it did not undertake a program to encourage the prophylactic use of antibiotics in rheumatic heart disease until 1955, years after their benefits had been demonstrated.[25]

Some physicians claimed, according to the *New York Times,* that support for rheumatic fever "is more difficult to enlist than that for other and more striking, if less serious, diseases—more difficult because we cannot see the infirmities it causes; its cripples do not limp." Yet in 1943 Don Gudakunst, a representative of the National Foundation for Infantile Paralysis, stated at a U.S. Children's Bureau conference that both rheumatic heart disease and polio required long periods of hospitalization and care by specially trained professionals and that both had the sympathy of the public:

We have learned that there is interest in these medical problems on the part of the public [which] can be directed toward and translated into service programs. I grant you that the picture of the crippled child has somewhat greater eye appeal than the picture of the child with heart disease, but it certainly has no greater emotional appeal to the heartstrings or the purse strings of the public. I have been very much concerned about the fact that we have not had, long before this, some national movement on a solid, widespread basis for the care of rheumatic heart disease and for the study of the problems involved therein. We have all the natural elements working for us—public interest, a corps of people with professional training. You don't need a lot more.[26]

The Metropolitan Life Insurance Company endeavored to arouse public interest in rheumatic heart disease by publishing advertisements in national magazines, distributing leaflets to policyholders and the public, and sending a clinical booklet to 40,000 physicians throughout the country. It also funded and published a major epidemiological study of the disease by John Paul in 1930 at the request of the AHA. In 1940 the company announced a major campaign to educate the public, teachers, health workers, and physicians by means of pamphlets, radio messages, newspapers, and lectures.[27] However, the Metropolitan, unlike the AHA, was not in a position to become a national leader in coordinating rheumatic heart disease programs.

The federal government became concerned with rheumatic heart disease in 1939 when Congress authorized the U.S. Children's Bureau to include children with rheumatic heart disease in its programs for crippled children. The programs were created as a result of the Social Security Act of 1935 and made funds available to states to develop services for handicapped children. By 1952, 603 special clinical centers existed for children with rheumatic heart disease and other cardiac diseases, but 282 of them were located in just four states. Programs for crippled children also cared for children with acute rheumatic fever and rheumatic heart disease in about thirty-six states, but only 8,000 children with the conditions were enrolled in them. Thus the federal government provided funding but no leadership.[28]

The local situation in 1960 was described in a report of the American Public Health Association and the American Heart Association. It concluded that "most communities have limited facilities and plans, that the full scope of rheumatic fever prevention is not yet appreciated by the majority of private medical practitioners, and that communities have not yet taken full advantage of available resources and opportunities to improve their services." In 1965, a presidential commission criticized the lack of coordination among federal agencies, state and local health departments, and state and local heart associations.[29]

Centralized leadership could make a significant contribution to the prevention and treatment of rheumatic heart disease. This was demonstrated by the armed forces, which were concerned with rheumatic fever because of the periodic outbreaks on military bases. Some leading experts on rheumatic fever were military physicians and a pioneering study of penicillin prophylaxis was carried out on a military base. The armed forces were among the first to employ large-scale antibiotic prophylaxis for streptococcal infections and to use antibiotics to treat soldiers who contracted rheumatic fever.[30]

Mortality rates from rheumatic fever and rheumatic heart disease declined steadily during the first half of the twentieth century, despite the absence of therapeutic and prophylactic measures. Among white Metropolitan Life Insurance Company industrial policyholders ages 1–74, the age-adjusted mortality rates from acute rheumatic fever per 1,000 policyholders declined from 6.2 in 1911–15 to 2.4 in 1931–35 and 1.4 in 1945. With regard to rheumatic heart disease, mortality rates for the same population from organic diseases of the heart (most of which were rheumatic heart disease) declined from 1.5 per 1,000 policyholders in 1911–15 to 1.2 in 1941–45. By the 1980s the disease had practically disappeared in the United States.[31]

New attacks in children with rheumatic heart disease were also declining, and they were also best explained by improvements in the standard of living. This was shown in a study of 782 children ages 2–20 registered with the Cardiac Rheumatic Clinic at the New York Hospital. In 1938–40, 32% had an attack within the previous two years; in 1941–45, only 20% had an attack within the same time period; and in 1952–56, 17% had an attack within the previous two years. Antibiotic therapy was first used prophylactically in the clinic in 1952, so it did not contribute to the declines in the preceding years. The study found that the decline over the period occurred only for children in families in "good" or "fair" socio-economic groups. No decline in recurrence rates occurred among children in families in "poor" socio-economic groups.[32]

Further evidence that improved social conditions were responsible for the decline in the rates of rheumatic fever and rheumatic heart disease is the continuing ubiquity of streptococcal infections in children. Many are so mild that they are unnoticed by parents or physicians and are not treated with antibiotics. The great change has therefore been the declining proportion of streptococcal infections that result in rheumatic fever. Another possible explanation for the decline, that the streptococcus has become less virulent, is contradicted by the consistently high rates of rheumatic fever in impoverished densely populated areas of underdeveloped nations.

Thus the management of rheumatic heart disease was marked by confusion, disorganization, and a lack of acceptance of the statistical evidence. These failures were to be repeated on a much larger scale with coronary heart disease, the great epidemic disease of the twentieth century.

11

THE EARLY YEARS OF THE CORONARY HEART DISEASE EPIDEMIC

Unlike other conditions in medicine, most sufferers from heart disease cannot be cured. The disease generally is a chronic one, and the purpose of intelligent care is the prolongation of life, the diminution of suffering and the increased mental and physical efficiency of the patient. . . . If the difference between correct and incorrect advice given to a patient with early heart failure is a matter of two to five years of added life, then proper treatment renders much more aid than most of the unhappy sufferers of cancer obtain from the thousands of surgical operations that are performed for their relief.

(Samuel Levine, 1938)[1]

The onset of the great coronary heart disease epidemic of the mid-twentieth century was marked by concern and confusion about this new and highly fatal disease. Clinical medicine and traditional public health measures provided few effective methods of treatment and prevention. The most useful knowledge came from vital statistics and the risk factors of the life insurance industry.

Disease Classification Systems

Severe chronic diseases, including heart disease, became more important causes of death in the early twentieth century as more people survived to old age. This produced a demand for accurate statistics about their incidence, prevalence, and trends, which in turn created new problems for the system of disease classification used for reporting deaths.

Statistical analyses of mortality patterns require a system of disease classification that enables physicians to file accurate and consistent death certificates. The first widely used system was devised by William Farr (1807–1883), an English public health official, after the inaugural International Statistical Conference at Brussels in 1853. It was later called the International List of Causes of Death and was revised at decadal intervals. The most significant revision occurred in 1893 and created a new classification of 161 diseases that, according to Lancaster, was a "synthesis of English, German and Swiss classifications used by the city of Paris and was based on the principle, introduced by Farr, for distinguishing between general diseases and those localized to a particular organ or anatomical site." This revision was adopted in almost all western nations, including the United States. Responsibility for subsequent revisions devolved successively on the French government, the League of Nations, and the World Health Organization. In 1949 the system was renamed the International Classification of Diseases.[2]

As heart diseases became more important causes of death, the number of categories used to classify them increased from four in 1900 to twenty in 1938 and forty in 1948. These included such new categories as congenital, infectious, degenerative, and hypertensive heart disease. The categories of the more inclusive "cardiovascular and renal disease" expanded from fifteen in 1900 to forty-two in 1938 and seventy-nine in 1948. With regard to the subcategory of coronary heart disease, the 1929 revision replaced "angina pectoris," which had been used since 1900, with "diseases of the coronary arteries and angina pectoris," the 1949 revision adopted "arteriosclerotic heart disease, including the coronary arteries," and the 1965 revision grouped those and other diseases under a new category, "ischemic heart disease." The revisions sometimes reassigned individual diseases or even groups of diseases to different categories, such as from heart disease to kidney disease, so that even the broadest categories could not be compared from revision to revision with complete accuracy.[3]

The classification of multiple causes of death in a single individual, which had never been clarified, became a more serious problem with the growing number of deaths from chronic diseases. Before 1900, a single cause of death usually sufficed because most deaths were caused by infectious diseases and occurred in persons who had not reached old age and were otherwise healthy. After 1900, more persons died at older ages when they were suffering from more than one serious illness. In 1914 the United States published a Manual of Joint Causes of Death, which was revised periodically to conform to changes in the International List of Causes of Death. The manual clarified several issues, according to Moriyama: "To many physicians the cause of death is the terminal disease or condition responsible for the death. To others it is the main or principal disease condition under treatment. For public health purposes, the cause of death . . . is the disease or injury that initiated the train of events leading to death." If a severe myocardial infarction incapacitated a patient who then contracted and died of pneumonia, the appropriate cause of death for vital statistics was the myocardial infarction. Many physicians, however, preferred to list pneumonia because it was the immediate cause of death.[4]

The need to list multiple causes of death produced changes in the death certificate, the basic reporting unit for information on cause of death. Early in the century, most death certificates in the United States required only the primary cause of death but permitted the listing of secondary and contributory causes. In 1925 a League of Nations report recommended replacing primary and contributory causes with a chronological approach using immediate and antecedent underlying causes. This was adopted in the United States in 1939, when all medical conditions involved in the death were to be listed in reverse chronological order. The condition listed last was considered to be the underlying cause. This approach required greater expertise of the certifying physician, and studies about 1950 showed that physicians in urban areas, who were better trained and had better diagnostic facilities, reported more causes of death than those in rural areas.[5]

From 1914 to 1949, the United States used arbitrary priority rules in the case of multiple causes of death, regardless of the physician's opinion as to the underlying cause. For example, before 1949 the cause of death in patients with both coronary heart disease and diabetes was attributed to diabetes (preferences were also given to cancer, nephritis, and some other diseases over coronary heart disease). Unfortunately for the analysis of trends, the periodic revisions sometimes reversed the priorities. In 1948, as part of a major revision in the International List of Causes of Death, the physician's judgment was accepted for the underlying cause of death. This did not eliminate the need for priority rules because a 1950 study found that as many as one-fourth of all death certificates were internally inconsistent and required recoding.[6]

Diseases of the circulatory system, including heart diseases, diseases of blood vessels, diseases of the lymphatic system, and renal (kidney) diseases, caused the most serious classification problems. Many of the diseases involved two or more organs simultaneously and heart failure occurs in all deaths. Woolsley and Moriyama observed in 1948 that "heart disease, as a mortality classification, has probably been abused more than any other cause-of-death category. It has frequently been a convenient statistical 'waste-paper basket' simply because the physician was hard put to it for a definite diagnosis, particularly when called in at the terminal phase of the illness."[7]

The Onset of the Coronary Heart Disease Epidemic

Coronary or ischemic heart disease is a condition in which the blood supply serving a part of the heart muscle (myocardium) becomes deficient because of narrowing or blockage of the hollow center (lumen) of the arteries that serves that particular region of the myocardium. The arteries are called coronary arteries because the early anatomists visualized them as enveloping the myocardium like a crown. In some cases the deficiency is asymptomatic, often called silent ischemia, and may never be discovered. If the narrowing of the lumen occurs gradually, collateral circulation can develop in other coronary arteries so that even the complete blockage of a major coronary artery may not produce symptoms.

The symptomatic forms of coronary heart disease have been graded by their effect on the heart muscle. In the mildest form, the narrowing of the lumen prevents the myocardium from receiving sufficient blood only under conditions of physical exertion or other extreme demands. This form, today called angina pectoris, produces chest pain that subsides when the conditions are relieved, typically by rest. In a more severe form, the blood flow deficiency produces pain even at rest, but the myocardium still receives enough blood to keep the cells alive. In the extreme case, when the blockage of a lumen deprives some part of the myocardium of sufficient blood for enough time, necrosis occurs in the tissue in the heart muscle served by that artery, called a myocardial infarction. The necrotic tissue, which can be as small as a few millimeters in diameter, may be replaced by connective scar tissue that enables the patient to live a relatively normal life. In the most severe case, death can ensue from complications such as rupture of the myocardium, fibrillation, or so much dead tissue that the heart muscle is unable to pump sufficient blood for survival.

Blockage or narrowing of the lumens of arteries can reduce blood flow in other parts of the body as well, a general condition called arteriosclerosis. The lumens of the arteries serving the brain can be blocked or narrowed and produce the death of brain cells, called cerebral infarction or stroke. The lumens of the arteries serving the leg muscles can be blocked or narrowed, a condition that can produce intermittent claudication (weakness) or cramping. One of the greatest enigmas in modern medicine is that arteriosclerosis in different parts of the body has different causes. This is clearly indicated by the steady decline in mortality rates from stroke in the United States and western Europe since 1900, while coronary heart disease mortality rates escalated dramatically during the middle decades of the century.

Coronary heart disease was first depicted and called angina pectoris in 1768 by an English physician, William Heberden (1710–1801). Heberden described some patients who experienced chest pain on physical exertion that subsided when they rested. Neither he nor others differentiated attacks in which the pain subsided quickly and those in which it subsided more slowly or only partially. In 1772 Edward Jenner discovered in autopsies of two cases of angina pectoris that the coronary arteries had become so calcified (he called them "bony canals") that they could not expand and increase the flow of blood to the myocardium. He thereupon attributed angina pectoris to calcification of the coronary arteries.[8]

Until well into the twentieth century the term angina pectoris was used for many conditions with chest pain as their predominant symptom, ranging from mild chest pain on exertion to the most severe forms of myocardial infarction. Luminal narrowing was considered only one possible cause because autopsies found that some patients did not have luminal narrowing or blockage and that others had no symptoms despite significant luminal narrowing or blockage of even major coronary arteries. Additional accepted causes included organic damage to the heart and stress. During the 1920s the term angina pectoris was gradually restricted to heart disease caused by inadequate oxygenation of the heart muscle due to blockage or narrowing of the lumens of the coronary arteries. This new concept was incorporated in the 1930 revision of the International List of Causes of Death. The 1949 and 1965 revisions further restricted angina pectoris to the mildest form of coronary heart disease.[9]

Because of the diagnostic and classificatory difficulties, trends in coronary heart disease rates have been the source of considerable controversy. Some have claimed that no real increase has occurred and cite a number of changes to explain the apparent increase, primarily the growing number of the elderly, new diagnostic tools, and more deaths in hospitals. On the other hand, an imposing array of statistical and other evidence substantiates the existence of a major pandemic of coronary heart disease in the early twentieth century in all westernized countries.

Coronary heart disease was extremely rare in the nineteenth and early twentieth centuries. Angina pectoris, used in its original inclusive sense, was not listed as a cause of death in English mortality statistics until 1856, almost ninety years after the condition was identified. In Hamburg, Germany, in 1845 angina pectoris was listed as the cause of three of 5,171 deaths, and in 1857 a German physician called it one of rarest symptoms of heart disease. In America, Austin Flint (1812–1886), a prominent physician and medical author, reported only fifteen cases of angina pectoris in 338 consecutive cases of heart disease. James Mackenzie (1853–1925), the leading heart specialist in England, stated in 1923 that during his career he had seen 380 cases of angina pectoris, about a dozen cases annually.[10]

The rarity of coronary heart disease in the nineteenth century has sometimes been attributed to misdiagnosis. Very mild chest pain can be and undoubtedly was confused with gastric symptoms like indigestion or dyspepsia, such as the condition called "acute indigestion" at the time. Maurice Cassidy, however, stated in his Harveyian oration of 1946 that most diagnoses of angina pectoris did not require complex technology and that eminent physicians at the beginning of the twentieth century "were at least as competent to diagnose angina pectoris as are physicians of this generation." Certainly the characteristics of a severe myocardial infarction were striking and distinctive. David Rogers, a prominent American physician and medical educator in the late twentieth century, in 1987 described his own myocardial infarction, which he first diagnosed as indigestion, as follows:

After the first fifteen to twenty minutes, when the pain was waxing and waning . . . I felt I must sit down very, very quietly. Despite doing so, the pain became a steadily expanding deep penetrating ache spreading from beneath mid breast bone, around the sides of my chest, up my neck into my lower jaw, and down the inner aspect of my left arm into my fourth and fifth fingers. . . . Sometimes it would seem most dreadful in my chest, then in my jaw and lower teeth, then in my left arm. . . . I felt . . . about two hours of what seemed absolutely intolerable pain. . . . I would guess it took about ten to twelve minutes to build to maximal intensity and there it stayed. During the entire period I sat absolutely still with my eyes closed, conscious of the fact that I was sweating profusely and that I probably looked very pale and very lousy. Although my wife was . . . in the kitchen not fifteen feet away, I said absolutely nothing, feeling that even moving my tongue or vocal chords was simply too much. There was no inclination to groan or cry out. . . .

There was absolutely no doubt in my mind that I was about to die. As the pain remained, I simply wished exodus would go ahead and happen. . . . The quality of the pain . . . was a dreadful, deep, nauseating ache. . . . [I]t was an

absolutely monstrously awful sensation and it was totally untouched by twenty
or thirty or forty milligrams of morphine given me over the next two hours.
That morphine gave so little relief has made me feel for the hundreds of
patients with the same disease I've treated with this drug.[11]

Had coronary heart disease been widespread in the nineteenth century, many physicians would have observed enough severe cases to be shocked
by their horrifying course. The patients who died within a few hours or
days would have led them to develop a disease category that would describe
at least severe coronary heart disease. Yet Samuel Levine, one of first American
specialists in cardiology, reported that the clinical picture of coronary heart
disease was not well enough understood to be described in textbooks of
medicine until the 1920s.[12]

Statistical analyses can also be used to evaluate misdiagnosis as an
explanation of the low rates of coronary heart disease before the 1920s. The
1915 annual report of the New York Department of Health cross-tabulated
the one "determining" and multiple "contributing" causes of the 55,355
deaths from selected causes in that year.[13] New York City physicians used
contributing causes only when they considered them appropriate, because
they appeared in only 13% of the 4,836 deaths whose determining cause
was cancer and in only 8% of the 8,825 deaths whose determining cause
was pulmonary tuberculosis. Those two diseases were also seldom used as
contributing causes.

Angina pectoris, as coronary heart disease was then called, was an
extremely rare determining cause of death and was listed in only 0.5%
(286 cases) of the deaths listed in the table and 0.4% of all 73,405 deaths
that occurred in that year. The accuracy of the diagnosis is supported by
the use of "diseases of arteries" as a contributing cause in 136 of these deaths
and "organic heart disease" in 40. Angina pectoris was listed as a contributing cause in 93 cases, with organic heart disease as the determining cause in
72 of them, again supporting the presence of coronary heart disease. "Diseases of arteries," which could have included the coronary arteries, was a
much more common cause of death, constituting 2,210 cases or 3% of all
deaths. However, the majority of these cases involved the cerebral arteries,
as shown by the most frequent contributing cause: "apoplexy" or stroke
(1,255 cases) and "paralysis" (42 cases), as compared to "organic heart disease" (25 cases), and "angina" (5 cases).

"Organic heart disease" was the most common cause of death in New
York City and was the determining cause in 10,383 deaths (14%). Organic
heart disease was a very broad category that included deaths from the val-

vular diseases produced by rheumatic fever, infections of the heart, and degenerative diseases, including coronary heart disease. Contributing causes included 2,708 cases of chronic nephritis, 1,190 cases of diseases of the arteries, but only 72 cases of angina pectoris. Had organic heart disease been another term for coronary heart disease, angina pectoris would have been used much more often as a contributing cause of diseases of the arteries. Organic heart disease was a contributing cause in 2,103 deaths, including 507 cases of chronic nephritis and 500 cases of pneumonia, but only 25 cases of diseases of the arteries and 40 of angina pectoris. The strong relationship between organic heart disease and chronic nephritis, which often resulted from the same streptococcal infections that caused rheumatic heart disease, suggests an infectious rather than arteriosclerotic origin of most cases of organic heart disease. This is supported by the statistics for chronic nephritis, which constituted a determining cause in 5,076 deaths (7%) and a contributing factor in 3,793 deaths. As a determining cause, it was accompanied by diseases of the arteries in 739 cases, by organic heart disease in 507, by apoplexy in 360, and angina pectoris in four.

These statistics indicate that coronary heart disease was a rare determining or contributing cause of death in New York City in 1915. Similar death rates from organic heart disease, kidney disease, and angina pectoris occurred in Philadelphia, Chicago, Boston, Cleveland, and Baltimore, which suggests a similar pattern for those cities.[14]

It has also been proposed that in the nineteenth century many persons who suffered from coronary heart disease died of infectious diseases, which were listed as the cause of death. After infectious disease mortality rates declined in the twentieth century, this group died of coronary heart disease, thereby increasing coronary heart disease mortality rates. Tuberculosis was the infectious disease that caused the greatest number of deaths among adults and also one that declined rapidly in the early twentieth century. In 1917, only 2.2% of tuberculosis deaths in the death registration area listed heart disease (all forms) as a contributing condition, which declined to 0.8% in 1940. In 1940, 2.5% of all infectious and parasitic disease deaths listed heart disease as a secondary cause.[15] Even if there was gross undercounting, the decline in infectious disease mortality rates could not have accounted for the increase in coronary heart disease mortality rates.

Expressions of concern and confusion by physicians during the 1920s indicate that they viewed coronary heart disease as a new and growing problem in medicine. Levy, Bruenn, and Kurtz observed in 1934: "The increasing death rate from cardiovascular disorders has fired the imagination of the laity and aroused concern in the minds of those whose function it is to conserve the public health. Coronary artery disease, due perhaps in part to the dramatic features of acute obstruction and the frequency with which it terminates the careers of prominent citizens by sudden death, has stimulated an unusual amount of general interest." Physicians expressed the need for more statistical and clinical information, as one observed in 1927: "geographical distribution, etiology, age relation, infectivity, heritability, therapeutics—wherever the subject is touched there is uncertainty."[16]

Autopsy studies were recognized as particularly useful because the heart and coronary arteries were observed directly. One autopsy study concerned with the accuracy of clinical diagnoses found that coronary heart disease was often misdiagnosed, but mostly as other forms of heart disease. The study compared pre- and post-mortem diagnoses of 8,080 autopsied cases between 1933 and 1937 in the Los Angeles County Hospital, with the cases comprising about 40% of all deaths in the hospital over that period. The pre-mortem diagnoses were less accurate than expected because many patients were unable to speak English or arrived moribund (38% had been in the hospital less than forty-eight hours before death). Coronary artery disease was verified at autopsy in only 66% of patients diagnosed with the condition before death, compared to 75% of the cases of stroke (hemorrhagic and thrombotic), 79% of all cases, and 88% or more of the cases of tuberculosis, diabetes, appendicitis, and some cancers. Yet most misdiagnoses of coronary artery disease were within the heart disease category. Ninety percent of the 972 cases diagnosed before death as some form of heart disease were also diagnosed as heart disease at autopsy.[17]

An autopsy study by Levy, Bruenn, and Kurtz of trends in coronary heart disease found an increase in its prevalence during life regardless of whether or not it was listed as the cause of death. The study identified 762 autopsies that mentioned diseases of the coronary arteries in a group of 2,877 total autopsies at Presbyterian Hospital in New York City from 1910 to 1931. The proportion of all autopsies that mentioned diseases of the coronary arteries increased from 12% in 1910–19 to 19% in 1920–31 for those ages 25–44, from 30% to 40% for those ages 45–64, and from 52% to 60% for those ages 65 and over. The proportion of men with coronary artery disease increased from 22% to 34%, while the proportion of women with the disease increased from 12% to 25%.[18]

Two autopsy studies estimated trends in the prevalence of coronary heart disease in patients who died of unrelated conditions. One, conducted at Grace-New Haven Hospital in Connecticut between 1935 and 1954, examined the presence of the disease in 2,731 autopsied white males ages

40 and above who died of cancer or accidents. During that period the hospital autopsied 59% of all patients who died there, and all autopsy findings were reviewed by at least two pathologists. The proportion of these cancer and accident victims who had coronary heart disease increased from 12% of 543 autopsies in 1935–39 to 18% of 835 autopsies in 1950–54. The proportion with at least 50% blockage of a coronary artery or a major branch of the artery increased for all age groups. A comparable study at Presbyterian Hospital in New York City examined consecutive autopsies of white males who died of an infectious disease from 1931 to 1935 and of automobile or industrial accidents from 1951 to 1955. It found "moderate or advanced" obstruction of the coronary arteries in 20 of 50 men ages 46–60 in the earlier period compared to 43 of 50 in the later period.[19]

In his impressive study of death certificates in Brookline, Massachusetts, Francis Denny examined all death certificates from 1900 to 1935 that listed heart disease as the cause of death and reclassified them to conform to the 1930 version of the international classification. The city, a suburb of Boston that grew from 20,000 to 50,000 inhabitants over the period, was one of the wealthiest communities in the nation. Its inhabitants had access to excellent health services and diagnoses were probably superior to the average. The proportion of the population ages 45 and over was a very high 26% in 1910 and increased to 33% in 1935, with women constituting 61% of those ages 45 and over in 1930. Denny found that in the 1930s many physicians switched from the old "angina pectoris" to the new "diseases of the coronary arteries" on the death certificates, indicating that they considered the two conditions equivalent. The reclassified death rates per 1,000 inhabitants from the combination of angina pectoris and diseases of the coronary arteries were 0.2 in 1900–04, 4.1 in 1920–24, and 17.8 in 1930–34. The death rates per 1,000 population from all forms of heart disease increased from 15.4 in 1900–04 to 32.7 in 1930–34. Thus the increase in deaths due to coronary heart disease far exceeded the increase in the proportion of the population ages 45 and rose from 10% to 55% of deaths from all heart diseases. Although women outnumbered men among those ages 45 and over, 65% of all coronary heart disease deaths occurred to men and the ratio was even higher for those under age 60.[20]

Anderson and LeRiche reclassified a sample of between 2,500 and 5,000 death certificates of men ages 45–64 in Ontario in each Canadian census year from 1901 to 1961. The authors used three definitions of heart disease: a narrow definition that included only some form of coronary heart disease, a broader definition that added nonspecific heart disease deaths, and the broadest possible definition that added other causes of death that might possibly have been confused with coronary heart disease. They found no consistent trend for any of the definitions from 1901 to 1921, a nine-fold increase for the narrow definition from 1921 to 1961, a three-fold increase for the broader definition from 1931 to 1961, and a doubling for the broadest definition from 1931 to 1961.[21]

Strong support for a real increase in coronary heart disease death rates is also provided by a different approach: if the increase was due to changes in physicians' diagnostic preferences, mortality rates must have declined in other disease categories that physicians were no longer using. This counter-balancing decline would have to be very large because coronary heart disease mortality rates were increasing significantly and overall mortality rates were declining. David Miller and two coworkers examined the issue and observed in 1956: "That death was mistakenly attributed to other causes is unlikely; no other cause of death with which coronary heart disease might be confused has shown a commensurate decrease."[22]

Last, support for a real increase is provided by the consistent finding that male death rates from coronary heart disease far exceed those for females, with the ratio being highest in the youngest age groups and decreasing with advancing age. The noted cardiologist Paul Dudley White said that a group of clinical studies in the 1920s and 1930s found that males constituted between 65% and 95% of coronary heart disease cases. Death rates from four major cardiovascular-renal diseases among Metropolitan Life Insurance Company industrial policyholders in 1931–35 show that the male-female ratio for the combination of coronary artery disease and angina pectoris was much greater than for any of the other diseases (see Table 11.1). The sex ratio decreased with age for coronary heart disease, while it generally increased with age for the other diseases. The authors attributed the increasing rates to the long-term effects of adverse working conditions on the men. Anderson found a similar pattern in 1961 for the male-female ratios of ischemic heart disease death rates in the vital statistics for Canada, the United States, and England and Wales. The male-female ratios in all three countries were more than 6 to 1 for the 35–44 year old group and declined steadily to 2 to 1 for the 65–74 year old group. Here also the ratio for coronary heart disease differed from the male-female ratio for all other cardiovascular-renal diseases combined and for stroke, which were less than 1.5 to 1.[23]

Anderson has observed that the distinctive sex ratio of coronary heart disease provides valuable evidence that coronary heart disease rates increased during the early twentieth century. Because the sex ratio for coronary heart disease differs strikingly from all other forms of cardiovascular-renal dis-

Table 11.1: Mortality Rates For Major Chronic Diseases by Age and Sex: Metropolitan
Life Insurance Company White Industrial Policyholders, 1931–1935

| | (annual death rates per 1,000 policies) | | | | | | | |
| Age | Coronary artery disease and angina pectoris | | Chronic nephritis | | Cerebral Hemorrhage/ Paralysis | | Chronic Myocardial Heart Disease | |
	M	F	M	F	M	F	M	F
35–44	0.3	0.1	0.4	0.3	0.2	0.2	0.3	0.2
45–54	1.0	0.3	1.0	0.9	0.8	0.8	1.6	0.9
55–64	2.1	0.8	2.7	2.2	2.6	2.3	4.7	3.2
65–74	3.4	1.9	7.3	6.3	6.9	6.1	12.2	9.9

Source: Louis I. Dublin and Alfred J. Lotka, *Twenty–Five Years of Health Progress* (New York: Metropolitan Life Insurance Company, 1937), 274, 288, 302, 262.

ease, any increase in the ratio of male to female deaths in the general category of heart disease is probably due to an increase in coronary heart disease. Vital statistics show that mortality rates for all forms of heart disease exhibited no sex difference early in the century, but the male-female ratio increased steadily subsequently. This can be explained only by an increase in coronary heart disease mortality rates.[24]

Thus a large number of studies using different methods and populations all found a real increase in coronary heart disease death rates that began around 1920. The increase also occurred at the same time in other westernized countries. Unquestionably, at that time coronary heart disease began its rise to become the great pandemic disease of the twentieth century in all advanced countries.[25]

By 1940 coronary heart disease was a major cause of death among older American men and women (see Table 11.2). It was the listed cause of death in U.S. vital statistics for 10% of deceased men and 2% of deceased women ages 35–44, rising to 14% of deceased men and 8% of deceased women ages 65–74.

Coronary heart disease was predominantly a disease of white rather than black men. Statistics of Metropolitan Life Insurance Company industrial policyholders early in the century are particularly valuable because both white and "colored" policyholders were urban, of lower socio-economic status, and resided in the same geographic regions. In 1931–35, "colored" Metropolitan Life Insurance Company male and female industrial policyholders had higher mortality rates or rates equal to their white counterparts from all causes of death and from chronic nephritis, chronic

Table 11.2: Mortality Rates for Major Chronic Diseases by Age and Sex, 1940

(death rates per 1,000 population)

Cause	Age			
	35–44	45–54	55–64	65–74
Male				
All	5.9	12.5	26.2	54.2
Coronary artery disease and angina pectoris	0.6	2.0	4.4	7.4
Other heart disease	0.7	2.5	6.9	17.3
Cancer	0.5	1.8	4.8	9.7
Stroke	0.2	0.7	2.2	5.9
Nephritis	0.3	0.8	2.0	5.1
Female				
All	4.5	8.6	18.1	41.9
Coronary artery disease and angina pectoris	0.1	0.5	1.5	3.5
Other heart disease	0.5	1.6	4.4	13.2
Cancer	0.9	2.4	4.6	7.7
Stroke	0.2	0.8	2.1	5.5
Nephritis	0.3	0.7	1.6	4.1

Source: Forrest E. Linder and Robert D. Grove, *Vital Statistics Rates in the United States, 1900–1940* (Washington, DC: U.S. GPO, 1943), 534–39.

myocardial disease, and cerebral hemorrhage and paralysis (stroke) (see Table 11.3). In striking contrast, white men had higher coronary heart disease mortality rates than "colored" men, while white and "colored" women had similar coronary heart disease rates that were lower than their male counterparts. The same pattern occurred in the 1950 U.S. vital statistics. Nonwhite men and women, who were predominantly black, had much higher death rates than their white counterparts for all causes of death and for hypertensive heart disease, chronic nephritis, and vascular lesions of the central nervous system (stroke). Here also, white men had the highest rates of arteriosclerotic (predominantly coronary) heart disease in the four race-sex groups, and the differences between white and nonwhite men increased with age, with rates per 1,000 population of 3.2 and 2.5 for white and nonwhite men ages 35–44 respectively rising to 16.1 and 9.4 for those ages 65–74. This growing disparity with age did not occur for the other diseases. The U.S. vital statistics for 1940 and 1960 show patterns that were very similar to those for 1950.

One possible explanation for the striking excess of white male deaths from coronary heart disease is physician diagnostic bias or misreporting. If

Table 11.3: Mortality Rates from Cardiovascular–Renal Diseases, Ages 55–64 by Sex and Race, 1931–1935 and 1950

	White (annual death rates per 1,000 policies)		"Colored"	
	male	female	male	female
All causes	33.0	23.0	42.4	35.4
Coronary artery disease and angina pectoris	2.1	0.8	1.0	0.7
Chronic myocardial disease	4.7	3.2	4.7	2.6
Chronic nephritis	2.7	2.2	5.5	4.7
Cerebral hemorrhage and paralysis	2.6	2.3	4.5	5.0

II.

U.S. Vital Statistics, 1950

(annual death rates per 1,000 persons)

	White		Nonwhite	
	male	female	male	female
All causes	23.0	12.9	34.8	27.6
Arteriosclerotic heart disease	8.1	2.7	5.5	3.7
Hypertensive heart disease	1.1	0.9	4.0	4.2
Chronic nephritis	0.3	0.2	1.0	0.9
Vascular lesions of central nervous system	1.8	1.6	4.8	5.0

Sources: Louis I. Dublin and Alfred J. Lotka, *Twenty–Five Years of Health Progress* (New York: Metropolitan Life Insurance Company, 1937), 16, 262, 274, 288, 302. Robert D. Grove and Alice M. Hetzle, *Vital Statistics Rates in the United States, 1940–1960* (Washington, DC: Department of Health, Education, and Welfare, 1968), 376–78, 457–59, 471–74, 476–78, 447–50.

overreporting of coronary heart disease deaths occurred among white men, underreporting of deaths must have occurred in other heart disease and related categories for white men relative to black men. Conversely, underreporting of coronary heart disease deaths among nonwhite men should produce overreporting elsewhere. An examination of the vital statistics death rates provides little support for either possibility. The only plausible conclusion is that coronary heart disease was primarily a disease of white men.

Many physicians before mid-century believed that coronary heart disease occurred primarily in the higher socio-economic groups, which they attributed to greater stress. The eminent physician William Osler noted in the 1914 edition of his internal medicine textbook: "Business men leading lives of great strain, and eating, drinking, and smoking to excess, form the large contingent of angina cases." Paul Dudley White, the leading heart specialist of his era, agreed in 1927: "The stress and strain of modern life, particularly fostered by strenuous business and professional methods, and by two 'conveniences'—the telephone and the automobile—are quite likely responsible for the marked increase in angina pectoris."[26]

Newspapers enthusiastically embraced the view that higher socio-economic groups had higher rates of coronary heart disease because they experienced greater stress. In 1931 the *New York Times* reported that "many of our ablest men and women have become incapacitated and their lives shortened" by heart disease. It stated that "doctors had become greatly concerned with such conditions as angina pectoris and hardening of the arteries [that] crippled or killed with increasing frequency persons during the prime of their lives. . . . [T]he stress, strain, and complexity of city life were important factors in the increase in heart disease incidence." In 1937 a headline in the newspaper stated: "Congress Warned Strain Brings 'Disease of the Intelligentsia,'" and the article noted that "coronary occlusion has been called the disease of the intelligentsia because of its frequent occurrence among the leaders in the business, professional, financial and political worlds." A U.S. Senator who had just died of heart disease was described as a "very typical example of the hard-working, high-tension, dynamic individual who is ever attentive to the day's work."[27]

The social-class distribution of coronary heart disease victims was examined in several statistical studies. A Massachusetts General Hospital study of 3,400 consecutive autopsies from 1925 to 1937 found that coronary atherosclerosis was "considerably greater" among the "economically well-to-do" private patients than the "economically less fortunate" ward patients. Other studies did not share this conclusion. In their hospital autopsy study in New York City, Levy, Bruenn, and Kurtz reported that, despite the claim that "business executives with greater responsibilities" are particularly vulnerable to coronary heart disease, "in this series at least, occupation has not seemed to play a highly selective part." A 1940 study of 1,215 cases of coronary heart disease among workers in New York City found that the occupational distribution of the cases was practically identical to those of all workers in the city. Last, two physicians who treated workers in the garment industry in New York City, all of whom were healthy enough to be employed and 84% of whom were under age 50, reported in 1932 that "coronary sclerosis, far from finding the majority of its victims among individuals of wealth and learning, cripples with especial frequency at least certain groups of workmen."[28]

Two Metropolitan Life Insurance Company studies of its industrial and ordinary policyholders provided the best statistics concerning the relationship between socio-economic status and heart disease. A 1935–39 study found that lower-income industrial policyholders in every age and sex group had significantly higher death rates than the higher-income ordinary policyholders overall and from many specific diseases, including diseases of the heart and arteries (see Table 11.4). Although the heart disease category included several types of heart disease, the very high male-female ratio indicated that coronary heart disease was the major component. A 1955 Metropolitan study found similar socio-economic differences for several categories of heart disease. The mortality rates per 1,000 white male indus-

Table 11.4: Mortality Rates by Cause, Age, and Sex: Metropolitan Life Insurance Company Industrial and Ordinary Policyholders, 1935–1939

	(rates per 1,000 policies)					
White Males	*36–45*		*46–55*		*56–65*	
	Ind.	Ord.	Ind.	Ord.	Ind.	Ord.
All causes	6.6	3.8	14.4	9.2	30.9	21.6
Pneumonia	0.5	0.3	1.0	0.5	1.8	0.9
Tuberculosis	0.9	0.4	1.3	0.5	1.4	0.6
Cancer	0.4	0.3	1.6	1.2	4.5	3.5
Cerebral hemorrhage	0.2	0.1	0.7	0.5	2.3	1.6
Heart, arteries	1.3	0.8	4.1	2.8	10.5	7.8
Chronic nephritis	0.3	0.2	0.8	0.5	2.0	1.5
White Females	*36–45*		*46–55*		*56–65*	
	Ind.	Ord.	Ind.	Ord.	Ind.	Ord.
All causes	4.4	3.3	9.0	6.6	20.9	14.7
Pneumonia	0.3	0.2	0.4	0.3	0.9	0.6
Tuberculosis	0.4	0.3	0.3	0.2	0.4	0.3
Cancer	0.8	0.8	2.1	2.0	4.2	4.1
Cerebral hemorrhage	0.2	0.1	0.8	0.5	2.2	1.4
Heart, arteries	0.7	0.4	2.0	1.2	5.9	4.1
Chronic nephritis	0.3	0.2	0.7	0.4	1.6	1.0

Source: Malvin E. Davis, *Industrial Life Insurance in the United States* (New York: McGraw–Hill, 1944), 318–19.

trial and ordinary policyholders respectively ages 55–64 were: all cardiovascular diseases 13.1 and 9.9; all heart diseases, 11.0 and 8.6; and arteriosclerotic and degenerative heart disease, 9.7 and 7.7. Similar differences occurred for policyholders in younger and older age groups.[29]

These studies showing higher rates of coronary heart disease in lower socio-economic groups were supported by both English studies of the time and later American studies. Coronary heart disease was similar to practically all other major causes of death in attacking the poor with greater frequency and severity than the rich.[30]

Some physicians rejected the belief that stress was more severe in upper socio-economic groups. An English physician, W. Melville Arnott, observed in 1954 that "most of the evidence adduced in its support is dubious and much of it is absurd." The proponents of the theory claimed that its "lethal influence consists of (a) the exacting character of sustained mental work accompanying intellectual occupations and posts involving heavy responsibility; (b) the emotional tension that frequently accompany business, professional, and intellectual life; and (c) the inheritance of an ambitious or conscientious personality pattern." If this were true, "the labouring classes in the wealthy countries and the great majority of the agrarian inhabitants of the Orient live some sort of idyllic existence, close to the soil, securely insulated from the fierce competitive, intellectual and emotional burdens which grind the life out of those unfortunates whose lot it is to think, direct, and govern." Yet the life of a professional in an advanced country was "surely much less stressful than that of a peasant in the Yangtse Valley, with the ever-present menace of flood, famine, pestilence, and war." The "stress and strain" theory was popular because "it nourishes the [self-esteem] of the believer and it is readily acceptable to the unfortunate victim and his relatives. It places ischemic heart disease in the position of being the unjust reward of virtue. How much nicer it is when stricken with a coronary thrombosis to be told it is all due to hard work, laudable ambition and selfless devotion to duty."[31]

A common opinion was that the rising coronary heart disease rates were an inevitable result of the steadily improving standard of living. Levy, Bruenn, and Kurtz observed in 1934 that the increase "is not to be regarded as a matter of concern. Rather it should be a source of satisfaction that, due largely to effective control of infectious diseases, men may survive to an age when disorders incident to senescence lead to the termination of life." The same philosophy concerning "chronic diseases of later life" was expressed in the 1938 annual report of the New York City health department: "After all, man's life span is limited. All health work can hope to do is to bring as many as possible of the new-born safely through the perils of early life to a ripe old age." The department cited as evidence of success the declining mortality rates below age 60 since 1900.[32]

The Treatment of Coronary Heart Disease

The treatment of severe coronary heart disease was particularly trouble-some for physicians. Laboratory experimentation, which was producing highly beneficial treatments for such non-infectious diseases as diabetes and pernicious anemia, could not be applied to coronary heart disease. Instead, clinical experience provided the basis for treatment.

The first important discovery was that coronary heart disease was not invariably fatal, which had been the accepted position until the early twentieth century. In 1912 James Herrick was among the first to report that patients survived acute myocardial infarctions and experienced complete functional recovery, but he reminisced in 1936 that his findings were disregarded for years. As late as 1920, according to White, physicians believed "that angina pectoris and coronary heart disease were very serious indeed and would not allow long survival, a few years at best." By 1930, White "realized that some of [his] patients had not only recovered but were in good health and back at work." The Metropolitan Life Insurance Company studied 166 male policyholders with coronary thrombosis who qualified for "total and permanent disability" between 1934 and 1936 and followed them up to 1947. Most were 45 to 60 years of age and none was over 65. Seventy percent survived for five years and 43% for twelve years. The ten-year survival rates by age were 57% of those admitted to disability in their 40s and 47% of those admitted in their 50s and 60s. A comparable later study found that 83% of the deaths were due to heart disease. The survival rates in the earlier study, although lower than for healthy persons, were significantly higher than for the seventy cases who had valvular heart disease, mostly rheumatic, of whom only 44% survived for five years, 27% for ten years, and 22% for twelve. Such findings soon led life insurance companies to insure persons who had recovered fully from myocardial infarctions.[33]

The treatment of patients with coronary heart disease remained practically unchanged from 1930 to 1955, according to a review by the cardiologist and medical historian W. Bruce Fye. Pain in mild cases was relieved temporarily by nitroglycerin or amyl nitrate, which dilated the arteries and increased blood flow but did not affect the underlying condition. Myocardial infarctions were treated with morphine for the pain and almost complete immobilization, under the theory that the formation of a firm scar over the dead heart cells took six weeks and the establishment of collateral circulation took even longer. In the 1944 edition of his extremely influential textbook White prescribed "one month of bed rest (the first fortnight very quiet), one month of gradually getting up and around (the first week in a chair a little more each day, the second week walking on the level increasing distance, the third week going slowly over the stairs once a day, and the fourth week going out for short daily rides, weather permitting, and a third month to consolidate the recovery nervously as well as otherwise." During the first month patients were even not allowed to feed themselves. Hospitalization was considered unnecessary except for specific reasons, such as oxygen therapy or laboratory tests.[34]

In the 1940s the public rebelled against the prolonged bed rest demanded by physicians. They complained that it produced despondency, medical complications like constipation and bed sores, physical weakness due to muscle atrophy, and lost earnings. Sympathetic physicians cited recent experimental evidence showing the adverse physiological consequences of physical immobilization. Most physicians defended bed rest, in part because they were less likely to be blamed if patients died while bedridden than when they were mobile. Public criticism had a gradual impact, however. In the 1938 edition of his textbook, Samuel Levine called for at least four to eight weeks of complete bed rest after a coronary thrombosis and a long convalescence thereafter; in 1951 he admitted that "one of the most common and harmful errors in the management of acute coronary thrombosis is to outline a lengthy period of invalidism and convalescence." Instead, many patients ought to be back to work on a part-time basis by eight weeks. On the other hand, Emanuel Goldberger in a 1951 textbook insisted on three months' convalescence before returning to work.[35]

The lifelong regimen prescribed for patients who recovered from myocardial infarctions or suffered from angina pectoris consisted of restraint in every aspect of life. Paul Dudley White observed in his 1931 heart disease textbook that a "very carefully controlled life may add a good many years to the expected limit." Yet he also believed that the decision ultimately belonged to the patient: "Always one must consider the happiness of the individual as well as the length of his life; he may justifiably prefer to live a moderately active life for 5 years than to live as a complete invalid for 10 or 15 years." Permanent restraint was particularly burdensome for men of lower socio-economic status with angina pectoris who could not avoid jobs that involved such mild exertion as climbing stairs.

Samuel Levine observed in 1938 that "too often the social and economic status of the patient is ruined without any significant gain in their health to compensate for this preventable loss."[36]

By the 1940s critics began to question the need for lifelong regimens of almost complete restraint. In 1946 the *New York Times* reported that William Stroud, a professor of cardiology and former president of the American Heart Association, complained that "even after patients had suffered heart attacks and the coronary occlusions had healed, . . . 'too many such patients' became 'total invalids unnecessarily' because they were not permitted to lead more or less normal lives." Other physicians contended that the patients themselves chose to become psychological "cardiac cripples." White said that some patients with coronary heart disease continued to lead active lives despite sporadic attacks of anginal pain while others were "badly crippled by fear more than by the symptom of oppression itself."[37]

The Prevention of Coronary Heart Disease

In the early years of the coronary heart disease epidemic, the absence of any modes of prevention perplexed public health officials and physicians. The 1916 annual report of the New York City Health Department observed: "The one discouraging feature in the statistics of the year was the continued increase in the death rate of the degenerative diseases," including heart disease. "The acute infectious diseases have been successfully combated, but the mortality of the chronic diseases of later life has received but scant attention from health officials." The annual report of the preceding year offered the simple platitude: "Diseases of the heart, kidneys and vascular system are for the most part avoidable by following simple rules of hygiene, to wit: moderation in work, food, and exercise." The report expressed the wistful hope that "as public opinion is awakened," mortality rates will decrease. Samuel Levine observed more cogently in his heart disease textbook in 1938:

> We are now constantly hearing the cry of prevention from the lay public and the medical profession. It seems that with our limited available information, too much is being promised by our medical brethren with regard to the prevention of heart disease. Although much is being said, little that is effective has as yet been accomplished, but the great importance of the subject warrants the tremendous agitation that is current.[38]

The identification of asymptomatic patients at high risk of coronary heart disease was especially important because, as William Osler observed in 1914, "many [heart disease] cases never come under treatment; the first are the final symptoms." The public was in advance of most physicians in recognizing the need for early identification, according to a 1932 medical textbook: "Many persons have besieged their doctors to examine them and to allay their fears of sudden death from heart failure. With the daily press constantly relating the sudden demise of some prominent citizen from causes said to be heart disease, the problem is more sharply brought to the attention of the newspaper readers approaching middle life." Unfortunately, physicians lacked the diagnostic tools to distinguish between "true disease and the normal progressive degenerative changes at the various age periods." The results were unsatisfactory for both patients and physicians.

> Having . . . assured [a patient] that his heart and blood-vessel system were normal, it becomes rather disconcerting to explain to the family the man's sudden death on his way home. This sad experience has unfortunately not been an infrequent one in the practice of many physicians; yet a reconsideration of all of the facts of the case made afterwards has not given the doctor any clue that would explain this accident.[39]

Early identification of myocardial infarction was revolutionized by the electrocardiograph, a machine that measures and graphically displays waveforms of the patterns of electrical impulses during the cycles of the heart. The electrocardiograph was invented in 1902, but units practical for office and hospital use were first manufactured in the 1920s. In 1926, five hundred electrocardiographs were in use in the United States, 46% in hospitals and 39% in private offices. By the 1930s, the life insurance industry was using electrocardiograms regularly in medical examinations of life insurance applicants, indicating that units were available in the offices of many physicians.[40]

Electrocardiograms required special expertise for their proper interpretation. This provided opportunities for the new cardiologists, who interpreted the waveforms for insurance companies, employers, cardiac clinics, and others. However, White complained in 1931 that electrocardiographs were often used by physicians "who are as yet insufficiently trained to make proper use of them." Stroud was quoted by the *New York Times* as stating in 1946 that many physicians "were taking tracings routinely and were unable to interpret the tracings accurately, with the result that 'too many doctors urge patients to give up their employment and become invalids on such minor electrocardiographic findings.'" As late as 1963 a study of three cardiologists, each of whom read 537 electrocardiograms, found that one of them made a diagnosis of coronary heart disease in 101 cases, two of them agreed on the diagnosis in 60 cases, and all three agreed in only 26 cases. The three cardiologists also sometimes changed their opinions when they reread the electrocardiograms without knowing their previous diagnoses.[41]

The greatest impetus for prevention was the acceptance of coronary heart disease as a disease, not an inevitable consequence of aging. Cohn had stated in 1927 that "if men are, as the old adage has it, as old as their arteries, it becomes an important consideration to learn how long [arteries] may live. If they live their full span of years, death from old age and death from circulatory defect may prove to be the same thing." In the 1940s cardiologists like Charles Friedberg deprecated "the fatalistic assumption that arteriosclerosis is an inevitable and inexorably progressive process. . . . It is more probable that [it] represents a disease process due to definite physical and chemical factors. More fruitful results will be obtained if concentrated efforts are directed toward discovering and mastering these etiologic elements." This new perspective became widely accepted when physicians began to see coronary heart disease in persons too young to be experiencing physiological degeneration. Furthermore, coronary arteriosclerosis was quite common and occurred in the early 1930s in 26% of 2,877 autopsies at Presbyterian Hospital in New York City and 28% of 5,060 autopsies at the Mayo clinic in Rochester, Minnesota.[42]

Neither clinical medicine nor public health offered new approaches that would help prevent coronary heart disease. Physicians continued to advise moderation in work and physical activity and avoidance of stress, amorphous recommendations that were difficult for patients to implement. Public health officials still focused on infectious diseases and programs for infants, children, and mothers.

The life insurance industry, on the other hand, had devised a new approach to the prevention of chronic disease in adults based on the risk factors that it was using to evaluate applicants for policies. Life insurance companies had a profound interest in the health of middle-aged persons, who constituted the bulk of their policyholders. When middle-aged policyholders died, the companies paid death benefits far in excess of the premiums they had received. The companies therefore assiduously sought to determine the personal characteristics of applicants that could be measured by medical examiners and increased the probability of premature death.

The tests and measurements used by the medical examiners of life insurance companies to evaluate the risk of premature death in applicants for policies were ideally suited to public health and community medicine. Most were inexpensive, simple enough to be performed by general practitioners, did not unduly inconvenience or endanger the applicants, required little time and effort, and produced reasonably accurate results. The predictive value of the tests was demonstrated in statistical studies that followed hundreds of thousands of policyholders for up to twenty years. The major criticism of the life insurance approach was that policyholders were healthier than the general population. Yet the clinical studies preferred by the critics used small samples of highly atypical patients at one or a few hospitals.

Insurance studies of coronary heart disease confirmed the importance of one of their earliest predictive risk factors: build. For example, one study of 200,000 policyholders for twenty years from 1909 to 1928 found that overweight male policyholders had higher mortality rates from coronary heart disease, as well as from stroke and kidney disease, than those who were of normal or below average weight.[43]

Based on these findings, the Metropolitan Life Insurance Company made significant efforts to educate the public about weight control. The company developed weight and height tables for specific age groups that became the national standard for health professionals, educators, and laypersons. Its pamphlets and popular magazine advertisements referred to overweight with great frequency, either as a health problem by itself or in conjunction with heart disease, diabetes, and other chronic diseases. A 1934 Metropolitan national magazine advertisement informed readers that "people past 45 who weigh 20% more than the average have a deathrate greater by one half than the average for their age. If they have a persistent 40% overweight, the rate is almost double that of the average." Readers were informed that overweight increased the likelihood of high blood pressure, heart disease, diabetes, and kidney disease. The advertisement concluded: "In nearly every case it is brought on by eating too much food and exercising too little. . . . [T]reat your overweight as you would a menacing disease. Give it immediate attention."[44]

Physicians began to take a serious interest in weight control in the 1910s and 1920s. Life insurance companies required them to measure height and weight in medical examinations. Patients began to ask their physicians about losing weight, primarily because slenderness had become important for the new middle-class fashions and lifestyles. As a result, physicians were increasingly expected to be able to make useful recommendations about weight control.[45]

The other medical condition brought to public attention by the life insurance industry was high blood pressure, which was associated with hypertensive heart disease, coronary heart disease, and stroke. Hypertensive heart disease was defined as enlargement of the myocardium's left ventricle, which pumps blood into the aorta to be circulated throughout the body. When the arterial blood pressure is high, the heart must pump with greater muscular exertion for the blood to circulate. This can enlarge the left ventricle (left ventricular hypertrophy), which in turn can reduce the pumping action and the quantity of blood pumped. The ultimate consequences can be congestive heart failure, stroke, or coronary heart disease.

Hypertension presented a complex health problem quite different from build. Laypersons could easily weigh themselves to determine if they were overweight, but they could not measure their own blood pressure. Laypersons could reduce their weight, but they could not lower their blood pressure. Hypertension usually produced no symptoms, so that the condition was frequently diagnosed coincidentally during the course of a routine or life insurance medical examination. Arthur M. Fishberg observed in 1930 that "such individuals have usually felt well or have had but trivial complaints, and are astounded to hear that they have the dreaded high blood pressure. Or the patient comes to the doctor because of symptoms of another disease . . . and his blood pressure is found to be elevated."[46] The problem was exacerbated because many physicians in the 1920s had only limited experience with the sphygmomanometer and could not take accurate blood pressure measurements or interpret them correctly.

The nature of hypertension as a medical problem was far from clear. Some physicians thought that it might be a beneficial response to the narrowing of the lumens of arteries by arteriosclerosis. High blood pressure could enable more blood to flow through the narrowed lumens, thereby reducing the risk of coronary heart disease or stroke. White observed in his 1931 textbook that "for aught we know, the hypertension may be an important compensatory mechanism which should not be tampered with even were we certain that we could control it." Most physicians believed that high blood pressure was a progressive medical problem. Theodore Janeway, a leading early investigator, thought that the extra work imposed on the heart by high blood pressure would always produce at least hypertensive heart disease.[47]

As physicians gained more experience with hypertension, they learned that it did not have an onset, symptoms, and a predictable course like most diseases. "Far more often," Fishberg noted, "after an insidious onset, essential hypertension runs an exquisitely chronic course extending over years, and there are many cases in which marked hypertension lasts for decades without ever doing the individual any discernable harm, until he finally dies of an unrelated disorder." During the 1920s and 1930s statistical studies demonstrated that many hypertensives lived to within a few years of their normal life expectancy. These findings led many physicians to conclude that hypertension was receiving undue attention and that it should not be treated unless absolutely necessary.[48]

One of the most perplexing issues for physicians was a numerical blood pressure level that defined essential hypertension. The level was not obvious because blood pressure varied among patients along a continuum. The issue was so controversial that most textbooks and articles refused to state a specific level as constituting essential hypertension. As a result physicians accepted life insurance values for hypertension in the same way that they accepted life insurance height and weight tables. Based on millions of observations, the life insurance industry agreed on upper limits of normal blood pressure of 140 to 145 mm Hg systolic and 90 to 95 mm Hg diastolic. Some physicians preferred higher levels because life insurance applicants tended to be younger and healthier than most of their patients.[49]

The treatment of essential hypertension posed significant difficulties for physicians. Sedatives like the barbiturates or vasodilators like nitroglycerine could not be used safely on a long-term basis. Nonmedical treatments like weight loss were difficult to achieve and maintain. The lack of effective treatments produced considerable anxiety among the public. Fishberg observed in 1930: "The general public, at least in the large cities, is entirely too well acquainted for its own good with the dangers of arterial hypertension. Almost everyone knows some unfortunate who had high blood pressure and died suddenly in the street, or is now paralyzed in half his body." Once the patient learned that he or she had the condition, "often enough, the peace of mind of the patient is gone, symptoms make their appearance, and there starts the troubles of the patient and, even more, of the family," and, it could be added, of the physician. Fishberg expressed a view that was widely shared among physicians: "Many individuals with essential hypertension not only need no treatment whatsoever, but are much better off without it. Many persons with asymptomatic hypertension would have been more fortunate if they had never learned of their hypertension." Yet physicians were reluctant to withhold the information from their patients, who might learn of it elsewhere and lose confidence in the physician.[50]

Given the ineffectiveness of medical treatment, many physicians fell back on the old clinical touchstone—avoiding stress. Fishberg urged physicians to advise patients: "Moderation in all things should be the watchword. . . . get them to take things more easily and face unpleasantness with equanimity. Excessive concentration on business should be stopped and the patient induced to devote a sufficient portion of his time to play and amusement." Because the recommendations were ineffective, a steady stream of new approaches ensued, including diet, rest, baths, and psychotherapy. White observed of them in 1931: "Each remedy in turn has been hailed as a specific therapy for high blood pressure, only to take its place after further trial as merely another measure of slight or of doubtful utility."[51]

Thus a new kind of disease posed new problems of prevention, control, and treatment that challenged traditional clinical medicine. The life insurance industry showed that statistical investigations, which were poorly understood by most physicians, provided the most useful results. The great challenge was that coronary heart disease was not simply another disease of the middle-aged and elderly; it had replaced tuberculosis as "the captain of all these men of death."

PART IV

Risk Factors and Coronary Heart Disease

12

CAUSES, CORRELATIONS, AND THE ETIOLOGY OF DISEASE

> Formerly the quantitative scientist could only think in terms of causation, now he can think also in terms of correlation. This has not only enormously widened the field in which quantitative and therefore mathematical methods can be applied, but it has at the same time modified our philosophy of science and even of life itself.
>
> (Karl Pearson)[1]

The rise of coronary heart disease and other chronic diseases led to greater recognition of the inapplicability of cause-and-effect models based on laboratory experiments involving bacterial diseases. A more suitable conceptual framework was correlation, a new method of finding associations rather than causes. Correlation was one of the most important new scientific concepts in the twentieth century and greatly expanded the methods that could be used to study the causes, prevention, and treatment of disease.

Bacteriology and the Doctrine of Specific Etiology[2]

Prior to the nineteenth century, disease causation was a highly flexible concept that involved attributes of both the individual, such as age, gender, occupation, and heredity, and the environment, including geographic location, climate, and characteristics of the population. The large number of causal factors and their many interrelationships made the numerous theories of disease etiology too complex to be useful in public health and clinical medicine.

The modern approach to disease etiology emerged in the early nineteenth century. Pathologists used autopsies to identify pathological lesions in the organs of deceased patients and related them to the patient's medical condition prior to death. This produced the principle that a precise causal relationship existed between changes in specific organs and the symptoms of a disease. The primary methodological limitation of the autopsy was that it occurred after death, making it impossible to demonstrate that the changes in the organs preceded the symptoms.[3]

In the late nineteenth century bacteriology provided a major impetus to etiological models because it surmounted most of the methodological limitations of the autopsy and drew its findings from tuberculosis and other important infectious diseases. Bacteriological experiments using laboratory animals demonstrated that: (1) virulent bacteria could be removed from the bodies of diseased animals and grown in cultures, thereby proving that they existed independently of the animal and were not part of the animal's constitution; (2) pure bacteria from the cultures could be introduced into healthy animals, which developed the same disease promptly; (3) the disease never developed without the presence of the bacteria in the animal. These "Koch's postulates," formulated by great bacteriologist Robert Koch (1843–1910), appeared to provide a method for establishing true causal relationships in medicine. They established a temporal ordering in which the introduction of the bacteria preceded the onset of clinical disease, and they eliminated all other possible causal factors by keeping two groups of animals under identical conditions and infecting only one group with the bacteria.

The many successes of bacteriological research led to the doctrine of specific etiology, which holds that (1) infectious diseases are caused by the introduction of specific microorganisms into the body, and (2) each disease produces a distinctive clinical pattern in infected patients. Thus a disease could be classified, diagnosed, and treated without reference to other personal characteristics of the patients. The doctrine of specific etiology seemed to solve the vexing problem of causation in medicine and reinforced the pathological concept of disease specificity. The great successes of bacteriology in public health and clinical medicine gave the doctrine, according to Robert Aronowitz, a "lasting preeminence" and made it the "prototype for explaining most diseases," even those that were not infectious.[4]

The greatest difficulty with the doctrine of specific etiology, according to Henrik R. Wulff, was that "it strengthened the false idea of the monocausal determination of diseases." In living organisms the development of infectious disease depends not only on the introduction of the bacterial pathogen into the body, but also on events that occur in the body after its introduction. Even Koch conceded that the presence of the tubercle bacilli, his greatest discovery, did not always produce clinical tuberculosis: "Often, a tuberculosis focus that has expanded significantly begins to shrink, to scar over, and to heal. This means . . . that a body that provided a suitable medium for invasion by tuberculosis bacilli, gradually lost the properties that favored the bacilli and changed into an unsuitable medium." This finding, which was confirmed by many thousands of human autopsies, provided incontrovertible evidence that the characteristics of the human host were as important as the tubercle bacillus in causing disease.[5]

The doctrine of specific etiology thus resulted from the methodology of laboratory research, not from evidence about the natural history of disease. According to the bacteriologist Rene Dubos, eminent researchers like Robert Koch and Louis Pasteur had the remarkable ability to design laboratory experiments in which a particular bacterial pathogen was not only necessary but also sufficient to produce the disease. They used species of laboratory animals that were highly susceptible to the disease and devised methods of introducing the bacteria into them that routinely produced the appropriate symptoms and pathological changes. They maintained the animals under laboratory conditions that facilitated this process. "Useful as this artificial system has been," Dubos observed, "it has led to the neglect— and indeed has often delayed the recognition—of the many other facts that are essential to the causation of disease under circumstances prevailing in the natural world—namely, the physiological characteristics of the host and the physicochemical as well as social environment."[6]

In the natural world the development of infectious disease depends on the relationships among the pathogen, the host, and the environment. During the past two centuries, most residents of large cities have been infected at some time by virulent pathogens, such as tubercle bacilli or an influenza virus, without contracting clinical disease. According to Dubos, "through a variety of adaptive mechanisms, man usually manages to reach a state of ecological equilibrium with the parasites ubiquitous at a given time in his communities. Infection is the rule and disease the exception." From a biological perspective, this situation can be tolerated by the host and the microorganism, because both survive whereas disease would cause one or both to die. However, the equilibrium is an unstable one; when an individual's resistance is weakened by deteriorating health or a declining standard of living, vulnerability to clinical disease increases. In the nineteenth century, the perilously low standard of living of much of the urban population, exacerbated by periodic economic depressions and social and natural catastrophes, produced high rates of infectious disease.[7]

During the twentieth century improved standards of living enabled more humans to resist infectious diseases or to experience milder cases of the disease. However, many virulent pathogens remained prevalent in advanced societies and reemerged with fatal consequences when social disruptions occurred. Tuberculosis death rates surged in Europe when living standards declined during the world wars. Typhoid fever reappeared in cities and towns when natural catastrophes caused breakdowns in social organization.

The doctrine of specific etiology has been accepted in bacterial diseases because it is not necessary to deal with all of the etiological factors to prevent or cure illness. Wulff has observed that "all events in and outside medicine are determined by numerous factors, and the selection of *the cause* is not a question of natural science; it depends on our interests which in medicine are often therapeutic or preventive." Even when a disease has multiple causes, "the clinician may still be able to interrupt the disease process if only he can eliminate one necessary factor in that complex."[8] Physicians can cure bacterial diseases with antibiotics and prevent some infectious diseases by immunization. Public health programs can remove bacterial pathogens from food and water supplies. However, these interventions must be carried out repeatedly because they rarely eliminate the diseases from the society.

The doctrine of specific etiology also dominates biomedical research, which is conducted primarily through laboratory investigations. According to Dubos,

> The great scientific institutions are geared for the analytical description of the body machine, which they approach in much the same spirit as they do simple inanimate objects. They pay little heed to the scientific study of man as a functioning entity. . . . Nor do they pay much attention to the environmental factors that condition the manifestations of human life. . . . [T]hrough its emphasis on oversimplified models, the scientific community is betraying the very spirit of its vocation—namely, its professed concern with reality.[9]

The limitations of specific etiology as a paradigm were clearly demonstrated in research on poliomyelitis, which became a significant health problem during the first half of the twentieth century. Based on clinical observations, poliomyelitis was believed to be a disease of children after infancy that produced a high rate of motor paralysis and muscular atrophy. A well-financed program of laboratory investigation was undertaken to find the responsible microorganism using the bacteriological model, but it failed to produce either a treatment or a method of prevention. In the 1930s some epidemiologists visited the homes of recent polio victims and discovered that other family members had experienced mild illnesses about the same time as the child who had developed polio. Using antibodies in the blood of the family members, they demonstrated that these mild illnesses were actually cases of poliomyelitis. Soon thereafter epidemiological research showed that in underdeveloped countries polio was a ubiquitous mild infection of infants that immunized them against the disease. The higher standard of living in advanced societies reduced the incidence of the disease among infants so that older children remained susceptible to it. This new concept of poliomyelitis, based on a knowledge of the disease in its natural environment, led to a polio vaccine in the early 1950s.[10]

Multifactorial Etiology in Chronic Diseases

Chronic and degenerative diseases, including coronary heart disease, stroke, and cancer, have as complex an etiology as infectious diseases. Both classes of disease result from multiple causal factors but differ in several key respects. No factor comparable to a bacterial pathogen is present in all persons who develop a particular chronic disease and some etiological factors, such as obesity, are not specific to a particular disease but are associated with several chronic diseases. Chronic diseases also differ from infectious diseases in the time lag between the first manifestations of the etiological factors and the onset of disease: most infectious diseases have a latency period of up to about ten days, rheumatic fever develops about a month after a streptococcal infection, but coronary heart disease and stroke develop years or decades after the onset of conditions like essential hypertension. This suggests a very complex etiological process in chronic disease.

The etiology of chronic diseases has not been amenable to traditional methods of medical research. Laboratory investigations are based on the premise of a direct relationship between specific causes and effects, which does not exist in chronic diseases. Also, many chronic diseases occur only in human beings and cannot be studied directly in the laboratory. Clinical observation is of limited benefit because chronic diseases develop very slowly and at advanced ages when many persons have more than one medical condition. Many of the factors associated with chronic diseases are not dichotomous, such as the presence or absence of a pathogen, but vary from low to high, such as body weight and blood pressure. Individual characteristics that vary continuously are difficult to evaluate as causes of disease.

The etiology of chronic disease is more amenable to investigations using correlation, a revolutionary new conceptual framework and statistical tool formulated at the turn of the twentieth century. The concept of correlation was devised by English biometricians who were studying heredity by examining human characteristics that varied from person to person, such as height. Because they had no specific theory of hereditary transmission, they simply compared the heights of genetically related individuals, such as fathers and sons. If many of the fathers and sons had similar heights, that characteristic could have a hereditary component. The studies found that most taller-than-average fathers had taller-than-average sons, most fathers of average height had sons of average height, and most shorter-than-average fathers had shorter-than-average sons.

The distinctive feature of these studies was that the unit of analysis was a pair of individuals who shared a particular characteristic, in this case the heights of fathers and sons. Knowledge of the height of a father was of no value unless it was matched to the height of his son. This differed from most research, which simply compared the average heights of groups of fathers and sons. While statistical tools existed for comparing averages, none were available for analyzing the correspondence between pairs. To fill this void, the greatest early biometrician, Francis Galton (1822–1911),[11] devised a method that he termed correlation. Correlation provided a range of numerical values that described the degree of correspondence between sets of pairs. Galton's formula has been superseded by one devised by a younger English colleague, Karl Pearson (1857–1936), and supplemented by others designed for specific types of data, but the basic principles remain the same. The Pearson product-moment correlation coefficient produces numerical values that range from +1.0 to -1.0. A coefficient of +1.0 exists when the scores of each pair have a positive perfect correspondence—for example, if every son was one inch taller than his father. A coefficient of -1.0 represents a negative perfect correspondence: essentially, the taller the father, the shorter the son. A coefficient of 0.0 indicates the absence of any correspondence between the heights of fathers and sons.

Correlations can also be applied to relationships between pairs of characteristics of the same individual, which is the most common situation in medicine and public health. For example, a positive correlation exists in western societies between the ages of persons and their blood pressure levels, such that most older persons have higher blood pressure levels and most younger persons have lower levels. Correlations can also relate characteristics of persons that are dichotomous, such as the presence or absence of diabetes, to other dichotomous characteristics of the same person, such as the presence or absence of coronary heart disease.

Correlation was a revolutionary new approach to the scientific study of human behavior. It created an alternative to the cause-and-effect models used in laboratory investigation. Its underlying principle—looking for correspondences between pairs rather than causes and effects—has become the conceptual foundation for all quantitative studies in natural environments that relate individual or social characteristics to each other. The statistics range from two-variable percentage tables to correlation coefficients to complex multivariate analyses. All researchers who use quantitative data gathered in natural environments now think in terms of correlations, even if their ultimate goal is causal inferences. This was Karl Pearson's meaning when he said that correlation has "modified our philosophy of science and even of life itself."

Correlation also freed quantitative studies of disease etiology from the constraints of the laboratory. Liberated from the bonds of cause-and-effect models, studies of characteristics of persons could be carried out in many kinds of natural settings and over durations of many years, yet quantified as rigorously as experimental data.

Correlations were soon found to be extremely useful in medicine and public health, even without the determination of causality. An example is a correlation between a directly observable personal characteristic and another that is not, such as the correlation between age and blood pressure level in western societies. The relationship is not causal, because unknown factors associated with aging are responsible for the rise. Yet knowledge of the correlation alerts every physician to be more concerned with blood pressure when examining older patients. The utility of noncausal relationships was recognized early in the twentieth century by the life insurance industry, which used easily measured risk factors to predict mortality rates without being concerned about causality.

In many cases it is desirable to move beyond correlations to causal inferences. The issues involved may be elucidated by comparing laboratory investigations and quantitative studies in natural environments. A causal relationship requires that the cause precede the effect, and laboratory experiments can introduce the causal factor and wait for the effect to appear. Studies in natural environments often measure the two factors at the same time or under other circumstances that preclude temporal ordering. Causality also requires removing the influence of all other factors that can influence the effect. Laboratory experiments are quite successful in this because they maintain both the experimental and the control groups of animals under identical conditions. In correlation studies in natural environments, the influence of only a few other factors can be identified and measured. On the other hand, laboratory experiments are artificial. Their rigorous control of all aspects of the study, according to Gio Batta Gori, "frequently introduce deliberate bias in order to enhance the probability of a positive response." Relationships based on such experiments can never be extrapolated directly to human beings and usually not to other species of animals.[12]

Inferring causality from statistical correlations requires corroborating evidence. One common type of evidence in medicine and public health consists of the effect of reversals in the hypothesized causal factor. For example, higher blood pressure levels are associated with higher rates of stroke. Lowering blood pressure levels in a group of hypertensive persons reduces the rate of strokes, from which it is inferred that blood pressure is one of the causal factor in strokes. Another type of evidence that is considered to support causality is the "dose-response" relationship. If higher levels of one factor produce higher levels of another factor, it is often inferred that the relationship is causal. In the relationship between blood pressure and stroke, groups with the highest blood pressure levels have the highest stroke rates, those with average blood pressure levels have average stroke rates, and those with the lowest blood pressure levels have the lowest stroke rates.[13]

One of the greatest contributions of statistical correlation is that more than one factor can be related to an outcome simultaneously. If a correlation between two factors is less than perfect, other factors must be involved and their identification and inclusion will increase the level of the correlation. As an example, most older persons in western societies have higher blood pressures than younger persons, but older persons also tend to gain weight, reduce their physical activity, and change their diets. The statistical correlation between age and blood pressure levels is only moderate, but adding other characteristics can increase the correlation. Multifactorial statistical techniques also permit measurement of the relative importance of each of the factors and their impact on each other. Multifactorial statistics are so valuable that A. Bradford Hill, the author of the first textbook of medical statistics in 1937, defined statistics as "methods specifically adapted to the elucidation of quantitative data affected to a marked extent by a multiplicity of causes."[14]

A multifactorial theory of disease etiology has very different consequences for clinical medicine and public health than does specific etiology.

From the perspective of specific etiology, once a factor is considered to be the sole or predominant cause of a disease, physicians and public health officials can disregard other possible factors. From a multifactorial perspective, if a relationship is found between one factor and a disease, it does not diminish the significance of other factors. Furthermore, as more factors related to a disease become known, the ability to predict the occurrence of the disease in an individual increases. Persons who have two of the etiological factors are more likely to develop the disease than persons with only one of them, and persons with three factors are more likely to develop the disease than those with two characteristics. Thus the knowledge of the number of factors present in an individual provides a much more useful assessment of the probability of contracting the disease than an approach based on each factor considered separately.

Correlation was adopted to varying degrees in different scientific disciplines. Public health and the social sciences made the concept of correlation—looking for relationships rather than causes—their core methodology and adopted it for both quantitative and qualitative models. In medicine, correlation was adopted primarily as a mathematical tool to supplement laboratory investigation and clinical observation. The concept of correlation has not been widely accepted because of the preference for mechanistic models and specific etiology. Another factor retarding acceptance has been the growing emphasis on reductionism, the belief that disease pathology can be best understood at the cellular and molecular levels. Yet most reductionist models are not true causal models but only explain the sequence of changes produced by disease.

Because correlation is treated in medicine as a tool rather than a conceptual framework, it has often been incorrectly used. Correlation, like all statistical and mathematical techniques, is an arbitrary method of describing a complex relationship in a highly simplified form based on a number of assumptions. The Pearson correlation coefficient assumes that the values of each of the two factors approximate a normal (also called a Gaussian) distribution. Using an oversimplified example, most persons have blood pressure levels at or close to the average. As blood pressure levels become more distant from the average, the number of persons with each blood pressure level decreases rapidly. Normal distributions are also symmetrical in that the distribution of persons is the same for blood pressure levels above and below the average.

If too many blood pressure readings are at the low or high extremes, called "outliers," the distribution will not be normal and the statistical correlation will be meaningless. The outlier problem occurred in the widely cited Intersalt study of the 1980s, which related blood pressure levels to sodium excretion in fifty-two centers in thirty-two countries. Four of the centers were small isolated tribal societies in Brazil, Kenya, and New Guinea with extremely low levels of both salt consumption and blood pressure. When a correlation coefficient was computed for all fifty-two centers, sodium excretion (used as a measure of salt consumption) had a statistically significant correlation with blood pressure level. When the four outlier centers were excluded, the correlation was not statistically significant. Nevertheless, in 1993 the American Heart Association used the invalid finding for all fifty-two centers to claim that salt consumption was related to blood pressure level.[15]

In some studies, the pairs used to compute correlations are groups rather than individuals and their characteristics are averages, rates, or other statistics rather than individual measurements. This type of analysis is called an "ecological correlation." The Intersalt study did not base its statistics on the blood pressure and sodium excretion levels of all of the individuals in the study. Rather, averages were computed for each center and used to calculate the correlations. The use of averages eliminated the variations in both sodium excretion and blood pressure levels among the individuals in each center, which could have nullified any correlation. Ecological data also cannot show that the specific individuals with the highest (or lowest) sodium excretion levels had the highest (or lowest) blood pressure levels. False conclusions from ecological correlations are so common that they have been termed "ecological fallacies."

Often the factors used in a correlation are selected arbitrarily, while others that are equally important are disregarded. The Intersalt and similar studies were based on the well-documented finding that some tribal societies that consume very small amounts of salt have very low blood pressure levels. Westernized societies consume much larger amounts of salt and have higher blood pressure levels. Based on this correlation between salt consumption and blood pressure, it was concluded that salt consumption is a causal factor in determining blood pressure levels. However, tribal societies differ from western societies in innumerable ways, such as being much more physically active, smaller and leaner, consuming a completely different diet, and not gaining weight with age. To single out salt consumption as a cause of high blood pressure under these conditions is completely unjustified.[16]

Because of the dominance of mechanistic models in medicine, many social and environmental factors that are amenable to analysis using correlations have been disregarded. Researchers studying the etiology of coronary heart disease have emphasized such physiological characteristics as blood pressure, body weight, age, and chronic diseases like diabetes. They have generally excluded social characteristics such as education, occupation, income, working conditions, living conditions, marital status, family structure, and source of health care. Yet each of these social factors has long been shown to be an important factor in disease etiology.

The use of correlation in medicine has not produced broad-based investigations of disease in the natural environment. Instead, as Aronowitz has observed of risk factors, the approach has served as a "modest corrective to, rather than a fundamental critique of, standard biomedical ideas and practices" that endeavor to identify "the specific localized pathogenetic processes that cause disease."[17] Individual responsibility for disease has been emphasized at the expense of underlying social and economic conditions. This is in striking contrast to the beliefs of earlier public health officials and physicians, who considered the patient's environment a basic factor in disease etiology and often the aspect that could be modified most readily.

Clinical Trials

The concept of correlation has been used most often in the branch of statistics known as inferential statistics. During the nineteenth century, descriptive statistics were gathered from an entire population, such as the vital statistics enumerated by governments, and statisticians agreed that complete enumerations of a population were essential to produce useful statistics.[18] Early in the twentieth century, English statisticians created inferential statistics, a new method of analysis in which data was obtained from a sample of the population and the findings generalized to the whole population. They developed techniques for determining suitable sample sizes and methods for drawing the samples. They devised new mathematical formulas to estimate the trustworthiness of generalizations from the samples to the population. Statistical sampling greatly reduced the cost and logistical problems of gathering quantitative data and led to many quantitative studies that had previously been impossible. Statistical sampling was first used in agriculture, the social sciences, education, and business.

Clinical trials use inferential statistics to examine diagnostic, treatment, and preventive measures in a sample and generalize the findings to the population of interest. The simplest form consists of two subgroups selected at random from a single sample: one subgroup receives the treatment or preventive measure in question and is called the intervention or treatment group; the other subgroup does not and is called the control group. The theory of clinical trials is that patient outcomes depend on multiple factors besides the intervention. For that reason some patients in both the intervention and control subgroups will have favorable outcomes and others will have unfavorable outcomes. If the intervention is beneficial, the intervention subgroup will have a higher rate of favorable outcomes than the control subgroup.

The purpose of randomized assignment to the intervention and control groups is to make the two groups as similar as possible in all respects except the intervention. Randomized assignment requires a formal method that gives each individual an equal or known probability of being included in either subgroup, comparable to tossing a coin to assign each participant to one of the groups. Randomization is essential in clinical trials because human selection always involves bias. For example, a clinical trial of a surgical procedure usually involves some risk from the operation itself, so that in nonrandomized trials surgeons prefer to assign the sickest patients to the control group to minimize the risks from the surgical procedure. This predisposes the control group to a worse average outcome than the surgery group.[19]

Clinical medication trials endeavor to ensure that the persons involved in the study do not know which individuals were selected for the control and intervention groups, because the knowledge can create a mindset that could affect the outcomes. In a single blind study participants in the control group receive a placebo, a substance identical in appearance to the active medication but without pharmacological effects. In a double blind study the health care providers who care for the patients do not know which patients are receiving the active drug and which the placebo. In practice, the side effects of the medications and other features of the study reveal the groups to which many of the persons were assigned.

Clinical trials were adopted in medicine in response to the introduction of many new treatments in the 1920s and 1930s. The resulting confusion, according to L. J. Witts, meant their "value could not be left to be determined by the slow processes of time and fashion as in the past." Although the earliest large-scale clinical trials were undertaken in the United States on the treatment of syphilis in the 1930s, the Second World War was the "great divide, after which it was no longer possible for the clinician, however distinguished, to discuss the prognosis and treatment of disease unless his words were supported by figures." The development of streptomycin as a treatment for tuberculosis led to major clinical trials in the Great Britain and the United States in the late 1940s, and these were soon followed by many others. In 1962 the United States Congress enacted legislation that required proof of efficacy of all drugs and authorized the Food and Drug Administration to establish appropriate regulations. Thereafter the controlled clinical trial became the method of testing drugs required by the United States government.[20]

Controlled clinical trials violate the requirements of inferential statistics in one crucial respect. The primary objective of clinical trials is to generalize the findings obtained from the study sample to some larger population of interest. Thus the first step is to specify the population of interest and use statistical methods to ensure that the sample is representative of that population. Randomized selection of samples from a population is just as important as randomized selection of individuals to intervention and control groups. Yet practically all clinical trials concerning chronic diseases recruit volunteers, under the assumption that drugs or lifestyle changes will have the same physiological effects on volunteers as on the population of interest. Any psychological effects will be taken into consideration by comparing the intervention group to a control group that has received a placebo.

Volunteers are never representative of any general population. They are more health conscious, as indicated by their willingness to volunteer, and they behave in different ways that often affect their health. The unrepresentativeness of volunteers was demonstrated in the largest study ever undertaken of lifestyles and coronary heart disease, the Multiple Risk Factor Intervention Trial (MRFIT), which screened more than 360,000 male volunteers ages 35–57 who wanted to participate in the trial. The investigators recruited only persons at very high risk and expected the volunteers to have considerably higher mortality rates than the general population. However, the overall mortality rates for the 360,000 volunteers during the five years after the screening, according to an analysis, was "approximately half that expected with the use of U.S. life tables. Even after adjustment for the incomplete death ascertainment based on the [Social Security Administration] file, the number of deaths is substantially lower than one would expect on the basis of U.S. life tables."[21]

Generalizations to a population of interest are also questionable because of other features of clinical trials. Many clinical trials use volunteers at high risk of the disease being studied because it is believed that changes in their risk levels will provide the most clear-cut evidence of the benefits of the interventions. This assumes that the difference between high-risk persons and those at slightly above average risk is one of degree, not of kind. Little evidence exists to support this widely held view; persons at high risk often differ in several ways, such as having genetic defects. In addition, the composition of the sample usually changes over the course of a clinical trial because persons are removed from the trial if their conditions deteriorate. These nonrandom losses from the sample change its characteristics and affect outcomes, because persons who experience adverse events after removal from the study are usually not counted.

In all clinical trials, especially those utilizing health-conscious volunteers, the outcomes can be affected by behaviors that are not being taken into consideration. This occurred in a large, randomized, double-blind clinical trial that compared the effect of a cholesterol-lowering drug and a placebo on mortality rates. No differences in mortality rates were found between the intervention and control groups over five years. The total sample was then divided into four subgroups: one that took its medication more conscientiously than the average; one that took its placebo more conscientiously; one that took its medication less conscientiously; and one that took its placebo less conscientiously. The more conscientious members of the medication group were expected to have the lowest mortality rates of the four subgroups. Instead, the groups of participants that took their medication *or their placebo* more conscientiously had equally lower mortality rates, while the groups that took their medicine or placebo less conscientiously had equally higher mortality rates. Some unidentified factors related to conscientiousness in drug-taking affected the differences in mortality rates.[22]

The widespread use of medications in chronic diseases has had a major impact on clinical trials. When no useful treatments were available for a condition, only the intervention group received medication, which provided relatively clear-cut evidence of its effects. The widespread use of drugs has led to the ethical principal that the control group should receive available treatments while the intervention group receives the new and unproven treatment. Interactions among the combinations of drugs being taken by the patients can affect the results, but most studies make no attempt to consider these.

Most outcomes in clinical trials of chronic diseases are serious ones such as deaths or myocardial infarctions, because they can be measured with the greatest accuracy. The small number of these outcomes in a three-to-five-year clinical trial produces differences of a few percentage points between the intervention and control groups. This difference could easily result from chance variations in the health of the specific persons assigned to the intervention and control groups. Investigators must therefore separate the effect of the intervention from the chance differences that always occur between intervention and control groups. Statistical techniques have been developed to address this problem. Most ask the same question: what is the probability that the difference between the rates or averages of the two groups could have occurred by chance? If the probability that the difference could have occurred by chance is high, that explanation must be accepted. If it is sufficiently low, the difference may have resulted from the intervention.

The numerical probability that a difference between two rates or averages could have occurred by chance can be determined mathematically, but the significance of the probability requires a judgment. Since the mid-twentieth century a probability of less than .05 has been adjudged sufficient evidence that the difference between the groups did not occur by chance. However, the samples in clinical trials are not randomly selected from the population of interest, so much greater scope should be allowed for chance variations. As evidence, in the early 1950s Hammond and Horn carried out a major study of 200,000 smokers and nonsmokers, using a value of .05 to decide that differences in disease rates between smokers and nonsmokers did not occur by chance. In 1984 Richard Doll examined the extent to which the study's findings were supported by subsequent research. Of the 15 findings that met the .05 criterion, 11 were still considered to be causal in 1984, 1 was considered to be unrelated, and the remaining 3 were uncertain. Of the 19 findings that did not meet this criterion and were concluded to be due to chance variations, 14 were still considered to be due to chance variations in 1984, 2 were now considered to be causal, and the remaining 3 were uncertain. Thus a strikingly large proportion of the conclusions based on the .05 criterion were reversed or not supported by subsequent research.[23]

Because clinical trials in chronic diseases normally take several years, individual participants in the study may experience spontaneous changes in their conditions that mimic the effects of the intervention. Some of these changes can be predicted by the principle of regression toward the mean, which was discovered by Francis Galton. One form of the principle is the tendency in large groups for those subgroups with unusually high or low average values of characteristics to move closer to the average of the whole group over time. A partial explanation is that any measurement of an individual, such as blood pressure, includes a "true" value plus or minus an "error" value consisting of factors like errors in measurement and temporary variations in blood pressure. When a study begins, the people with the highest (or lowest) true values plus the highest (or lowest) errors are placed in the extreme groups. When their blood pressure levels are remeasured, the true values remain the same but the errors usually return to normal levels. This causes the average values of the extreme groups to move closer to the overall average for all participants.[24]

Regression toward the mean has been repeatedly demonstrated with regard to blood pressure, as shown in the rigorous Framingham Heart Study (see Table 12.1). At the beginning of the study, a baseline diastolic blood pressure level was recorded for a large number of people, who were then placed in five groups: a group with below average blood pressure (less than 80 mm Hg); a group with average blood pressure (80–89 mm Hg); and three groups with above average pressures. The diastolic blood pressures of the participants were remeasured after two years and again after four years. Over the four years, the average blood pressure of the original group with the lowest diastolic blood pressure rose from 70.8 to 76.2 mm Hg, while that of the original group with the highest diastolic blood pressure declined from 116.4 to 104.7. The averages for the two other above average groups also declined. Most of the decline occurred during the first two years. A comparable six-year Finnish study of 3,701 persons found very similar changes in the blood pressure levels of the groups.[25]

Regression toward the mean has great significance for clinical trials. When a large number of persons with different blood pressure levels are followed for a long period of time, regression toward the mean will occur in the subgroups with the highest and lowest blood pressure levels. The reduction in the blood pressure levels of the highest groups can easily be misattributed to treatment. For example, one study administered a placebo to 1,119 subjects with high blood pressure for three years. Their original baseline blood pressure readings averaged 157 mm Hg systolic and 102 diastolic. After four months the average levels had dropped to 145 and 92,

Table 12.1: Diastolic Blood Pressure Levels Over Four Years: Framingham Heart Study

Diastolic Blood Pressure	Number of Cases	Baseline	After Two Years	After Four years
	(Blood pressure in mm Hg)			
		Group averages		
Less than 80	1,719	70.8	75.7	76.2
80–89	1,213	83.6	83.0	83.9
90–99	566	93.5	91.2	91.3
100–109	186	103.4	99.2	98.5
110 or greater	92	116.4	107.3	104.7

Source: Stephen MacMahon, et al., "Blood Pressure, Stroke, and Coronary Heart Disease," *Lancet* 335 (1990): 767.

where they remained until the termination of the study after 36 months. According to the investigator, the decline was "not influenced by age, by family history of hypertension or stroke, by smoking, or by serum cholesterol level."[26]

This analysis has described the complexity of research involving statistical correlations and the multiple opportunities for methodological errors. Many of these errors have been repeatedly found in investigations of coronary heart disease, as the following chapters will show.

13

CIGARETTE SMOKING AND STATISTICAL CORRELATIONS

> We believe the campaign against tobacco is based on statistical inferences unsupported by clinical findings.
>
> (Chairman of R. J. Reynolds, 1981)[1]

> We have acknowledged that smoking is a risk factor in the development of lung cancer and certain other human diseases, because a statistical relationship exists between smoking and the occurrence of these diseases.
>
> (Annual Report of Philip Morris, 1990)[2]

The use of statistical correlations to establish etiological relationships experienced its greatest challenge with cigarette smoking. Biomedical scientists and physicians who were committed to laboratory investigation refused to accept statistical correlations in epidemiological studies as compelling evidence that smoking caused disease. Their views were adopted by the cigarette industry and shared by many health-related government agencies and voluntary associations. The general public and government agencies not concerned with health were much more receptive to evidence provided by statistical correlations.

Statistical Relationships Between Smoking and Disease

Popular wisdom has long associated tobacco consumption with ill health and premature mortality. The popular American term for a cigarette, "coffin nail," dates back to the nineteenth century. Yet smoking has also been associated with alcohol consumption, debauchery, riotous living, and moral debasement. In order to prove that smoking itself caused disease, its effects had to be separated from other behaviors of smokers.

Before mid-century most physicians did not believe that smoking adversely affected overall health. In his pioneering 1914 text on occupational diseases, W. Gilman Thompson observed that smoking (cigars, pipes, and chewing tobacco) was harmful when used to excess but it was "a great solace to many a workman whose pleasures are few, and, used in proper moderation, it neither shortens life nor impairs health, as is often claimed for it, provided it is not used in boyhood or early youth." In 1950 an editorial in *JAMA,* the flagship journal of the American Medical Association, claimed that "more can be said in behalf of smoking as a form of escape from tension than against it. . . . [T]here does not seem to be any preponderance of evidence that would indicate the abolition of the use of tobacco as a substance contrary to the public health."[3]

Smoking was often mentioned in connection with the growing coronary heart disease epidemic, but most physicians believed that it was, if anything, one of a multitude of causal or aggravating factors. In his 1931 textbook, *Heart Disease,* Paul Dudley White wrote that tobacco "causes no actual heart disease," but can "precipitate or . . . aggravate angina pectoris" in "a few people with coronary disease." In 1937 the *New York Times* stated that White and two other physicians reported to the American Medical Association convention that "inheritance, ancestral longevity, racial factors, urban life, occupations of a professional or business nature, overeating, excessive use of tobacco and increased nervous sensitivity and strain all figure prominently in young persons afflicted with heart disease, but alcohol does not seem to play an important part." In his 1949 heart disease textbook, Charles Friedberg concluded that "there is no significant evidence that excessive smoking or overindulgence in alcoholic drinks contributes to the development of advanced coronary artery disease or acute coronary occlusion," although he prohibited the use of tobacco in the "acute phase" of myocardial infarction and curtailed it thereafter. In 1935 *Fortune* magazine reported that while "some physicians view tobacco with deep suspicion, the majority concede that it is not a cause of arteriosclerosis, at most a possible contributing factor, but even they play safe after angina pains have occurred or coronary occlusion has developed and forbid smoking."[4]

The first disease to be associated with cigarette smoking was lung cancer, which was extremely rare before the twentieth century but increased significantly in the 1920s. In 1939 the *Statistical Bulletin* of the Metropolitan Life Insurance Company reported that between 1917–18 and 1937–38 the age-standardized lung cancer rates per 1,000 industrial policyholders ages 45–74 rose with "startling rapidity" from 2.6 to 15.0. The rates for men increased from 4 to 23 while those for women rose from 2.5 to 8. Considering possible explanations for the increase, the report rejected improved diagnosis and inhaled substances such as "exposure to dust from tarred roads, the inhalation of polluted air, and the smoking of tobacco."[5]

Cancer textbooks of the period were divided about the effect of smoking on lung cancer. In their 1947 text, Lauren V. Ackerman and Juan A. del Regato stated that the rapid increase in new cases of lung cancer was much greater than for other cancers and far exceeded that expected from better diagnosis and the growing proportion of the elderly. They doubted that smoking was a major reason for the increase. R. A. Willis, author of an English textbook, observed that "every known inhaled substance and almost every known infection of the lungs has, by one writer or another, been claimed or suggested as a possible factor in the causation of pulmonary carcinoma. The subject is then confused and confusing." Epidemiological research did "afford strong grounds for suspecting the carcinogenic result of smoking" but it did not constitute "incontrovertible proof—especially in the eyes of smokers themselves!"[6]

By mid-century lung cancer had become a serious national health problem, especially among men. National vital statistics showed that the age-adjusted death rates from lung cancer per 100,000 men increased from 11.1 in 1940 to 21.3 in 1950 and 34.8 in 1960, while those per 100,000 women rose from 3.4 in 1940 to 4.6 in 1950 and 5.2 in 1960.[7]

Laboratory investigations were employed to test the relationship between smoking and lung cancer. In the early 1950s, adopting a traditional method for determining the carcinogenic properties of chemicals, the backs of mice were shaved and tobacco smoke condensate (tobacco tar) was applied to them. This produced skin tumors, but so did many other chemicals, including some that were innocuous and widely used in humans. Efforts to force animals to inhale cigarette smoke failed because animals breathe through their noses, which filter out most of the harmful agents in the smoke. In 1967, investigators induced smoking in beagles by inserting tubes in holes cut in their necks. They found microscopic tumors in the lungs of some of them, but the findings were inconclusive. The tobacco industry and biomedical scientists frequently cited these negative or ambiguous laboratory findings as the strongest evidence that smoking did not cause lung cancer.[8]

Studies of human lung tissues in the 1950s did suggest a relationship between smoking and disease. Oscar Auerbach and his co-workers examined many thousands of lung tissue samples from 1,500 cadavers without prior knowledge of their smoking status or causes of death. Using statistical analyses, they found a much higher rate of changes that often preceded or increased susceptibility to diseases such as lung cancer in the lungs of smokers than nonsmokers. Postmortem findings, however, could never prove that smoking caused lung cancer.[9]

Clinical observation and vital statistics provided the most seminal evidence relating smoking and lung cancer. Most physicians agreed that the etiological agent was inhaled rather than circulated to the lungs through the bloodstream and that lung cancers developed very slowly. Vital statistics showed that lung cancer rates were much higher among men than women and in urban than rural areas in the United States and western Europe. These findings led to a search for environmental factors that urban men inhaled in low levels over a long period of time.[10]

Occupation was the first factor considered because of the long history of occupational lung cancer. Fatal lung diseases were identified in underground miners in the Erz mountains between Dresden and Prague in the sixteenth century, diagnosed as lung cancer at the turn of the twentieth century, and finally explained by exposure to radiation in the mines in the mid-twentieth. During the early twentieth century the growth of employment in metal mining, smelting, and manufacturing led to the identification of such pulmonary carcinogens as arsenic (which was also used in agricultural pesticides), nickel, asbestos, and certain chromium compounds. However, a 1959 review concluded that the "population exposed to established industrial carcinogens is small, and these agents cannot account for the increasing lung-cancer risk in the remainder of the population." Nevertheless, any local study of lung cancer needed to ascertain the occupations of the participants to determine their exposure to industrial pulmonary carcinogens, because the locality might contain industries that use carcinogens.[11]

It was soon found that cigarette smoking patterns produced the best fit with lung cancer rates. The temporal relationship was appropriate. More efficient manufacturing processes and national advertising led to a enormous increase in cigarette sales prior to the great increase in lung cancer rates, from 49 cigarettes per person ages fifteen and over in 1900 to 611 in 1920 and 3,322 in 1950. Cigarette smoking, like lung cancer, was also more common among men than women. In 1955, 50% of men smoked cigarettes regularly compared to 23% of women, and at that time few women had smoked for enough years to develop lung cancer.[12]

Based on these findings, epidemiological surveys modeled after social surveys began to examine the relationship between smoking and lung cancer. The recently invented social survey was designed to gather information from a sample of people via questionnaires that were self-administered or administered by trained interviewers. Unlike earlier surveys, social surveys used formal sampling procedures to ensure that the sample was representative of the population of interest. They also required respondents to select among predetermined response categories rather than answer questions in their own words. The number of respondents who selected each response category could then be tabulated for the whole sample and for gender, age, education, and other subgroups.

Social surveys were first used on a large scale in the 1930s and 1940s. The federal government conducted surveys to examine the impact of New Deal programs on farmers and other groups. During the Second World War the Office of War Information surveyed the American population to measure reactions to civilian programs related to the war effort. The War Department surveyed soldiers to determine their attitudes and needs and disseminated the findings to officers in the field. Most government survey researchers later taught in universities and trained their students in survey research methods. Public opinion polls were started in the 1930s by George Gallup, Elmo Roper, and others to measure consumer attitudes and predict election results. They came to public attention in 1948 when the major polls predicted erroneously that Governor Thomas Dewey of New York would defeat President Harry Truman in the presidential election. The resulting publicity aroused considerable interest in social surveys.[13]

Epidemiological surveys about smoking required expertise in social survey research methodology. The samples had to be representative of the population of interest. Large samples were necessary because in 1950 one-fourth of 25–year old men died before reaching age 60, which meant that many smokers died of other diseases before they developed lung cancer. The surveys needed to consider gender and urban-rural differences in smoking patterns, occupational exposure to pulmonary carcinogens, the amount of tobacco consumed daily, the number of years smoked, and the smoking method, whether pipes, cigars, or cigarettes.[14] The construction of the questionnaire required considerable expertise. Yet none of the physicians or medical scientists who conducted the early surveys had more than a rudimentary knowledge of social survey methodology.

The first smoking surveys were retrospective studies that compared the smoking rates of hospital patients with and without lung cancer. In the most famous of these, which was co-authored by Ernst Wynder and Evarts Graham and published in *JAMA* in 1950, Wynder used interviews to determine the smoking patterns of lung cancer patients at a surgical service in a New York City hospital. He compared them to the smoking patterns of hospital patients without lung cancer in the chest unit of a hospital in St. Louis, Missouri. Wynder later added miscellaneous cases from other hospitals around the country to both the lung cancer and non-lung cancer groups. Wynder found that lung cancer patients had higher smoking rates than the other patients, which he said could not be explained by their occupations.[15]

Retrospective studies like Wynder's suffered from serious methodological problems, particularly the practical impossibility of selecting an appropriate comparison group without lung cancer. Wynder's use of a smoking group in one city and a nonsmoking group in a different city and his adding other cases to both groups exacerbated the problem. Furthermore, hospital patients were among the worst possible comparison groups because smoking contributes to so many diseases that hospital patients were more likely to be smokers than the general population, which Wynder suspected at the time.[16]

A superior method, prospective studies, selected a group of healthy smokers and nonsmokers and followed them for a period of time. It then compared the two groups to see whether more smokers than nonsmokers died or developed diseases. Prospective studies have the overwhelming advantages of starting with a single group of healthy persons and observing their rates of death or disease. They also have several disadvantages: they are time-consuming and expensive; some persons refuse to participate or drop out during the study and always differ from the participants in important respects; and they measure smoking only at the beginning of the study, thereby disregarding changes in smoking behavior during the study.

The most influential American prospective study of the effects of cigarette smoking was carried out by E. Cuyler Hammond and Daniel Horn and published in *JAMA* in 1954. The sample's 187,766 white males ages 50–69 were selected by 22,000 volunteers of the American Cancer Society, who were trained to administer a carefully pre-tested questionnaire that obtained information about age, address, and smoking history. Each volunteer was instructed to "ask the cooperation only of men with whom she expected to be in contact for the next several years," so that the sample consisted primarily of friends and relatives of the interviewers. This probably biased the sample toward participants with more education and higher incomes. Interviewers were told to select men who were not seriously ill so that the sample had a lower mortality rate than the general population early in the study. The study benefited from an extremely large and geographically diverse sample and careful verification of the cause of death. Over a period of almost two years, it found that cigarette smokers ages 50–59 had overall mortality rates that were 60% higher than comparable nonsmokers. The higher death rates were from more diseases than had been suspected previously, including several forms of cancer and coronary heart disease. Pipe and cigar smokers had mortality rates only slightly above those of nonsmokers. The findings occurred for men who lived in both urban and rural areas.[17]

The Hammond-Horn study was so widely publicized that national public opinion polls as early as 1954 found that 90% of the respondents had heard stories linking smoking and lung cancer. On the other hand, a 1962 poll found that only 38% of the respondents believed that smoking caused lung cancer. The study also enhanced the credibility of statistical correlations in establishing disease etiology. In 1957 the *New York Times,* reported that Hammond and Horn "viewed their report as a triumph of biometrics, the study of disease by statistical analysis. With the development of medical statistics as a tool, biometrics has come a long way."[18]

Harold F. Dorn used superior sampling methods in his study of veterans, mostly from the First World War, who purchased U.S. Government life insurance policies between 1917 and 1940. The policyholders were reasonably representative of the millions of men who met the induction standards of the U.S. Armed Forces. They were fairly homogeneous because all had a certain minimum level of education and were in good physical and mental health at the time of their induction. In 1954 Dorn mailed all policyholders a questionnaire asking about their smoking behavior and received replies from 199,000 policyholders, 68% of the total. Dorn had access to practically complete death records because proof of death was required for payment of life insurance claims. Over the next thirty months he found that cigarette smokers had overall mortality rates that were 58% higher than nonsmokers and higher death rates from a variety of diseases.[19]

The most methodologically sophisticated early study was carried out in England by Richard Doll and Austin B. Hill, who was a pioneer in the use of statistics in medicine. In 1951 they mailed questionnaires about smoking behavior (but not type of smoking) to the 59,600 physicians on the Medical Register and received usable replies from 40,701 or 68%, whom they followed for fifty-three months. The sample consisted of members of a very homogeneous profession with respect to education, income, lifestyles, and other factors, which greatly reduced the number of factors other than smoking that could have produced any differences in lung cancer rates. The investigators also had little difficulty obtaining accurate cause-of-death information. The age-standardized mortality rate of the respondents in the second year of the study was only 63% of that of all physicians on the Medical Register, but rose to 93% after four years. A 1961 resurvey of 261 of the original respondents and 179 of the nonrespondents found that only 15% of the respondents smoked at least 15 cigarettes daily compared to 28% of the nonrespondents. Overall annual age standardized death rates per 1,000 men ages 35 and over were 13 for nonsmokers and 19 for those who smoked 25 or more grams per day. The greatest difference by disease occurred for lung cancer, with death rates per 1,000 of .07 for nonsmokers compared to 1.7 for men who smoked 25 grams per day. The findings were greatly strengthened as the study progressed.[20]

The correlation between smoking and lung cancer was not proof of causation, because some unknown factors that were more prevalent in smokers could be responsible for their higher lung cancer rates. Yet the dose-response relationship in every study strongly implied a causal relationship: the more cigarettes smoked, the higher the death rate. The Dorn study found that compared to nonsmokers, the mortality rates over thirty months were 29% higher for those who smoked 1–9 cigarettes per day, 66% higher for those who smoked 10–20 cigarettes per day, 77% higher for those who smoked 21–39 cigarettes daily, and 99% higher for those who smoked 40 or more daily. In the Hammond and Horn study, the mortality rates per 1,000 persons ages 55–59 were 2.1 for those who smoked 1–9 cigarettes daily, 2.5 for those who smoked 10–19 cigarettes daily, and 3.1 for those who smoked 20 or more cigarettes daily. Similar trends occurred in every other age group.[21]

The dose-response relationship appeared in other measures of the amount of smoking. For groups who smoked a certain number of cigarettes per day, the more years that they smoked, measured by the age when they started smoke, the higher their mortality rates. Ex-smokers consistently had lower mortality rates than current smokers. The only exception to the dose-response relationship occurred in studies that measured smoke inhalation into the lungs, which should increase dosage and therefore mortality rates. One English study reported that "many of the patients did not understand what was meant by inhaling" or misinterpreted the term. They concluded that their answers to this question were so "unreliable" as to be worthless.[22]

The dose-response relationship occurred for a variety of diseases and groups. Dorn found that smokers of 1–9, 10–20, and 21 or more cigarettes per day had mortality rates from lung cancer that were 5.5, 10.0, and 15.8 times respectively the rates of nonsmokers. The mortality rates for the three groups of smokers from coronary heart disease were 1.3, 1.8, and 1.8 times the rates for nonsmokers respectively. Other studies showed that the dose-response relationship between smoking and lung cancer occurred for urban men, for rural men, and for women.[23]

The consistency of the dose-response relationship essentially eliminated any possibility that some unknown factors more prevalent in smokers were the true cause of their greater risk of lung cancer. Hammond noted in 1960 that any such "predisposition" would have to increase in direct proportion to the number of cigarettes smoked or the number of years smoked and to decrease in ex-smokers in proportion to the length of time since smoking cessation. Furthermore, the dose-response relationship was an accepted scientific methodology devised in the late nineteenth century to understand the carcinogenic properties of industrial substances like lead and radium. By 1950 it was widely used in industry to set worker threshold and maximum exposures limits.[24]

Scientific Responses to the Statistical Evidence

Despite the unequivocal findings of the dose-response evidence, many biomedical scientists and physicians insisted that causal inferences could never be based on statistical correlations. A 1959 report of a conference on smoking observed that some medical scientists opposed the findings on the grounds "that the relationship between cigarette smoking and lung cancer is based exclusively on 'statistics' and lacks 'experimental' evidence." The committee report remonstrated that "the differentiation between various methods of scientific inquiry escapes us as being a valid basis for the acceptance or the rejection of facts."[25]

The issue of causality raised by the scientists greatly influenced media reporting about smoking, as shown in articles in the *New York Times*. In 1954 the newspaper reported that the retiring president of the American Medical Association "voiced the belief that the case linking cigarettes and cancer had 'not been proven.'" The article stated that his successor believed that smoking was "a probable cancer-inciting agent" for lung cancer, but he "was not convinced that there was a cause-and-effect relationship between cigarette smoking and forms of cancer other than that of the lungs."

He was reported as believing that "tremendously important constitutional factors," probably "glandular disturbances," might both cause people to smoke and develop cancer. Howard Rusk, a highly regarded physician-columnist, reported that the Hammond-Horn study "should not be interpreted to mean that there is definite proof that cigarette smoking is a primary cause of [heart disease and lung cancer]. There is no single piece of evidence that bears out this thesis, but there are many bits of evidence that link cigarette smoking with high mortality." The newspaper's science reporter wrote in 1954 that E. Cuyler Hammond accepted a cause-and-effect relationship while the director of the American Cancer Society was not convinced. The reporter concluded that the "cause-and-effect relationship . . . needs more proof."[26]

The tobacco industry used laboratory research to rebut the statistical evidence. In 1957, the Tobacco Industry Research Council described a conference report as "another review of studies made by others [that] places heavy reliance on statistical associations that have been widely publicized for several years and widely questioned by other scientists as to their significance." It rejected the findings of the Hammond and Horn study, according to an article in the *New York Times,* stating that the "basic origins of cancer and heart disease will eventually be learned by careful laboratory and clinical study, not through statistical reports that are subject to different interpretations from the innumerable variables involved." The function of statistical studies "is to suggest possible areas for further and more definitive investigation using experimental techniques. They do not prove cause-and-effect relationships."[27]

The controversies about the health effects of smoking led the Surgeon General of the U.S. Public Health Service, Luther L. Terry, to convene an advisory committee of scientists in 1962 to review the evidence. The decision was also influenced by a 1962 report of the Royal College of Physicians in England which concluded that smoking caused lung cancer. The committee was carefully designed to placate the tobacco industry: five of the ten members were smokers and the tobacco industry, health groups, and federal agencies were all allowed to veto appointees. The committee reviewed three thousand articles concerning the health effects of cigarette smoking published between 1952 and 1964.[28]

The committee's 1964 report, *Smoking and Health,* was a landmark in publicizing the adverse health effects of smoking, but its conclusions were greatly influenced by an ideological commitment to the methodology of laboratory investigation. The report stated that "various meanings and conceptions of the term *cause* were discussed vigorously at a number of meetings of the Committee and its subcommittees." It recognized the need for a specific term and considered the words factors, determinants, and causes. The "committee agreed that while a factor could be a source of variation, not all sources of variation are causes" and that "often the coexistence of several factors is required for the occurrence of a disease, and that one of the factors may play a determinant role, i.e., without it the other factors . . . are impotent."[29] Thus the committee applied to chronic diseases the doctrine of specific etiology, which holds that specific bacterial pathogens are necessary causes of individual bacterial diseases. It rejected the accepted position that most chronic diseases are produced by multiple factors and that no one factor is present in all cases of the disease.

The committee decided that "the word *cause* is the one in general usage in connection with matters considered in this study, and it is capable of conveying the notion of a significant, effectual, relationship between an agent and an associated disorder or disease in the host." Here also the committee's language was grounded in the methods of the laboratory sciences. Statisticians would have stressed that multiple factors were responsible for the development of any disease and that smoking should be evaluated as one possible factor.[30]

The panel examined several types of evidence to determine the nature of the relationship between smoking and lung cancer. It reviewed the laboratory experiments and concluded that attempts to induce pulmonary carcinomas in experimental animals had not produced convincing results. It found that autopsy studies of humans were only suggestive. Ultimately the committee relied on statistical correlations as the basis of its conclusions. It placed great emphasis on the strong dose-response relationship, the extreme differences in lung cancer mortality rates between smokers and nonsmokers, and the very high extra risk of lung cancer due to smoking compared to the extra risk due to other pulmonary carcinogens. The panel stated: "The array of information from the prospective and retrospective studies of smokers and nonsmokers clearly establishes an association between cigarette smoking and substantially higher death rates." Conceding the absence of causality in this statement, it added: "It is recognized that no simple cause-and-effect relationship is likely to exist between a complex product like tobacco smoke and a specific disease in the variable human organism." The committee did not observe that no simple cause-and-effect relationship exists between any etiological factor, including bacterial pathogens, and a disease.[31]

Many of the committee's conclusions reflected its ambivalence about statistical correlations. It concluded that "cigarette smoking is causally related to lung cancer in men" and cited the dose-response relationship: "The risk of developing lung cancer increases with duration of smoking and the number of cigarettes smoked per day, and is diminished by discontinuing smoking." It then stated that "the data for women, although less extensive, point in the same direction," but did not explain why the statistical findings for men could not be generalized to women. The committee's difficulties were exacerbated in its conclusions regarding coronary heart disease, where it refused to accept causal relationships:

> It is established that male cigarette smokers have a higher death rate from coronary artery disease than non-smoking males. Although the causative role of cigarette smoking in deaths from coronary heart disease is not proven, the Committee considers it more prudent from the public health viewpoint to assume that the established association has causative meaning than to suspend judgment until no uncertainty remains.[32]

Subsequent Surgeon General's committees on smoking were more receptive to statistical correlations and even borrowed the concept of the risk factor from life insurance in order to stress the multifactorial nature of disease etiology. The Surgeon General's second report in 1967 evaluated developments in the three years since the first report:

> Prospective morbidity studies confirm the relationship between cigarette smoking and coronary heart disease. These studies also provide the opportunity to evaluate the effect of smoking independently and in combination with other known "risk factors," such as high blood pressure and high serum cholesterol that are also important in the pathogenesis of coronary heart disease. It has been demonstrated that cigarette smoking not only operates as an independent "risk factor" but that it may combine with other "risk factors" to produce even greater effects on cardiovascular health.[33]

The 1968 report went even further: "The acceptance of a multiple factor causation hypothesis for coronary heart disease emphasizes the need for more sophisticated statistical analyses of appropriate data." It added new risk factors for coronary heart disease, including "sociological, psychological, and personality variables," as well as "genetic and constitutional factors." The 1968 report included new kinds of statistical analyses and the 1971 report extended the concept of risk factors to peripheral vascular disease and other diseases associated with smoking.[34]

A multifactorial concept of disease etiology dominated the 1986 U.S. Public Health Service report, *The Health Consequences of Involuntary Smoking*, which concerned the inhalation of tobacco fumes released into the air by burning cigarettes. Based on statistical dose-response relationships, the report concluded that "involuntary smoking is a cause of disease, including lung cancer, in healthy nonsmokers." Concepts of causality were not mentioned and the legitimacy of epidemiological and statistical research methods never questioned. The transformation in concepts of disease etiology between the 1964 and the 1986 reports was as great as that produced by the germ theory of disease a century earlier.[35]

Public Policies Concerning Smoking

For many years government health agencies, voluntary health associations, and the health professions also believed that statistics could not establish a causal relationship between smoking and disease. Wynder, who was a leader in the anti-smoking movement, reminisced in 1988: "In retrospect, it is difficult to comprehend why it took health professionals and society so long to grasp the full extent of the causative association between lung cancer and smoking." Recognizing the importance of economic interests, he continued: "The position of the tobacco industry is understandable as is its influence on groups depending on its financial support, such as the media, and even governments." But, he insisted, economic interests could not explain why most of those directly involved in health activities failed to act.[36]

　　The political and economic influence of the tobacco industry was a significant obstacle for the anti-smoking movement. About 1970, tobacco farming was a $1 billion industry and tobacco sales a $10 billion consumer product that produced $4 billion in tax revenues to federal, state, and local governments. Tobacco farming and cigarette production were concentrated in a few states, which increased their political power. Cigarette sales contributed to the earnings of hundreds of thousands of retailers. Tobacco advertising was a major source of revenue for newspapers, magazines, billboards, and radio, and generated 8% of television advertising revenues about 1970. Advertising agencies remained loyal to the industry: in 1969 19 of 23 New York agencies without cigarette accounts said they would unhesitatingly accept them. The leading voluntary health associations relied on the mass media to present their messages without cost and received support from companies that benefited from cigarette sales. Medical societies at the national, state, and local levels were sensitive to economic interests.[37]

　　The cigarette industry was a highly cohesive economic and political force dominated by six firms. The larger companies established pricing policies that were adopted by the smaller ones, assuring high profits for all.

Competition occurred primarily through advertising and the introduction of new brands and products. The patterns of close cooperation enabled the companies to adopt a unified strategy in contesting the evidence.[38]

The tobacco industry appealed to the ideological views of many biomedical scientists and physicians by funding laboratory investigations and denigrating epidemiological studies. In 1954 it created the Tobacco Industry Research Committee (renamed the Council for Tobacco Research in 1964) to sponsor research, and its director promised "complete freedom of thought and action" to investigators. The committee proposed "glandular disturbances" as causes of both heavy smoking and cancer, a hypothesis comfortably amenable to years of futile but well-funded laboratory investigation by credulous biomedical scientists. In the next decade, the Council spent $7 million supporting research, most of it concerned with unrelated aspects of cancer and heart disease. In 1964 the *New York Times* stated that the Council for Tobacco Research reported that "studies made in the last ten years have found no laboratory evidence linking lung cancer or fatal heart disease with cigarette smoking." According to the *Wall Street Journal* in 1993, "the Council for Tobacco Research . . . has been the hub of a massive effort to cast doubt on the links between smoking and disease [and] has spent millions of dollars advancing sympathetic science. At the same time, it has sometimes disregarded, or even cut off, studies of its own that implicated smoking as a health hazard."[39]

The tobacco industry had great influence on the federal government, as shown by the exclusion of tobacco products from relevant legislation. The 1963 Clean Air Act applied only to the outdoors and therefore had no significance for smoking. Smoking was specifically excluded from the 1966 Fair Labeling and Packaging Act; the 1970 Controlled Substances Act; the 1972 Consumer Product Safety Act; and the 1976 Toxic Substances Act. President Jimmy Carter did not support most anti-smoking programs and Presidents Ronald Reagan and his successor George Bush were outspoken advocates of the tobacco industry and impeded the anti-smoking programs of federal government agencies. President Bill Clinton, who was elected in 1992, was the first president to ban smoking in the White House and to support the regulation of cigarettes by federal government agencies.[40]

Until the 1980s, most federal agencies whose missions involved the nation's health avoided dealing with the health effects of smoking and sometimes openly sided with tobacco interests. They did so even though public opinion polls in 1964 and 1966 found that between 70% and 75% of the respondents agreed that "cigarette smoking is enough of a health hazard for something to be done about it."[41]

Although the U.S. Public Health Service appointed the advisory committee that issued the 1964 report on smoking, its parent agency, the Department of Health, Education, and Welfare, opposed federal government action at that time to inform the public about the health hazards of cigarette smoking. In 1965 the Public Health Service established a National Clearinghouse on Smoking and Health to collect research findings and educate the public. Its activities, which were always limited, steadily diminished until the late 1970s when Joseph Califano, Secretary of Health, Education, and Welfare, reinvigorated it as the Office on Smoking and Health.[42]

The Department of Agriculture and its Tobacco Division were described by U.S. Senator Maurine Neuberger in 1963 as "at the very bottom of the list" of federal agencies concerned with smoking as a health problem. The introduction of filter tip cigarettes in the 1950s produced a demand by cigarette manufacturers for darker and stronger varieties of tobacco. In order "to furnish the manufacturers with a greater proportion of stronger-flavored tobaccos—with correspondingly higher quantities of tars and nicotine—the Department cut the price supports on several varieties of mild, bright leaf Virginia tobaccos to fifty percent of their former levels, thereby forcing the farmer to switch to the cultivation of stronger varieties." In the 1960s the Agriculture Department opposed warning labels on cigarettes and in the 1970s the elimination of price supports on tobacco leaf.[43]

The Food and Drug Administration, according to Neuberger in 1963, provided "a fair sampling of the overriding timidity and inertia that have plagued nearly every governmental response to the smoking problem." A Supreme Court decision stated in 2000: "In the 41 years since the promulgation of the modern Food, Drug, and Cosmetic Act, the FDA has repeatedly informed Congress that cigarettes are beyond the scope of the statute absent health claims establishing a therapeutic intent on behalf of the manufacturer or vender." The FDA maintained this position even though it approved as a drug a chewing gum that contained nicotine. In 1996 the FDA began to regulate cigarette sales to minors on the grounds that cigarettes serve as a delivery system for a drug, nicotine. The Supreme Court overturned this policy in 2000 in large measure because "as the FDA concedes, it never asserted authority to regulate tobacco products as customarily marketed until" 1996.[44]

Critics of the National Cancer Institute (NCI), according to James T. Patterson, claimed that it "moved gingerly on the smoking issue" and showed little interest in smoking research or control. For many years it emphasized research topics preferred by clinical researchers and biomedical scientists, including cancer treatments and laboratory investigations of the mechanisms by which cancer produced changes within the body. According to Robert N. Proctor, "the NCI's annual plan for 1977–81 failed even to mention tobacco or cigarette smoking in its discussion of the origins and impact of cancer." Among the most egregious of the NCI's actions was its establishment of the Less Hazardous Cigarette Working Group in 1968. This project, later called the Tobacco Working Group at the insistence of the tobacco industry, spent millions of dollars of public funds in a futile attempt to develop a safer cigarette. The project transferred the cost of the research from the tobacco companies to the taxpayers and deliberately misled the public into believing that a safe cigarette was possible. In the early 1980s the NCI developed a Smoking and Tobacco Control Program, which conducted research on methods of smoking control but never established any programs to implement the research.[45] The other relevant institute in the National Institutes of Health, the National Heart Institute, displayed little interest in smoking, instead emphasizing dietary factors as causes of coronary heart disease.

Yet some federal agencies not concerned with health disregarded the political pressures and moved aggressively against smoking. From the early 1930s through the 1950s, the Federal Trade Commission (FTC) brought approximately twenty actions against cigarette companies for misleading advertising, many of which involved fraudulent health claims. In 1964 it proposed and in 1965 required that health warnings be placed on all cigarette packages and that no advertising be directed at youth. In 1967 the Federal Communications Commission (FCC), which had been considered a pawn of radio and television stations, applied the "fairness doctrine" to cigarette advertising, even though the doctrine was designed to provide equal time to individuals exposed to personal attack. Stations were required to provide free time for opponents of smoking to reply to cigarette advertisements. In 1969 the FCC announced a plan to prohibit all cigarette advertising on radio and television, a policy then in force in some European countries.[46]

The tobacco industry quickly convinced the U.S. Congress to nullify many of the FTC regulations. In 1965 Congress enacted the Cigarette Labeling and Advertising Act, which required health warning labels on cigarette packages but voided the FTC's authority over smoking regulations for several years and preempted state and local regulations. The 1970 Public Health Cigarette Smoking Act banned cigarette advertising on radio and television, which had the effect of denying free air time to opponents of smoking. These laws so diluted the FTC and FCC regulations that they were unopposed by the tobacco industry. One journalist said of the 1965 legislation, "The bill is not, as its sponsors suggest, an example of congressional initiative to protect public health; it is an unashamed act to protect private industry from government regulation."[47]

Other government agencies not concerned with health continued to be undeterred by the tobacco industry and issued regulations based on statistical studies in the 1960s showing that involuntary smoking posed health risks to nonsmokers. Despite bitter disagreements about the causal relationships among health professionals, in the early 1970s the Civil Aeronautics Board (and its successor the Federal Aviation Administration) and the Interstate Commerce Commission required airlines, buses, and railroads to provide separate smoking and nonsmoking sections. These were soon followed by municipal ordinances, state laws, and administrative rulings that restricted or banned smoking in many buildings and other places of public congregation. The federal government was among the last to restrict smoking in the 1990s.[48]

Given the inaction of federal health agencies, responsibility for national health leadership devolved on the American Cancer Society (ACS) and the American Heart Association (AHA), the largest voluntary health associations of their kind. Prior to the Second World War, both were small organizations led by researchers and clinical specialists that published scientific journals and provided continuing education to physicians. After the war both associations became mass organizations of physicians, scientists, and laypersons that undertook large-scale public education and fund-raising campaigns. The American Heart Association increased its income from $100,000 in 1946 to $23 million in 1958.[49]

The American Cancer Society (ACS) pursued certain aspects of the problem and avoided others. It sponsored the Wynder and Graham and the Hammond and Horn epidemiological studies as its first original research studies. Based on the latter, it adopted a noncausal resolution in 1954: "The American Cancer Society emphasizes to the American people that the presently available evidence indicates an association between smoking, and particularly cigarette smoking, and lung cancer and to a lesser degree other forms of cancer. Our smoking study further revealed an association between smoking and heart disease." Its only action was to recommend a conference of health officials and to undertake further research. In 1960 the ACS finally concluded that "beyond a reasonable doubt cigarette smoking is the major cause of the unprecedented increase in lung cancer" and produced educational materials for schools. In 1961 it joined with the AHA and other societies to emphasize the seriousness of the problem to the president and the surgeon general of the Public Health Service. It did not strongly support warning labels on cigarettes and refused to support equal time for anti-smoking messages on radio and television. But subsequently, the ACS did move vigorously against smoking.[50]

The AHA was even more unwilling to recommend smoking cessation. In 1956, Irvine H. Page, the president and chair of an AHA committee that reviewed the smoking evidence, told the *New York Times* that "much greater knowledge is needed before any conclusion can be drawn concerning relationships between smoking and increased death rates from coronary heart disease." In 1958, another AHA president said that "the association always is being needled to take a stand about tobacco," but even if a link between smoking and lung cancer "were proven, as some think it has been, . . . what is the effect of stopping the smoking of cigarettes on heart disease? We don't know what the effect is." In 1959, according to a history of the association, the "medical leadership" rejected a policy statement on smoking because some of them thought that the "statistical association [between cigarette smoking and heart disease] might be coincidental rather than causal." In 1963 the association began a educational program to discourage smoking in conjunction with other agencies, which the *New York Times* reported was "the first time the association . . . has decided to wage a public campaign on smoking." However, the AHA did not oppose all smoking: it stated that the statistical evidence showed "that heavy cigarette smoking contributed to or accelerated the development of coronary heart disease based on the statistical relationship between smoking and mortality from coronary artery disease." The AHA's policies became less equivocal in the 1970s.[51]

The American Medical Association (AMA), the nation's largest and most influential medical society, also failed to provide leadership on the smoking issue. Most physicians in the 1950s and 1960s looked to the AMA for medical leadership and many politicians at all levels of government were greatly influenced by its recommendations. In matters internal to the association, the AMA accepted the evidence and its journals published some major research findings. In 1953, partly in reaction to disingenuous references to the AMA in some cigarette advertisements, it discontinued cigarette advertisements in its journals and prohibited cigarette exhibits at its scientific meetings.[52]

In matters external to the association, the AMA followed an entirely different policy. In 1963, its major legislative body, the House of Delegates, called for additional research on the relation between smoking and disease to "probe beyond statistical evidence." The AMA then accepted $18 million from six major tobacco companies for smoking research. In 1964 the

House of Delegates, under pressure to take a stand on the Surgeon General's report, approved a noncausal statement that smoking had a "significant relation to lung cancer." According to Patterson, the smoking research project "dragged on into the 1970s without producing a hint of structured findings." A final report entitled *Tobacco and Health* was issued in 1978 and concluded that smoking was a danger to those with preexisting coronary heart disease and contributed to chronic obstructive pulmonary disease. The report did not mention cancer.[53]

When informing the public directly, the association was especially evasive. In 1964, the AMA published a leaflet, *Smoking: Facts You Should Know,* which emphasized the dangers of cigarette burns and fires caused by cigarettes. It called the health risks "suspected health hazards" and claimed that qualified researchers disagreed about them. Twenty years later, the AMA wrote a special supplement on personal health care for *Newsweek* magazine. Smoking was not mentioned at all because the magazine opposed the topic. In 1985 the AMA approved several resolutions that urged stronger public policies against smoking and established more vigorous anti-smoking activities within the association.[54]

The AMA's position in the 1960s and 1970s was strongly influenced by its need for congressional allies who shared its opposition to Medicare, national health insurance, and similar health legislation. Many congressmen from tobacco growing states had views that were practically identical to those of the AMA on these matters. In 1964, the AMA's executive vice president (its chief executive) opposed any administrative regulations by the federal government concerning the labeling and advertising of cigarettes. The AMA preferred that Congress enact any legislation, fully aware that congressmen from tobacco states would influence its content. In 1971, a Tobacco Institute executive wrote a memorandum after a meeting with the AMA executive vice president stating that the AMA was "most anxious to avoid any incident which will create displeasure with the AMA among tobacco area Congressmen—he said AMA needs their support urgently." In 1982 another AMA executive vice president wrote a confidential memorandum to the editor of its leading journal, in which he "pointed out the existence of some particularly sensitive political questions and urged that we exercise appropriate caution in our *JAMA* publication on these subjects. They are: tobacco and control of tobacco use, nuclear war, abortion." Even though the AMA eventually adopted formal policies opposing smoking, Wolinsky and Brune observed in 1995 that its "failure to use its political leverage to fight tobacco interests is legendary among antitobacco lobbyists and congressional staffers."[55]

Changes in Smoking Behavior

Despite the lack of leadership of federal government health agencies and health and medical associations, the public accepted the statistical evidence concerning smoking with surprising celerity, according to Gallup public opinion polls. As early as 1954 40% of respondents thought that cigarette smoking was "one of the causes of lung cancer," which increased to 70% about 1970 and exceeded 90% in the 1990s. In the 1990s about 80% of the respondents thought that "second-hand smoke" was "very" or "some-what harmful" to adults and more than 90% wanted restrictions on smoking in workplaces, restaurants, and hotels and motels. Among smokers, the proportion who would "like to give up smoking" increased from 66% about 1980 to 75% in the late 1990s.[56]

The decline in smoking rates varied among groups in the population. By gender, the proportion of men who smoked leveled off at about 50% in the 1950s and early 1960s and then declined to 27% in 1995. Among women the proportion of smokers increased from 25% in 1955 to 34% in 1966, then declined to about 23% in 1995. By educational level, in 1974 about one-half of men and one-third of women with no more than a high school education smoked, compared to 29% of men and 26% of women with four or more years of college education. By 1995 about 35% of the men and 29% of the women in the high-school group smoked compared to 14% of both sexes of the college group.[57]

Practically all physicians came to accept the statistical evidence on smoking. Two surveys of primary care physicians and cardiologists in the mid-1980s found that 90% said that refraining from smoking would have a large effect on reducing the risk of coronary heart disease. Even more salient, the 60% of physicians who smoked in 1949 declined to 30% in 1964, and in 1989 only 6% considered themselves daily smokers.[58]

The behavior of physicians in assisting patients to stop smoking has been examined in several studies. The 1991–95 National Ambulatory Medical Care Survey conducted by the U.S. National Center for Health Statistics examined thousands of individual patient visits using forms completed by a random sample of all office-based physicians. Physicians identified the smoking status of the patients at only 59% of visits of new patients and counseled the patient about smoking at only 25% of the visits of new patients who smoked. Very similar proportions occurred for patients who made return visits. A 1994 survey limited to family physicians in Indiana with a low response rate of 37% found that 86% of the physicians asked all new patients if they smoked. A 1989–90 Texas survey of family physicians with a response rate of 51% found that 99% of the physicians asked their patients if they smoked cigarettes. Over 90% of the physicians in state-wide surveys advised smoking patients to stop smoking. From the patient's perspective, one survey of Michigan patients in the early 1980s found that "only 44% of smokers reported ever having received a physician's advice to quit," a proportion slightly higher than a 1975 national survey. Another survey of midwestern patients in the early 1990s found that 78% of the patients who smoked in the last two years reported being advised to stop smoking by their physicians.[59]

Many studies have found that physicians seldom go beyond simply advising patients to stop smoking. For example, surveys of patients filling prescriptions for nicotine patches in 1992 found that 60% to 80% of them requested the patch from their physicians. Other studies found that only small minorities of smoking patients reported being referred to smoking cessation programs by their physicians. These findings reflect the uncertainties of many physicians about their efforts. One 1981 study of Massachusetts physicians in primary care specialties found that only 3% considered themselves "very successful" in helping their smoking patients stop smoking and only 14% were reported as "optimistic about their ability to help patients . . . stop smoking." Another study of 208 California internists about the same time found that more than 70% of them agreed that "counseling about smoking is frustrating."[60]

In the 1960s the cigarette companies recognized that the smoking rates of the American public would decline steadily. They marketed cigarettes more aggressively in other countries, diversified by purchasing companies in other industries, and removed the word "tobacco" from their names. In 1990, the annual report of the nation's largest cigarette company, Philip Morris, conceded the health risks of smoking: "We have acknowledged that smoking is a risk factor in the development of lung cancer and certain other human diseases, because a statistical relationship exists between smoking and the occurrence of these diseases. According, we insist that the decision to smoke, like many other lifestyle decisions, should be made by informed adults. We believe that smokers around the world are well aware of the potential risks associated with tobacco use, and have the knowledge necessary to make an informed decision."[61]

Thus the cigarette companies justified their sales and advertising by claiming that adults understood the risks of smoking and made informed decisions. However, three Gallup Polls in the 1990s found that about 70% of smokers began smoking before age nineteen. Furthermore, a study of the brand loyalty of smokers in the 1980s found that so few smokers changed from a brand sold by one company to a brand sold by another company that "brand- switching alone could never justify the enormous advertising and promotion expenditures" of the cigarette companies.[62]

The political influence of the tobacco industry waned. A public opinion poll in 1997 found that 92% of the respondents believed that "tobacco companies know it causes cancer even if they do not admit it" and 80% believed "that some tobacco companies market their products deliberately to young people." According to the *New York Times* in 1997, nonsmokers obtained state and local legislation that restricted smoking over the opposition of the tobacco, liquor, and restaurant industries because "intimidation by the tobacco industry is not as effective as it once was." The tobacco industry's main strategy in the 1990s was to convince state legislatures to enact laws that preempted more restrictive local ordinances and to convince Congress, where their influence was greatest, to enact even milder laws that preempted state laws.[63]

Thus cigarette smoking served as the great battlefield over the use of statistical correlations to establish causal relationships. Ultimately, a new generation of physicians and biomedical scientists acknowledged the value of statistical correlations as scientific evidence.

14

BLOOD PRESSURE AND THE BENEFITS OF TREATMENT

> Of all the measurable functions of the body no other has caused greater controversy in the past than that of blood pressure, leading often to violent disagreement between the pure clinician and the life [insurance] underwriter, and even between clinicians themselves. The source of the trouble is that the correlation between blood pressure and mortality is statistical rather than individual.[1]

> The one glaring difference [among national and international guidelines for treating hypertension] is their stance on the management of uncomplicated mild hypertension. This may seem a minor matter considering the numerous points of agreement, but of course subjects with mild hypertension far outnumber all other hypertensive patients because of the distribution of blood pressure in the population.[2]

High blood pressure rose to prominence as a health concern with the development of effective antihypertensive drugs. One issue for public health has been methods of preventing hypertension. Another has been the minimum blood pressure level that warrants medical treatment, which affects millions of persons and can have a significant impact on health care costs.

The Statistical Distribution of Blood Pressure Levels

As male coronary heart disease morbidity and mortality rates continued their relentless climb during the 1940s and 1950s, its prevention became the most compelling health problem of the twentieth century. In 1950 about 1.1% of men ages 45–54 and 2.4% of men ages 55–64 died annually. Close to one-third of the deaths in each age group resulted from coronary heart disease compared to 4% from lung cancer and 16% from all cancers combined.[3] Many of the victims were seemingly healthy married men in their forties and fifties. Their deaths left their widows with heavy family and financial obligations, their children without fathers, and their work organizations and communities without their experience and skills. The enormous void created by the loss of so many men at the ages when they made their greatest contributions to society produced a sense of urgency unmatched by any other disease.

At mid-century the most useful predictors of coronary heart disease in healthy individuals were a family history of the disease and blood pressure level. Physicians had used family history to predict disease for centuries, but their use of blood pressure resulted from the demands of life insurance companies, as one physician observed in 1950:

> When an instrument for measuring blood pressure was introduced, it was almost immediately put to use by the doctor in every town and hamlet who was required in the course of his insurance examinations to furnish a blood pressure reading. (It may be remarked that while patients may have benefited little from blood pressure determinations, insurance companies have profited to the extent of untold millions.) Seldom has a new and somewhat expensive method of clinical diagnosis been so promptly put to use by the entire body of physicians.[4]

Life insurance companies found that blood pressure levels had very high statistical correlations with mortality rates, as shown by a study of twenty-six life insurance companies from 1935 to 1954 when no effective treatments existed. Men and women age 45 with a blood pressure level of 120/80 mm Hg had life expectancies of an additional 32 and 37 years respectively. A blood pressure level of 130/90 mm Hg reduced the life expectancy of men by 4 years and of women by 1.5 years. A level of 140/95 mm Hg reduced it by 9 years for men and 5 years for women, and a level of 150/100 mm Hg reduced it by 11.5 years for men and 8.5 years for women. Having a blood pressure level less than 120/80 increased a person's life expectancy. The percentage reductions in life expectancy for men were greater for persons younger than 45 years of age and less for persons older than 45 years of age.[5]

During the middle of the century, a debate developed over whether essential (having no known cause) hypertension was a disease. George Pickering, a leading English physician, asserted that essential hypertension was not a disease because it had the same normal distribution in the population as many other human characteristics, such as weight. It was also not a disease of aging because blood pressure levels tend to rise and become more varied with age in all western societies. A sample of males age 16 had an average systolic blood pressure of 118 mm Hg and two-thirds of them had levels between 106 and 131, a spread of 25 mm Hg. The average for males ages 60–64 was 142 mm Hg and two-thirds of them had levels between 121 and 163, a spread of 42 mm Hg. The pattern for females was similar. Pickering also stated that essential hypertension has no "unique cause" that differentiated the diseased from the healthy. Its alleged symptoms were questionable because "iatrogenic disease is extremely common in essential hypertension." The doctor's attitude "is communicated to the patient and is enhanced by articles in the public press. . . . Hence, it is the physician himself who, in applying to the patient the grim label of hypertension, produces the patient's symptoms."[6]

Pickering believed that the so-called disease of essential hypertension resulted from the needs of clinical decision-making. "When a doctor sees a patient his first concern is to establish a diagnosis: is the patient healthy or diseased and, if diseased, which disease?" The physician "is chiefly concerned with the transition from normal to abnormal, from physiological to pathological, from health to disease, from normotension to hypertension. His attention is firmly fixed on the moment when the line dividing normal pressure from hypertension is crossed."[7]

In 1955 Pickering defined essential hypertension as "that section of the population with arterial pressures above a certain value, selected on arbitrary grounds, and in whom there is no other disease to which the high pressure can be attributed." This perspective was shared by many physicians. A 1951 symposium observed: "There is considerable reluctance to regard a state that prevails in so large a portion of the population as abnormal, when . . . no impairment of longevity is necessarily implied for a great many of the cases." Physicians were also concerned about labeling essential hypertension a disease. "The emotional effects upon the patient of a finding of elevated pressure being what they are, it has seemed to some that it is preferable to have a broad rather than a narrow, range of normal pressure."[8]

Others claimed that essential hypertension was a symptom of a disease. A 1952 textbook observed that most diseases were diagnosed only when several signs or symptoms were present, yet "such a sound approach has been bypassed in cases of hypertension."

> Too much attention is often paid to the height of the blood pressure, and not enough to the clinical picture as a whole. In clinical medicine, the blood pressure level is not as important as is the absence or presence of underlying vascular disease. Increased blood pressure, in itself, is not a disease. It is a sign of some underlying disorder.[9]

Whether or not essential hypertension was a disease, its association with higher mortality rates led to many unsuccessful efforts to reduce blood pressure. The failures produced a fatalistic attitude among many physicians. Medical textbooks predicted an untimely end for the hapless patient, who was all but advised to prepare a will and select a good mortician. Irvine Page proposed the following for patients with essential hypertension in 1950:

> (1) Cultivating serenity; (2) coming to terms with the inevitable; (3) living a life of moderation; (4) participating only in those affairs which one can influence; (5) avoiding fatigue; (6) having more frequent periods of rest; (7) avoiding obesity; (8) avoiding food fads and eating a well-balanced diet more frequently than usual; and (9) selecting a physician in whom the patient can place full responsibility for wise counsel.[10]

As always, fads prevailed in the absence of useful therapies. The most famous was a diet of rice and fruit with no salt and very little fat introduced in 1948 by Walter Kempner. About 60 percent of the patients lowered their blood pressure levels, which Kempner attributed to reduced sodium consumption despite the lack of a control group. However, the unpalatable diet caused many patients to lose weight, which often lowers blood pressure levels, and its extreme nature made generalizations to moderate salt reduction doubtful.[11]

Drug Treatment of Essential Hypertension

During the 1950s several medications to reduced blood pressure were developed. One was an alkaloid extract of an Indian herb, rauwolfia, but it produced unacceptable side effects in many patients. In 1958, the first of several thiazide diuretics was derived from sulfa drugs and became a practical long-term antihypertensive drug with few unmanageable side effects.[12]

Clinical trials were immediately conducted to determine whether blood pressure reduction decreased mortality rates. Edward Freis, an investigator in the pioneering Veterans Administration study, observed:

> It has been stated, on good authority, for many years, that hypertension is a symptom only, an insignificant manifestation of an underlying vascular disease which proceeds inexorably regardless of the level of blood pressure. Therefore, reduction of blood pressure . . . is not a rational procedure because the vascular damage proceeds nevertheless. Such a nihilistic attitude was quite permissible 20 years ago when there were no effective methods for reducing and controlling hypertension. The whole question was academic anyway, and if physicians could be dissuaded from giving worthless and presumably dangerous medications, so much the better.[13]

Patients with varying levels of hypertension were given thiazide drugs to measure the impact on mortality rates. In persons with malignant hypertension, defined as extremely high blood pressure levels that produced very high mortality rates, the drugs lowered mortality rates so much that clinical trials were considered unnecessary. In persons with moderate and mild essential hypertension, who had lower disease and death rates, the lack of equally dramatic results led to clinical trials. The trials differed in fundamental ways from traditional drug trials: they used healthy rather than sick persons, required more participants because of the low death rates, and were conducted for many months or years in order to accumulate enough cases of death or disease.

The first major clinical trials of antihypertensive medication were begun in 1963 by the Veterans Administration using veterans who were receiving VA care. The two studies excluded patients who had severe hypertensive damage or serious diseases and eliminated participants who failed to take their medications conscientiously during a brief trial period. The study of moderate hypertension (diastolic blood pressure 115–129 mm Hg) found that the average blood pressure level of the treatment group dropped from 121 to about 90 mm Hg during the study while the placebo group remained unchanged. Of the 73 patients in the treatment group, none died and only 1 had to be removed from the study. Of the 70 patients in the placebo group, 4 died and 17 developed serious medical problems that caused their removal from the study. The results were so impressive that the study was terminated prematurely and all patients were placed on drug therapy.[14]

The study of mild hypertension (diastolic pressure 90–114 mm Hg) involved patients at much lower risk. In order to accumulate enough events, the investigators enrolled 380 persons, included less serious outcomes, and continued the trial for 5.5 years, although patients averaged only 3.3 years. The average diastolic blood pressure of the treatment group dropped 17 mm Hg during the trial, while that of the placebo group rose 1 mm Hg. The study found that the benefits of drug treatment varied by age. Among those ages 50 and over, 43% of the 95 placebo patients had "morbid events" compared to 18% of the 84 thiazide patients, a difference of 27%; among those under age 50, 15% of the 99 placebo patients had morbid events compared to 7% of the 102 thiazide patients, a difference of only 8%. Another factor was blood pressure level. For diastolic blood pressures of 105–114 mm Hg, 32% of the 110 placebo patients had morbid events compared to 8% of the 100 thiazide patients, a difference of 24%; for diastolic blood pressures of 90–104 mm Hg, 25% of the 84 placebo patients had morbid events compared to 16% of the 86 thiazide patients, a difference of only 9%. Similar findings occurred for the groups with systolic blood pressure levels below and above 165 mm Hg.[15]

The Veterans' Administration studies, according to Hart, "became the classical evidence on which virtually all treatment policies claimed to be based." Yet the patients were quite atypical of the general population: they were all male veterans who received care at Veterans Administration hospitals and Hart observed that they had "much more organ damage and a far higher complication rate than one would expect from a population sample of the same age and pressure." The study eliminated so "many uncooperative and unreliable patients," according to the authors of the study, that "treatment obviously would not have been as effective in a group of patients less carefully selected with regard to their desire to cooperate."[16]

Antihypertensive drugs were quickly adopted by physicians. Essential hypertension was well suited to the economics of private practice: it could be diagnosed and treated only by a physician; it required regular patient visits and medical tests that were not time consuming and were covered by health insurance; the treatments posed few difficulties or dangers; and return visits led to other medical services. By 1977–78, according to a survey, hypertension was involved in about 7% of ambulatory care visits to general practitioners and family physicians, 12% of visits to specialists in internal medicine, and 10% of visits to cardiologists.[17]

Antihypertensive medication also increased the use of periodic medical examinations. Medical examinations of healthy persons first became common early in the twentieth century with examinations of life insurance applicants and draftees during the First World War. In the 1920s the periodic medical examination became a standard medical procedure. Charap has observed that it is based on three assumptions: asymptomatic individuals can harbor serious diseases; the diseases can be detected in their early stages during an examination; and once detected in their early stages, the diseases can be controlled, reversed, or cured. Diseases that are widespread and progress slowly are most suitable. The thiazide diuretics made high blood pressure the first common medical condition that met every one of these assumptions.[18]

Minimum Blood Pressure Levels Appropriate for Treatment

The development of antihypertensive medication led to the important public health issue of the minimum blood pressure level that benefits from treatment. Unnecessary treatment can expose patients to adverse reactions, squander the financial resources of patients and health insurance systems, and divert physicians from more pressing responsibilities.

Because the lowest levels of hypertension are many times more common than the highest levels, every reduction in the minimum level for treatment adds millions of persons. Using data from the 1980s, treating all those with a minimum diastolic blood pressure level of 110 mm Hg would have included 4% of men and 3% of women ages 35–44 and 7% of men and 5% of women ages 45–64. A reduction of the minimum level to 90 mm Hg diastolic would have included 33% of men and 22% of women ages 35–44, 43% of men and 30% of women ages 45–54, and 43% of men and 41% of women ages 55–64. A study of the diastolic blood pressures of 159,000 men ages 30–69 found that 3% had levels greater 110 mm Hg, 5% had levels greater than 105, 8% had levels greater than 100, 15% had levels greater 95, and 25% had levels greater than 90 mm Hg.[19]

One of the greatest problems in determining blood pressure levels appropriate for treatment is that they vary greatly in individual patients in both the short and long run. In the short run, blood pressure levels change with the patient's emotional and physical state. As an example, measurements taken at the patients' homes tend to be lower and better predictors of risk than those taken in a health care facility.[20]

In the long run, blood pressure is much more variable than many other human characteristics. A study measured blood pressure levels in 1948 and every five years thereafter for thirty years in a group of 3,983 healthy and well-educated men who were found fit for the Royal Canadian Air Force pilot training program during the Second World War. Men who started antihypertensive medication were removed from the study, but this was uncommon during most of this period. As expected, the average blood pressure levels of the men rose steadily as they grew older: for example, among men who were 30–34 years of age in 1948, the average systolic blood pressure was 121 mm Hg in 1948, 124 in 1958, 130 in 1968, and 134 in 1978.[21]

The sample members with the highest blood pressures when they were young experienced a slower than average rise in their blood pressures as they aged. In the 30–34 year old group, of those in the top one-sixth in terms of their systolic blood pressure in 1948, only 35% were still in the top one-sixth in 1958, 28% were in that group in 1968, and 22% in 1978. For diastolic pressures, the proportions were 29% in 1958, 22% in 1968, and 18% in 1968. Similar patterns occurred in the top one-sixth of the other age groups: 20–24, 25–29, and 35–39. The consistency of this trend over twenty years makes it highly unlikely that it resulted primarily from regression toward the mean.[22]

The blood pressures of the men in 1948 were poor predictors of their blood pressures in the next thirty years. The Pearson correlation coefficients between the systolic blood pressures of the men at entry in 1948 and ten years later were low, from a minimum of 0.22 for the 20–24–year-old group to a maximum of 0.33 for the 35–39–year-old group. Between entry and twenty years later the coefficients were even lower, 0.18 and 0.31 respectively, and between entry and thirty years later they were quite low, at 0.13 and 0.16 respectively. The blood pressures of older groups were as unstable as those of younger groups. The correlation coefficient between the blood pressures of men age 50–54 and their levels ten years later was 0.36, which means that only 13% of the individual variations in blood pressure levels at ages 60–64 were explained by their levels at ages 50–54.[23]

The determination of the minimum blood pressure levels appropriate for medication have been based on clinical trials, but most trials in mild and moderate hypertension have had unsatisfactory control groups. Ethical constraints prevented them from using true placebo groups, so the participants were divided into special-treatment groups that received a new antihypertensive drug and usual-care groups that were taking older antihypertensive drugs. As an example, the four-year Treatment of Mild Hypertension Study in the early 1990s divided the 902 participants ages 45–69 into a placebo group and five different medication groups. Sixty percent of the participants in every group, including the placebo group, were taking antihypertensive medication prior to the start of the study.[24] Such studies cannot compare antihypertensive medication to no medication and do not even know the unmedicated blood pressure levels of the participants.

Two large-scale studies of mild hypertension in the 1970s merit detailed examination because they used placebo groups. The 1973 Australian mild hypertension study defined mild hypertension as a diastolic blood pressure of 95–109 mm Hg and a systolic pressure of less than 200 mm Hg, the latter level much higher than in American studies. It screened 104,000 community volunteers to obtain a sample of 3,427 persons ages 30–69 who did not have a history of heart disease or stroke and were not on antihypertensive medication. One-half of the participants were given drug treatment and one-half given placebos for an average duration of three years. The treatment and placebo groups were very similar: each group had the same proportion of men, 63%; the same average age, 50 years; the same average initial blood pressure level, 158/100 mm Hg; and the same proportions of smokers, a very high 75%. The treatment group experienced a drop in diastolic blood pressure between 10 and 17 mm Hg, depending on initial level, and the placebo group 5 to 9 mm Hg. Deaths due to unrelated diseases were practically identical for the two groups. The results were described as events per 100 person-years, which is comparable to the percentage of persons who experienced an event in one year of the trial. Per 100 person-years of exposure during the study, 1.7 of those in the treatment group experienced cardiovascular disease (coronary heart disease, stroke, and some other diseases) or death, compared to 2.5 of those in the placebo group. This was a difference of 0.8 events per 100 person-years in a group of persons with an average age of 50 years. The mortality rates of both groups were unusually high, probably because of the very large proportion of smokers.[25]

The other large drug and placebo study of mild hypertension, the 1977 British Medical Research Council study, used as a definition of mild hypertension a diastolic blood pressure of 90–109 mm Hg and a systolic blood pressure of less than 200 mm Hg. More than 500,000 persons were screened to obtain a very large sample of 9,048 men and 8,306 women volunteers ages 35–64 who did not have certain diseases and were not on antihypertensive medication. The men had an average age of 51 years and 31% were smokers, while the women had an average age of 53 years and 26% were smokers. The average blood pressure level of the men was 155/97 mm Hg and of the women was 158/97 mm Hg. The sample was divided into three groups that received one of two different drugs or a placebo for an average of 5.5 years beginning in 1977. Per 100 person-years of exposure during the study, the number of "cardiovascular events" (coronary heart disease, stroke, and some other conditions) were 0.66 and 0.67 for the two drug groups and 0.82 for the placebo group, a very small difference of about 0.16 cardiovascular events per 100 participants per year. The number of coronary events (myocardial infarction and sudden death) per 100 person-years was 0.52 for the drug groups and 0.54 for the placebo groups, a negligible difference. The largest difference between the drug and placebo groups was 0.14 compared to 0.44 strokes per 100 person years, which occurred in the group with the highest diastolic blood pressure:105–9 mm Hg.[26]

Both studies found a probability of less than .01 that the differences in cardiovascular events between the treatment and placebo groups could have occurred by chance. However, statistical tests are designed to give great weight to the size of the sample and both of these samples were extremely large. Statistical tests also require that the sample be chosen at random from the population of interest in order to make a valid generalization to that population. This was not done in either study; indeed, the authors of the British study stated that the participants "were clearly not a random sample of all people aged 35–64 with mild hypertension."[27] The very large samples and the lack of randomization indicate that chance variations should be considered the most likely explanation of the very small differences between the treatment and placebo groups in the two studies.

One common explanation for the small differences between treatment and placebo groups in these kinds of studies is the so-called "placebo effect," blood pressure reductions in the placebo group due to psychological factors. In the Australian study the average diastolic blood pressure level of the placebo group fell by 6.6 mm Hg compared to an average drop of 12.2 mm Hg in the treatment group. However, a placebo effect exists only if the placebo group experiences a greater decline in blood pressure than a third group that received neither placebo nor treatment. Such a group was used in the Australian study and the decline in its average blood pressure was generally greater than in the placebo group, just the opposite of what the placebo effect theory would predict. Thus the placebo effect cannot be used to explain the failure of the Australian study to produce meaningful differences between the drug and placebo groups.[28]

The Australian and British studies were the only two large-scale, long-term, drug and placebo trials undertaken in the twentieth century that used diastolic blood pressures of less than 110 mm Hg. Both studies used drugs that continued to be popular decades after the termination of the studies. Both studies had very large samples of healthy volunteers who were not taking antihypertensive medication prior to the trial. Both studies undoubtedly had excellent compliance with the therapeutic regimens because of the careful screening used to select the volunteer participants. Yet neither study produced meaningful differences in death and disease rates between treatment and placebo groups.

The Australian, British, and Veterans Administration trials, as well as every other clinical trial, found that lowering blood pressure with antihypertensive medication did not reduce a group's overall death and disease rates to the level of groups with that blood pressure level normally. In all studies, antihypertensive treatment produced much smaller benefits for coronary heart disease than stroke. However, coronary heart disease occurred much more frequently in the study groups, as it does in the general population. For example, coronary heart disease caused three times as many deaths as stroke in the United States in the 1970s. Because of the limited benefits of antihypertensive medication for coronary heart disease, persons whose blood pressures were lowered by medication will always have higher overall death and disease rates than persons with the same blood pressures normally.[29]

Even though the benefits of antihypertensive medication are small in cases of lower levels of mild hypertension, they may be worthwhile if they do not affect the patient's health adversely. However, antihypertensive medications produce serious side effects in many patients. The British study found that adverse drug reactions forced 15% to 23% of the participants, depending on the specific treatment group, to change their regimens. In the American Treatment of Mild Hypertension Study, side effects forced 14% of those in the treatment groups to discontinue their medication within one year. These numbers do not include the much larger proportion of patients who experienced less severe side effects.[30]

Government Recommendations for Minimum Treatment Levels

Because of the importance of essential hypertension as a health problem, The U.S. National Institutes of Health established a Joint National Committee on Detection, Evaluation, and Treatment of High Blood Pressure that has made periodic public pronouncements concerning minimum blood pressure levels appropriate for treatment. Each revision has reduced the minimum blood pressure levels and added millions of persons to the group needing treatment. In 1984 the committee lowered the diastolic blood pressure for mild hypertension from 95 to 90 mm Hg, which nearly doubled the number of hypertensives. According to the *New York Times,* critics said that the "very definition of this range has been shifting with dizzying speed" and that it was "stretched too far." The 1988 report went further and de-

fined "mild hypertension" as 90–104 mm Hg and "moderate hypertension" as 105–114 mm Hg diastolic; the 1993 report reduced the mild range
to 90–99 mm Hg and the moderate range to 100–109 mm Hg diastolic.
The minimum systolic pressure for mild hypertension was 140–159 mm
Hg when the diastolic pressure was not elevated. In 1997 this range was
called Stage 1 hypertension.[31]

The committee has proposed more aggressive measures to treat high
blood pressure in each succeeding report. In its 1988, 1993, and 1997
reports, the committee recommended observation and lifestyle changes for
a period of months in mild hypertension to see if the level returned to
normal without drugs. Lifestyle changes included weight reduction, physical activity, smoking cessation, alcohol restriction, and reduced consumption of dietary sodium. In 1988 drug treatment in addition to lifestyle
changes was recommended for all those with diastolic blood pressures of
95 mm Hg or higher and those with levels of 90–94 mm Hg who were at
higher risk, plus anyone else the physician chose. In 1993, drug therapy
was recommended for all those with blood pressures of 140/90 mm Hg or
higher, although it recognized that some physicians may elect to use a higher
value. In 1997 the option of selecting a higher value was omitted, and drug
treatment was also recommended for those with blood pressures of 130–
139 systolic and 85–89 mm Hg who had certain serious illnesses.[32]

The committee has consistently underestimated the benefits of smoking cessation compared to hypertension reduction. The British Medical
Research Council study observed in 1988: "Probably the best advice which
can be given to patients with mild hypertension is that they should not
smoke." The director of the Framingham Heart Study, one of the most
important long-term studies of coronary heart disease, observed in 1990
that "getting a hypertensive patient to quit smoking confers more immediate benefit than any known antihypertensive drug against coronary heart
disease." Yet as late as 1988 the Joint National Committee stated only that
"smoking cessation is strongly recommended." In 1993 and 1997 the committee made smoking cessation "essential," but did not compare its benefits to antihypertensive medication.[33]

The committee has never examined the economic consequences of
its proposals. In 1988 it recognized that drug therapy could impose a "burdensome financial obligation" on individual patients and urged physicians
to "minimize these expenses." In 1993 it conceded that "lifelong antihypertensive therapy represents a significant component of the nation's financial commitment to health. . . . [F]or individual as well as societal reasons,

minimizing cost must be an essential component of the health care provider's responsibility." In 1997, in a new section on "managed care," it claimed that the cost of managing hypertension was lower than the cost of treating the associated diseases but did not provide evidence to support the claim. It is very unlikely that the benefits of drug treatment for the very low levels of mild hypertension specified by the committee exceed the costs.[34]

The Joint National Committee recommendations may be contrasted with the higher blood pressure levels recommended for treatment by commissions in other countries. In 1989 the British Hypertension Society Working Party proposed that drug treatment be used for patients under age 80 with a diastolic blood pressure of at least 100 mm Hg. Those with diastolic blood pressures of 95–99 mm Hg were to be observed every three to six months. The working party was particularly concerned with "the economic costs and exposure to adverse drug reactions" that would occur at lower blood pressure levels. A second working party in 1993 stressed the importance of using factors other than blood pressure to decide on drug treatment, a policy that was adopted by the Joint National Committee in 1997. It claimed that drug treatment in patients with diastolic blood pressures of 90–99 mm Hg and who were not otherwise at risk was "controversial" and that the "potential benefit of drug treatment to individual patients may be relatively small. The evidence of benefit from therapeutic intervention in all classes of patients is not universally accepted." Drug treatment was recommended for patients at that level who had additional risks. In 1989 a Canadian group presented similar recommendations.[35]

In 1993, the World Health Organization-International Society of Hypertension proposed a minimum diastolic level of 95 mm Hg for treatment regardless of other risks. The group disagreed with the Joint National Committee's use of a category called "high normal," defined as 130–39 systolic and 85–89 mm Hg diastolic, stating that the category "does not seem justified at the moment."[36]

Little information is available on physicians' adoption of the Joint National Committee guidelines, but a 1986 study of 131 California physicians who managed blood pressure found that they prescribed medication only to patients who had higher blood pressure levels than recommended by the committee. When asked if patients need drug therapy at various diastolic blood pressure levels, 3% cited 90–94 mm Hg, 32% cited 95–99, 78% 100–04, and 92% 105–9. Sixty-one percent said that drug treatment of blood pressure in the elderly created more adverse reactions than benefits, contrary to the committee's recommendations.[37]

The Prevention of Hypertension

When antihypertensive drugs became widely available in the 1960s, public health departments organized programs to educate the public in order to identify all hypertensives. In 1972, the National Heart, Lung and Blood Institute established the National High Blood Pressure Education Program, a cooperative venture of federal agencies and voluntary health associations that soon included about 150 national organizations and practically all state health departments.[38]

One major problem in the 1970s was the large number of people who needed education about blood pressure, known as the "rule of halves": about half of those with essential hypertension were ignorant of the fact, half of those who were aware of their condition were not taking medication, and half of those taking medication did not have their blood pressure levels under control. The proportion of persons who knew their blood pressure levels increased significantly in the 1980s and 1990s. In 1976–80, 51% of a sample in the National Health and Nutrition Examination Survey were aware that they were hypertensive, 31% were being treated, and 10% had their blood pressures under control. By 1991–94, the proportions had increased to 68%, 53%, and 27% respectively. The latter study used low definitions of essential hypertension (140 mm Hg systolic or 90 mm Hg diastolic or on antihypertensive medication).[39]

Another public health education initiative has been to discover lifestyle changes that can prevent the development of essential hypertension. Stress reduction has been proposed more ardently than any other behavior change, because blood pressures rise with emotional and mental stimuli. (Blood pressure also rises with physical exertion, but no one has claimed that essential hypertension is more prevalent among professional athletes or workers engaged in arduous physical labor.) Despite a multitude of studies, no evidence exists that stress contributes to the development of essential hypertension. One problem is the lack of agreement as to the meaning of stress, according to a 1982 study by the Institute of Medicine of the National Academy of Sciences: "No one has formulated a definition of stress that satisfies even a majority of stress researchers. . . . 'stress' may mean a stimulus, the reaction to that stimulus, or the result of that reaction." Nevertheless, in 1988 the Joint National Committee advocated stress reduction and called "relaxation and biofeedback therapies" "promising," but said that "rigorous clinical trial evaluations" were needed. In its 1997 report the committee decided that relaxation therapy was not a "definitive therapy for prevention of hypertension."[40]

Reduction in salt consumption has been the most popular public health education initiative to prevent hypertension. This is based in part on the "pressure diuresis phenomenon" in the kidneys that reduces fluctuations in blood pressure levels. During periods of elevated blood pressure, such as emotional stress or physical exertion, the kidneys excrete more water and salt (and other electrolytes) into the urine in order to lower the blood pressure. During periods of low blood pressure, such as sleep, they excrete less water and salt in order to maintain or raise it. In persons with essential hypertension, less water and salt are excreted at every blood pressure level. Pressure diuresis is more affected by fluid than by salt intake. Sodium is so critical to human physiology that the body has several mechanisms to stabilize internal sodium balance regardless of variations in salt consumption.[41]

Interest in salt reduction also resulted from studies of the blood pressure levels of more than twenty hunter-gatherer societies. One study from 1929 through the 1960s of the native populations of Kenya and Uganda found that their blood pressure levels were very low and did not increase with age and that coronary heart disease was practically nonexistent among them. The tribes consumed very small amounts of salt because it was not locally available. When individual Kenyans became acculturated to western society, their blood pressures rose to western levels and increased with age. The authors of the study concluded that "ethnic groups who do not add common salt to their food have lifelong low blood pressure; no exception to this generalization has been traced." However, Muntzel and Drueke have observed: "Primitive cultures generally consume relatively large amounts of potassium, drink little or no alcohol, and are primarily vegetarian; fiber intake is greater and consumption of saturated fats is much less. Unacculturated people also tend to be smaller, leaner, and more physically active than their acculturated counterparts; and importantly, they do not gain weight with age." The studies never explained why only consumption of less salt was responsible for the lower blood pressure levels.[42]

Salt consumption has had a major role in the diets of western societies historically and has shown no increase in the last century that corresponded to the increase in coronary heart disease rates. Salting and smoking, especially of pork and fish, were the primary methods of preserving animal protein foods from at least Roman times until the modern era. Tannahill has observed that for most of the medieval era, "salt and smoke were the predominant flavors in the European kitchen for the whole of the winter and spring seasons; it must have been like living today on nothing but cheap factory bacon for half the year." Salt was also used to pickle vegetables and preserve milk in the form of cheese and butter. Many common vegetables, including legumes and potatoes, became popular largely because they neutralized the taste of salt. Europeans reduced their salt consumption somewhat in the late nineteenth century, when improved methods of transportation provided them with fresh meats, fish, grains, fruits, and vegetables from North and South America, Australia, and New Zealand.[43]

In the twentieth century canning, freezing, and refrigeration have practically eliminated the need for salt as a preservative, but salt consumption has remained high. Americans consume an average of about 9,000 milligrams (about 4.5 teaspoons) of salt daily, of which an estimated 75% is introduced during commercial food processing, 15% is added in cooking or at the table, and only 10% comes from salt found naturally in foods. Large amounts of salt are used in processed meats, canned fish, pickled vegetables, "salty snacks" like potato chips, and commercial baked products, including breakfast cereals and pastries. Salt is added to most canned, frozen, and restaurant foods. Other forms of sodium, such as baking powder and baking soda, are also widely used in modern food processing, but only salt (sodium chloride) has been found to affect blood pressure levels.[44]

One theory of the relationship between salt consumption and blood pressure is "salt sensitivity," which states that the ingestion of a given amount of salt raises the blood pressures of some individuals much more than others. Salt sensitivity received its greatest impetus from the researches of Lewis K. Dahl, who bred and studied strains of salt-sensitive and salt-insensitive rats. Salt sensitivity occurs in both normotensive and hypertensive humans and thus is not primarily a characteristic of persons with essential hypertension. Studies of salt sensitivity in humans have suffered from ignorance of such key issues as methods for identifying salt sensitive people, their distribution in the population, the size and duration of the increase in blood pressure necessary to constitute salt sensitivity, the amount of salt required to raise blood pressure, the long-term persistence of salt sensitivity in individuals, and its relationship to cardiovascular disease.[45]

The effect of salt restriction on blood pressure has been examined in short-term experimental studies, which have found that salt deprivation is more likely to reduce blood pressure than salt loading is to raise blood pressure. Most controlled studies of moderate low-salt diets have found that both normotensive and hypertensive participants vary in their responses to a low-salt diet. Three studies of sodium restriction of 2–4 weeks duration that used 119 participants with mild hypertension found almost as many increases as decreases in blood pressure: 26 of the subjects experienced a decrease in their mean arterial pressures of at least 5 mm Hg, 17 experienced an increase of at least 5 mm Hg, and 76 were between the two limits.[46]

The relationship between salt consumption and blood pressure has also been examined in "free-living" populations. Some of the studies examined the relationship between the average salt consumption and the average blood pressure of a number of groups of people, usually without considering other personal characteristics such as age. This method disregards variations in salt consumption and blood pressure in individuals within each group and cannot ascertain whether individuals who are high salt-users have high blood pressures and individuals who are low salt-users have low blood pressures. The groups were not randomly chosen, and sometimes they were selected because they fit the theory. The studies have rarely found a meaningful relationship between salt consumption and blood pressure. Alderman and Lamport observed about the largest of these studies, the 1980s Intersalt study of 52 centers in 32 countries (as discussed in chapter 12), which also examined the relationship between salt consumption and blood pressure in the individuals in each center: "The remarkable findings were that sodium intake varied so little in the vast majority of countries, and that within this 'unusual' range, little relation to pressure could be discerned."[47]

More useful studies examined the relationship between the blood pressure levels of free-living individuals and their dietary sodium consumption, measured by 24–hour urine sodium excretion or dietary histories. Muntzel and Drueke reviewed the studies involving urine sodium excretion, which is considered the superior measure, and concluded that they "indicate little if any association between blood pressure and dietary sodium intake." One of the most thorough and rigorous studies, the Framingham Heart Study, measured salt consumption by both dietary interviews and urine sodium secretion and found no relationship between either measure and blood pressure levels.[48]

Thus many studies using different methods have failed to find a statistical correlation between salt consumption and blood pressure level. Pickering noted that the most striking overall finding is "the remarkable ability of the human body to regulate the sodium content of its plasma despite enormous changes in sodium intake." Drastic reductions in salt intake do reduce blood pressure in the short run, but are unpalatable to most people and require special diets because most salt is added during food processing. A moderate reduction in salt consumption has been demonstrated to be beneficial in many patients who are taking antihypertensive medication because it increases the efficacy of the drugs and permits lower doses.[49]

Despite the lack of evidence, major health organizations have gradually agreed to support a population-wide reduction in salt consumption. In 1977, a U.S. Senate Select Committee held hearings on proposing dietary guidelines for the American population, during which the American Medical Association (AMA) opposed salt guidelines, in part "because of the tremendous range of biologic tolerance in normal human beings, the widely different levels of salt appetite, and the cultural significance which salt has in relation to food." In 1979 the AMA recommended consumption of less than 12,000 mg of salt daily, which was greater than the average intake and therefore meaningless. The American Heart Association (AHA) was cited in the statement of the Salt Institute at the hearings as favoring sodium-restricted diets only in patients with "congestive heart failure and uncontrolled hypertension," preferring the use of diuretics in others with essential hypertension. In 1978 the AHA recommended salt reduction and by 1993 a maximum daily intake of 7,500 milligrams. It acknowledged that in studies of individuals in the same populations "correlations of blood pressure with intake of sodium chloride are modest or nonexistent," that there was "limited or no proven benefit of such restriction for a large segment of the population," and that the "potential benefit is restricted to salt-sensitive hypertensive people." In 1996 the AHA reduced the maximum to 6,000 milligrams of salt per day to conform to federal government guidelines, but conceded that "the recommended guideline is an admittedly arbitrary recommendation for avoiding excessive salt intake rather than an attempt to impose low salt intake."[50]

Federal government and quasi-government agencies have been the most enthusiastic proponents of salt consumption guidelines. Public interest in the subject was shown in 1970 when commercial infant food companies were found to add salt to baby foods solely to make them more palatable to adults. The adverse publicity forced the companies to remove the added salt, even though the American Medical Association and the American Academy of Pediatrics supported the companies. About 1980, the Food and Drug Administration established its Sodium Initiative to reduce salt consumption in the population, claiming that the concept had the support of "most of the leading health and medical experts." In the same year the Food and Nutrition Board of the National Academy of Sciences stated: "The Board believes that sodium chloride intakes of many people in this country are excessive . . . . There is no reason to believe that reduction of sodium chloride intake to levels of [3000 mg] per day would be harmful for healthy persons, and it may be helpful for the prevention of hypertension in susceptible individuals for whom salt is a permissive factor."[51]

Disagreements among health organizations about the benefits of salt reduction was shown in two reports of the National Academy of Sciences. In 1989 its Food and Nutrition Board issued a lengthy report, *Diet and Health,* which stated, "there is still some controversy about the importance of salt in regulation of blood pressure [and] the desirability of recommending to the public that dietary sodium intake should be restricted." It nevertheless recommended that salt consumption be limited to 6,000 mg per day, citing "studies in human populations in different parts of the world" that produced ecological correlations showing that greater consumption "is associated with elevated blood pressure." Two years later the Academy's Institute of Medicine issued its report, *Improving America's Diet and Health,* which agreed with the recommendation but stated that "susceptibility to salt-induced hypertension is probably genetically determined" by unknown factors and that excess salt intake poses a risk only for salt-sensitive people. It also observed that "the salt-sensitive individuals who are likely to benefit most from this recommendation cannot yet be identified." The committee accepted the recommendation of the Food and Nutrition Board only because it believed it would have "no detrimental effect on the general population."[52]

The implementation of the 1990 Nutrition Labeling and Education Act by the Food and Drug Administration, which will be discussed in a later chapter, required the amount of sodium to be listed on the food nutrition label and permitted health claims to be used by food producers. The proposed "model claim statement" read: "Diets low in sodium may reduce the risk of high blood pressure, a disease associated with many factors."[53] Curiously, both the label and the claim disregarded the overwhelming evidence that only sodium chloride, not other forms of dietary sodium, affects blood pressure.

Thus many questions arise when statistical correlations demonstrate a gradient in risk for human characteristics that vary along a continuum. The findings are extremely valuable in characteristics like smoking, which can be eliminated entirely, but they pose major difficulties when the characteristic is physiological, such as blood pressure.

15

THE FRAMINGHAM HEART STUDY AND THE RISK FACTOR

The indication that personal habits and environment are related to the development of coronary heart disease provides a more hopeful outlook than the concept of the disease as an inevitable consequence of genetic make-up or the aging process. Environmental influences are more subject to change, and an unhealthful way of life can be manipulated.

(William Kannel, et al, 1962)[1]

The growing demand for preventive measures for coronary heart disease led to greater use of statistical correlations that related personal characteristics to future mortality rates. This model was applied most successfully in the renowned Framingham Heart Study, a unique long-term epidemiological community study. The Framingham study introduced the life insurance risk factor into research in medicine and public health, but restricted its scope by excluding the many social factors used by the life insurance industry.

As coronary heart disease reached epidemic proportions in the late 1940s, epidemiological studies were undertaken to better understand the etiology of the disease. Most of the studies examined workers in specific occupations or firms, including the Minnesota Business and Professional Men's study, the Albany Cardiovascular Health Study of New York State civil servants, the Chicago Peoples Gas Company study, the Tecumseh (Michigan) Health Study, and the Chicago Western Electric Company study. All used a methodology that had been devised in the late nineteenth century by the life insurance industry: they gave medical examinations to a sample of persons who were free of coronary heart disease and followed them for a number of years to determine the personal characteristics that were associated with higher rates of the disease.[2]

In 1947 the U.S. Public Health Service undertook planning for the Framingham (Massachusetts) Heart Study as a community epidemiological study and in 1949 assigned it to the newly created National Heart Institute of the National Institutes of Health.[3] The unique feature of the Framingham Heart Study was that physicians repeated the medical examinations of participants every two years. The follow-up examinations provided information about illnesses and changes in medical conditions and personal behaviors since the previous examination. The examinations also provided accurate information on all manifestations of coronary heart disease, not just deaths or myocardial infarctions. Study physicians provided no medical care to the participants, except in emergencies, but referred them to their regular sources of care.[4]

Framingham, Massachusetts, was a compact and autonomous industrial and trading center of 28,000 residents located twenty miles west of Boston. Almost all residents were of European ancestry, with more than one-half of Italian or Irish extraction. Framingham was selected because of its political autonomy, the annual town census, nearby medical centers in Boston, the participation of the state health department, and the town's experience with the 1917–23 tuberculosis study described in chapter 7. In order to enlist community support, the study staff organized committees of local citizens and health professionals, used the media to keep the citizens informed, and conducted seminars for local physicians.[5]

Formal sampling procedures based on the town's annual censuses were used to draw a sample of families ages 29–62. Of the 6,507 persons drawn in the sample, only 4,467 (69%) agreed to participate and were also free of coronary heart disease. A supplementary group of 704 volunteers free of coronary heart disease was added. The final sample free of coronary heart disease consisted of 5,127 residents, 55% of whom were women. The self-selection of the supplementary group raised concerns about the representativeness of the sample, but no important differences were found between the supplementary and the original groups.[6]

The Framingham study produced valuable evidence about methodological problems in longitudinal research on the health status of volunteers. Of the original sample, those who agreed to participate were healthier than those who refused as shown by their lower mortality rates for at least six years. Enthusiastic participants were much less likely to withdraw from the study than reluctant ones. After fourteen years, only 2% of the supplementary group of volunteers had dropped out due to refusal to participate. Of the original sample members, 2% of those who were enthusiastic enough to be among the first thousand to receive their initial medical examinations dropped out for the same reason, compared to 11% of the fourth thousand and 16% of the last 469 to be examined. Biennial re-examination rates of those remaining in the study were very high, with 75% of those still alive taking the first eight periodic medical examinations. Clearly, the Framingham study participants were not a representative sample of the city's population.[7]

The study also evaluated the accuracy of reports of causes of death. A panel of study physicians compared its own determination of cause of death for 2,683 participants ages 45 and over to their death certificates through 1988. The study physicians could determine no underlying cause of death for 124 persons (5%). Coronary heart disease was listed as the underlying cause of death on 942 death certificates, but the panel verified only 635 (67%) of them. It added another 123 deaths that were listed on the death certificates as due to other causes, producing 758 deaths from coronary heart disease (30% of deaths from known causes). Agreement was strongly related to age at death: for those dying at ages 45–64, coronary heart was listed on 245 death certificates and 230 of the panel's assessments; for those dying at ages 75 and over, coronary heart disease was the underlying cause of death on 383 death certificates compared to only 262 of the panel's assessments.[8]

The study concluded that coronary heart disease was "a disease which is extremely common and highly lethal, which frequently attacks without warning, and in which the first symptoms are all too often the very last. Also, it is a disease which can be silent even in its most dangerous form." In the study's first fourteen years, 102 men and 18 women died of coronary heart disease before reaching their 65th year. Of the 120 deaths, 66 occurred within one hour of the precipitating events and 78 occurred outside the hospital. Few warning signs preceded these deaths, because 53 of them had no "previous clinical evidence of coronary heart disease" at any time prior to their death. The investigators concluded that "a substantial part of [coronary heart disease] mortality casts only the faintest shadow before it, and that for most persons who died of [coronary heart disease] before age 65, the progression from nil or inapparent disease to death appears to be very swift."[9]

The study also found that both patients and their physicians often failed to recognize myocardial infarctions that occurred between examinations until they were diagnosed electrocardiographically at the next biennial examination. Thirty years of Framingham experience found that 28% of the 469 initial myocardial infarctions in men and 35% of the 239 in women were unrecognized. About one-half produced no symptoms at all and the remainder produced highly atypical symptoms. The proportion of all myocardial infarctions that were unrecognized increased steadily with both blood pressure levels and age for men, but only with blood pressure levels for women. The great danger of an unrecognized myocardial infarction was that it increased the patient's risk of future heart disease as much as a recognized myocardial infarction.[10]

Based on these somber findings, the investigators concluded that prevention was the only practical way to reduce the incidence of coronary heart disease. The physician should use epidemiological findings "to identify disease-prone individuals in his practice, often many years before the occurrence of clinically recognizable disease." If physicians could identify the "environmental and host factors associated with the development of disease," they might be able to prevent or delay the onset of the disease.[11]

The life insurance industry had devised the concept of the "risk factor" in the late nineteenth century precisely for this purpose. The term, defined as a characteristic of an applicant that produced a meaningful increase in the probability of premature death, became identified with the industry. For example, at a symposium on essential hypertension sponsored by the Commonwealth of Massachusetts in 1951, John Morsell observed that "data from life insurance experience constitute a large part of the material on which our knowledge of average [blood] pressures is based, and the hypertensive level has often, as a consequence, been set at the point which is associated with an abnormal mortality experience. . . . For the insurance company this constitutes a significant risk factor."[12]

A concept similar to the risk factor had been used since the 1930s by cancer researchers: the carcinogen. The Office of Science and Technology Policy defined a chemical carcinogen in 1984 as a substance "which either significantly increases the incidence of cancer in animals or humans or significantly decreases the time it takes a naturally-occurring (spontaneous) tumor to develop relative to an appropriate background or control group." Two aspects of risk factors and carcinogens are similar: (1) the comparison of probabilities of future disease occurrence between groups with and without the factors; and (2) an asymptomatic latency period between the presence of the factor and the onset of disease. The carcinogen concept added a third component rarely used in coronary heart disease: the briefer the latency period before a carcinogen produced disease, the greater its carcinogenic properties.[13]

In the 1950s the Framingham researchers adopted the risk factor concept and term directly from the life insurance industry, according to George Mann, one of the original researchers. In 1951, they recognized the importance of its underlying principle of multifactorial etiology: "arteriosclerotic and hypertensive cardiovascular disease . . . do not each have a single cause (as is the case in most infectious diseases), but . . . are the result of multiple causes which work slowly within the individual." In 1959 they referred to "factors believed to be important in the development of coronary heart disease." The term risk factor first appeared in study publications in 1961 as "factors of risk" or "risk factors" that could be identified by the practicing clinician.[14]

Age and sex were the most important risk factors for coronary heart disease in the Framingham sample. Older men and women had significantly higher coronary heart disease rates than younger men and women; men had much higher rates at each age than women; sex differences were greatest in the youngest and least in the oldest age groups; and men had more severe forms of the disease than women. After eight years of the study, 2.4% of men but only 0.1% of women who were ages 30–39 at the beginning of the study had experienced some form of coronary heart disease, including angina pectoris, coronary insufficiency, myocardial infarction, and sudden or other relevant death. The same events occurred in 6.6% of men and 2.0% of women ages 40–49 and 13.1% of men and 6.7% of women ages 50–59. Of the men with coronary heart disease, 63% suffered its most severe forms, death or myocardial infarction, compared to 24% of the women, of whom 67% experienced its mildest form, angina pectoris. The sex differences were not the result of men having higher blood pressures, serum cholesterol levels, or relative weights than women. At every level of each of these factors, coronary heart disease was more prevalent and more severe in men than in women.[15]

The Framingham study also confirmed a number of previously identified risk factors for coronary heart disease in healthy individuals, including blood pressure, serum (blood) cholesterol and other lipids, body weight, and smoking. The Framingham study was among the first to emphasize the dangers of smoking for coronary heart disease. It also found that diabetes, abnormal enlargement of the left ventricle of the heart muscle (left ventricular hypertrophy), and electrocardiographic abnormalities were strongly related to coronary heart disease.[16]

The study examined the effect of diet on blood cholesterol and blood pressure. From 1957 to 1960, the diets of 912 healthy participants, including the wives of the male participants, were studied with much greater care and thoroughness than in most dietary studies. Over the four-year period many participants changed their diets significantly, which indicated that past dietary preferences were poor predictors of present or future preferences. No relationship was found between blood cholesterol levels and the consumption of total calories, dietary cholesterol, animal fats, total fat, and percent of calories from fat, either for men or women. No relationship was found between blood pressure levels and urine sodium excretion or self-reported salt intake, either for men or women.[17]

The Framingham study carried out a one-time examination of physical activity that included both occupational and recreational activities. Questionnaires were used to obtain the information about the activities, but no measurements were made of their intensity or duration. Using these admittedly crude measures, sedentary men were found to be at somewhat greater risk of coronary heart disease than active men, but the benefits were "considerably weaker" than for other major risk factors.[18]

At least one early report examined social risk factors for coronary heart disease. Comparing men of the same ages, after six years less educated men had higher coronary heart disease rates than more educated men, and native-born men had higher coronary heart disease rates than foreign-born men. Blood pressure was examined in relation to occupation, number of jobs, and self-employment, but no consistent differences were found.[19]

One of the Framingham study's most important findings concerned multiple risk factors in the same individual. Persons with multiple risk factors had much higher coronary heart disease rates than indicated by the sum of the risks produced by each factor alone. This was shown by combinations of smoking (21 or more cigarettes daily), high serum cholesterol (250 mg/dl or higher), and high blood pressure (160/95 mm Hg or higher). After eight years of the study, men ages 30–59 with none of the three risk factors had a risk of developing coronary heart disease (excluding angina pectoris) that was one-half of the average of their age group; those with one of the characteristics had a risk slightly above the average of their age group; those with two of the factors had a risk twice that of their age group; and the very few men with all three characteristics had a risk five times that of their age group.[20]

William Kannel, the director of the Framingham study for many years, observed that these findings helped demonstrate that coronary heart disease "is a multifactorial process with no one factor strictly determinative, essential, or sufficient alone to produce the disease." Equally important, the clinical significance of each risk factor depended on the state of other risk factors. Physicians and public health officials needed to be concerned with the combination of risk factors in patients, not with each factor considered in isolation.[21]

Framingham investigators had a much more restricted concept of risk factors than did the life insurance industry or cancer researchers. This resulted from their early decision to make risk factors useful to the practicing physician.[22] Despite some promising early findings, they disregarded social characteristics such as education, income, occupation, living conditions, usual sources of health care, marital status, place of birth, and family structure. Yet social characteristics are as important as physiological ones in clinical decisions. Furthermore, the Framingham Heart Study was an epidemiological study, with all that implied concerning social and environmental causes of disease. The narrow focus of this pioneering study established a unfortunate precedent for most subsequent studies.

Several basic differences existed between the old life insurance risk factor and the new medical risk factor popularized by the Framingham study. The life insurance risk factor was conceived in terms of a gradient of risk depending on its level, while medical risk factors were often dichotomized into healthy and unhealthy levels. Each life insurance risk factor was related to all other risk factors, while each of the new medical risk factors was usually considered separately. Last, the life insurance risk factor emphasized both the social and medical characteristics of the applicant, while the medical risk factor was restricted to medical characteristics. The more restrictive concept of the medical risk factor created numerous difficulties as the concept became more widely used.

16

THEORIES OF THE CAUSES OF CORONARY HEART DISEASE

> Medicine is widely held to be a science, but many medical decisions do not rely on a strong scientific foundation, simply because such a foundation has yet to be fully explored and developed. Hence, what often happens in the decision-making process is a complicated inter-action of scientific evidence, patient desire, doctor preferences and all sorts of exogenous influences, some of which may be quite irrelevant.[1]

The analysis thus far has concerned risk factors that are associated with a number of diseases besides coronary heart disease. Risk factors specific to coronary heart disease are based on theories of the vascular changes that reduce blood flow to the heart muscle, with each theory being associated with different types of treatments.

Coronary Atherosclerosis and Coronary Thrombosis

All theories of the etiology of coronary heart disease seek to explain its defining characteristic, the diminution of blood flow to the heart muscle. Early in the twentieth century, the primary cause was considered to be a thrombus (clot) in one of the coronary arteries. A thrombus can form on the inner wall of the coronary artery and block or reduce blood flow at that point or it can form elsewhere, break loose, and flow in the bloodstream until it becomes lodged in the lumen (hollow center) of a coronary artery. The obstruction can produce sudden death, myocardial infarction, angina pectoris, or other forms of coronary heart disease.[2]

The coronary thrombosis theory focused on the obstruction because it considered subsequent events like myocardial infarctions to be consequences. However, evidence soon accumulated that coronary heart disease could develop without the presence of a fresh thrombus and that thrombosis did not produce coronary heart disease when collateral circulation had developed in other coronary arteries.[3]

Beginning in the 1940s, coronary atherosclerosis became accepted as the primary cause of the growing coronary heart disease epidemic. Atherosclerosis is the buildup inside an artery wall of an atheroma, a gelatinous plaque composed of cholesterol and other blood components. Atherosclerosis diminishes blood flow by making the artery wall less elastic and reducing the size of the lumen. Coronary atherosclerosis was found in many cases of coronary heart disease and was most common in the elderly, who had the highest rates of the disease. The greatest impetus for the coronary atherosclerosis theory resulted from an autopsy study reported in 1953. Two physicians in the Armed Forces Institute of Pathology described three hundred autopsies of American soldiers, almost all under age 33, who were killed in action in the Korean War. Coronary atherosclerosis was observed in many of these young men, which shocked the medical and public health communities. The findings suggested that the coronary heart disease epidemic was expanding beyond the elderly to threaten the entire adult male population.[4]

This inference was not supported by the statistical findings of the study. Only 3% of the Korean War soldiers experienced total blockage of one or more coronary arteries and another 8% experienced blockages of 70% or more. The sample size was so small that another sample could have produced quite different rates. The personal and social characteristics of the soldiers were not examined to see if they were representative of Korean War soldiers or American young men.

Furthermore, the history of atherosclerosis indicates that coronary atherosclerosis was equally prevalent in autopsy studies undertaken decades earlier. Atherosclerosis is a form of arteriosclerosis, a term coined about 1830 to describe thickening and loss of elasticity of arterial walls. The term atherosclerosis was created in 1904, but was not widely used for many years. During the Franco-Prussian War of 1871–72, German pathologists were surprised to find coronary arteriosclerosis, mostly atherosclerosis, in autopsies of deceased young soldiers. Their successors therefore carefully investigated the coronary and other arteries of deceased German soldiers in the First World War (1914–18). About 30% of autopsied soldiers under age 20 had arteriosclerosis in some artery in the body, as did 50% to 90% of those ages 30–45. One study found arteriosclerosis in the coronary arteries of 11% of soldiers ages 15–25, 23% of those ages 25–30, and 27% of those ages 30–35. These rates were similar to those found in the Korean War soldiers.[5]

American autopsy studies in the early twentieth century also discovered that coronary atherosclerosis was common among the young. One study found coronary atherosclerosis in 18% of 575 autopsies of men and women ages 21–40 in Boston, Massachusetts between 1925 and 1937, with 75% of the cases occurring in men. Autopsies of a very small sample of male cancer and accident patients ages 40–49 in New Haven, Connecticut, found coronary atherosclerosis in 34% of 53 cases in 1935–44 and 58% of 36 cases in 1945–54. Much later, an autopsy study about 1970 of 105 American soldiers killed in the Vietnam War found some degree of coronary atherosclerosis in 45% of the soldiers and "severe" atherosclerosis in 5%.[6]

The atherosclerosis theory of coronary heart disease is based on the physical properties of arteries. The thicker outer and middle layers of arteries contain muscle tissue and elastic fibers that enable the artery to expand and contract when the pulsating blood flows through it. Arteries are so elastic that the lumen must be narrowed to about one-third of its original diameter to produce significant restriction of blood flow. The outer layer also contains blood vessels that supply the artery with blood and agents used for repair when injury occurs. The inner layer contains an elastic membrane and the endothelium or inner lining of the artery wall, which consists of smooth cells that prevent platelets in the flowing blood from adhering to it. Atheromas develop in the inner layer adjoining the endothelium. Atheromas in the coronary arteries are especially likely to obstruct blood flow because their lumens are less than one-eighth inch in diameter. Yet coronary arteries are so elastic that fewer than one-third of adults with coronary atherosclerosis develop coronary heart disease.[7]

The physical structure of arteries makes the determination of atherosclerosis surprisingly difficult. The great majority of atheromas are benign and not associated with coronary heart disease. These are soft and fatty yellowish spots or streaks containing mostly cholesterol that can cover as much as one-fourth of the inner surface of the artery. One study of 1,600 autopsies in New Orleans beginning in the 1950s found streaks in the aortas of many children under age 3 and in all children above that age. Benign atheromas rarely occurred in the coronary arteries of children under age 10, but were present in more than 90% of the coronary arteries of both men and women ages 20 and above. These kinds of atheromas were first reported in 1837 and have been found in nonwestern societies where coronary heart disease is rare. Atherosclerosis can also be confused with normal changes in artery walls. During the first fifty years of life artery walls gradually become thicker, stronger, and less elastic due to an increase of muscle and elastic material in the middle and outer layers and finally additional inelastic fibrous connective tissue. These changes can produce a stiffening and a sinuous narrowing of the lumen that resemble atherosclerosis.[8]

The causes of atherosclerosis have received considerable attention. The most widely accepted theory is that atherosclerosis is produced by an excessive amount of cholesterol and other lipids circulating in the blood. The excess cholesterol adheres to the artery wall and forms atheromas. The strongest evidence in support of this process is familial hypercholesterolemia, a hereditary condition characterized by extremely high blood cholesterol levels. Persons with this condition have very high rates of atherosclerosis and coronary heart disease and often nodules composed largely of cholesterol (xanthomas) under the skin.

A contrasting theory holds that atherosclerosis is caused by a defective repair of damage to some part of the endothelium, the inside lining of the artery wall. This theory was proposed by the great German pathologist Rudolph Virchow (1821–1902) and extended in 1946 by the English physician J. B. Duguid. The endothelium sometime becomes damaged and ulcerates due to wear and tear from blood flow and other factors. A clot or thrombus, an easily crumbled mass of fibrin and blood platelets from the bloodstream, adheres to the ulcer to repair the damage. If the repaired site has an insufficient blood flow to carry away the damaged material, the thrombus can enlarge by accumulating cholesterol, platelets, dead cells, collagen, and fibrous material. New endothelial cells can then form over the thrombus so that it becomes part of the inner layer of the artery. Its contents gradually break down into "semi-fluid or paste-like" atheromas that "persist as areas of fatty degeneration," according to Duguid.[9]

Some blood vessels, including coronary arteries, are especially susceptible to ulceration because of the fluid dynamics of blood flow. Atherosclerosis occurs most often in arteries where blood flows under high pressure, less often in arteries subject to moderate blood pressure, and rarely in veins, where blood pressure is lowest. This is shown in coronary artery bypass grafts, where veins are grafted in place of damaged coronary arteries. The veins are subjected to much higher than normal blood pressures and develop atheromas frequently and quickly. The grafting process does not cause the atheromas, because arteries that are used as grafts rarely develop them. Higher blood pressures and greater ulceration occur where arteries curve, taper, bifurcate, and branch. Coronary arteries are particularly vulnerable because they undergo bending and twisting dozens of times each minute with every beat of the heart muscle.[10]

Supporters of the thrombus theory have observed that coronary thrombi observed in autopsies often look like atheromas because the thrombi begin to lose their red color after a few days. Patients who were autopsied some time after a fatal myocardial infarction can appear to have coronary atherosclerosis when they actually experienced thrombosis. Older coronary thrombi that have lost their red color can also be confused with atherosclerosis at autopsy. Some experts claim that this mistaken identification has been very common.[11]

Treatment Controversies in Coronary Heart Disease

The thrombosis and atherosclerosis theories have produced different treatments for coronary heart disease. The early popularity of the thrombosis theory produced the first treatments in the late 1930s, the anticoagulants heparin and dicumerol. Anticoagulants can prevent clots from forming but do not dissolve preexisting clots and can produce bleeding complications. Regardless, they were soon used to treat preexisting clots in myocardial infarction without success and with frequent adverse consequences. Subsequent studies found them to be appropriate preventive measures in patients with a high risk of future thrombosis.[12]

The first thrombolytic drug that dissolved clots, streptokinase, was discovered in the 1930s and found in the 1940s to dissolve preexisting clots in coronary arteries. By the late 1950s improved preparations produced fewer adverse reactions, although the risks of bleeding and other serious complications remained. Between 1959 and 1979 more than twenty randomized clinical trials were conducted, most in Europe. Some of them showed benefits from the drug, but the findings were far from conclusive. Nevertheless, in his 1994 history of cardiology, Louis J. Acierno called thrombolytic therapy "one of the most exciting advances during the twentieth century." Yet thrombolytic therapy became widely used only in the 1980s. In 1994 a panel of experts in emergency medicine recommended that all patients with myocardial infarctions receive thrombolytic drugs within thirty minutes of arrival in an emergency room.[13]

The slow acceptance of thrombolytic therapy, followed by its rather abrupt adoption, is a puzzling issue in the history of the treatment of coronary heart disease. Thrombolytic drugs had to be administered within a few hours of the myocardial infarction and sometimes caused bleeding or failed to dissolve clots or prevent reocclusion, but these problems remained when the drugs became popular. The early clinical trials of thrombolytic drugs produced mixed results, but equally inconclusive clinical trials of drugs to treat mild hypertension did not delay their adoption. Streptokinase was not patented and pharmaceutical firms did not promote its use, but other sources of information were readily available. A controversy developed over whether thrombi preceded or followed myocardial infarctions, but leading pathologists consistently insisted that thrombosis caused infarctions.[14]

The most plausible explanation is the preference of American surgeons and invasive cardiologists for the atherosclerosis theory. In the 1950s and 1960s a number of technical innovations made surgery on the heart and arteries feasible. In the late 1960s surgeons first performed coronary artery bypass graft surgery, in which the sternum was split in two, the heart was stopped, and sections of one or more atherosclerotic coronary arteries were bypassed using veins surgically removed from the patient's leg. The procedure was originally intended to relieve a severe form of angina pectoris in patients who were otherwise healthy and able to survive the operation. According to Thomas Killip, early coronary artery bypass graft surgery increased blood flow and relieved symptoms in "properly selected cases" and was "received enthusiastically, and often uncritically." It was soon extended to other forms of coronary atherosclerosis and in 1980 more than 110,000 operations were performed. In 1996, 666,000 operations were performed, twice the per capita rate of 1990, at a cost of many billions of dollars.[15]

Beginning in the late 1970s, critics claimed that coronary artery bypass surgery was being used excessively and inappropriately in the United States. American surgeons performed 58% of all coronary bypass operations worldwide in 1988. The procedure had operative mortality rates ranging from 1%–2% to 5%–6% at different medical centers in the late 1970s, and myocardial infarctions sometimes occurred in other patients. From 12% to 20% of the grafted veins developed atherosclerosis within a year. A 1984 study found that when the blockage in an artery was less than 50%, the replacement vein would probably become occluded sooner than the artery it replaced. In addition, safer and less expensive drug therapy was available for the milder forms of coronary heart disease.[16]

As an alternative to bypass surgery, cardiologists adopted another procedure based on the atherosclerosis theory, called angioplasty or balloon angioplasty. In 1977 a German cardiologist devised a method of inserting a catheter with a balloon tip in an artery and guiding it into the atherosclerotic coronary artery. The balloon was then inflated to dilate the lumen and increase blood flow through it. Angioplasty was designed for severe forms of angina pectoris, but it was soon used for other forms of coronary heart disease, including myocardial infarctions. It was safer than bypass surgery, but within six months one-third of the arteries were sufficiently reoccluded to require either another angioplasty or a bypass operation. The procedure quickly became extremely popular, largely because cardiologists saw the patients first and could perform an angioplasty instead of referring them to surgeons for bypass surgery. The number of angioplasties increased from 10,000 in 1981 to almost 400,000 in 1992, at a total annual cost of $10 billion for the angioplasties and procedures to correct subsequent blockages. American cardiologists performed 68% of all angioplasties worldwide in 1988.[17]

Thus by the 1980s three different treatments were available for coronary heart disease: drugs for the milder cases and coronary artery bypass graft surgery and angioplasty for the more severe cases. The most vexing social and economic problems were the enormous cost of the latter two, which were performed on many patients who could have been treated with drugs. The costs included both the direct costs of the procedures and the indirect costs of the reocclusions or related heart conditions that occurred in the majority of both kinds of patients.[18]

Clinical trials were soon undertaken to produce statistical comparisons of the benefits of the procedures. The ensuing debates were widely publicized in the mass media, such as these headlines in the *New York Times*: In 1988, "Findings are in Conflict on Value of Coronary Bypass Operations" and "Report Assails Emergency Heart Procedures" (angioplasty); in 1990, "Many Men with Angina Don't Need Bypass Surgery"; in 1993, "Study Finds Angioplasty as Good as Heart Bypass" and "Experts Split on Two Ways to Treat Heart Attack"; and in 1996, "No Difference Seen in Death Rates for 2 Heart Attack Treatments" (angioplasty and thrombolytic drugs).[19]

The most acrimonious debates concerned the validity of the statistical comparisons. As an example, the first controlled clinical trial that compared coronary bypass surgery and medication in the late 1970s found no differences in survival rates between the two groups except for patients with one specific condition. Surgeons complained that the findings were obsolete by the time the study was published because new operative techniques had improved bypass surgery. They protested that the hospitals used in the study lacked the expertise of the best centers. They belittled the statistical comparisons by describing short-term improvements in carefully selected patients.[20]

In order to resolve the controversies, expert panels and studies endeavored to identify the specific forms of coronary heart disease most appropriate for each method of treatment. In 1980 a federal advisory panel concluded that coronary artery bypass surgery was a "major advance" but that patients with mild symptoms could be treated with drugs at less risk and cost. In 1988, the American Heart Association and the American College of Cardiology recommended angioplasty for treating angina pectoris in men younger than age 65 without high blood pressure or diabetes, who had blockage in a small uncalcified single coronary artery. A 1991 committee of the British Cardiac Society recommended angioplasty when the blockages were "discrete, short, proximal enough to be reached by the balloon catheter, and preferably not in the immediate vicinity of acute bends or large side branches." A 1990 study of patients with angina pectoris found that coronary artery bypass surgery was superior to drugs where the heart's pumping action was weakened by previous myocardial infarctions.[21]

Many specialists disregarded the recommendations and continued to press for the broadest possible use of their own procedures. In 1995 the *New York Times* reported that a "rancorous debate" over the benefits of angioplasty and thrombolytic drugs divided cardiologists at the annual meeting of the American College of Cardiology. A 1994 recommendation concerning emergency room treatment of myocardial infarction was designed partly to "eliminate jurisdictional battles and disputes among emergency doctors, cardiologists, internists, family doctors, and other medical specialists who compete to care for heart attack patients," according to an article in the *New York Times*. The economic stakes were enormous: in the mid-1990s coronary artery bypass surgery was the most frequently performed major operation in the country and cardiologists who performed angioplasties earned considerably more than other cardiologists.[22]

Surgeons and cardiologists also extended the use of coronary artery bypass surgery and angioplasty to the very old, who had previously been considered unsuitable for such aggressive interventions. The new policy was justified by improvements in the procedures and the risks of no treatment, but another factor was the availability of fewer younger patients as coronary heart disease rates declined. A 1994 study concluded that both procedures were often performed on elderly persons who could have been treated as effectively and much more safely with drugs.[23]

Thus the atherosclerosis theory emerged as the primary basis for the treatment of serious coronary heart disease. It had equally significant consequences for the prevention of all forms of coronary heart disease.

17

THE DIET-HEART HYPOTHESIS

> This is a time when great pressure is being put on physicians to do
> something about the reported increased death rate from heart attacks
> in relatively young people. People want to know whether they are eat-
> ing themselves into premature heart disease.
>
> (Nutrition Committee, American Heart Association, 1957)[1]

The diet-heart or lipid hypothesis, based on the atherosclerosis theory of coronary heart disease, consists of a sequence of events involving dietary cholesterol
and fats, blood cholesterol, atherosclerosis, and ultimately coronary heart disease. The most rigorous statistical studies have shown very weak or nonexistent
relationships between diet or blood cholesterol and coronary heart disease.

Blood Cholesterol Levels and
Coronary Heart Disease Rates

The underlying factor in the atherosclerosis theory of coronary heart disease is cholesterol in the human body. Cholesterol is found in all cell mem-
branes and is especially prevalent in organs like the brain, liver, and kidneys; it plays a key role in the production of some hormones, steroids, and
vitamin D; and it is converted to bile that is essential for digestion. Choles-

terol tends to accumulate in atheromas because it is a lipid, a fatty or greasy compound that does not dissolve in water or blood and so cannot be removed by circulating blood. Cholesterol was identified and labeled in the early nineteenth century and its presence in atheromas was noted a century later.

Cholesterol in the human body is obtained from both external and internal sources. About one-third of the cholesterol found in the intestine comes from the consumption of animal foods, primarily meat, eggs, and dairy products. Two-thirds comes from internal synthesis in the intestines and liver. The human body regulates the total amount of its blood cholesterol by balancing internal synthesis and dietary intake.[2]

Cholesterol is transported from its sources in the intestine and liver to cells by flowing through the blood as lipoproteins, a soluble chemical combination of cholesterol and certain proteins. About 1950 John Gofman and his coworkers differentiated several types of lipoproteins according to their densities. The low density lipoproteins (LDL) transport 60%–70% of the cholesterol through the blood, the high density lipoproteins (HDL) transport 20%–30%, and the very low density lipoproteins (VLDL) transport 10%–15%. LDL contain 40%–45% cholesterol, VLDL contain 10%–20%, and HDL contain 18%. Each type of lipoprotein also contains varying amounts of protein and two other lipids, triglycerides and phospholipids. HDL is believed to remove excess cholesterol from the blood, but the evidence has been inconclusive.[3]

The atherosclerosis theory of coronary heart disease consists of a three step process: high levels of cholesterol in the blood lead to its accumulation in the arteries as atherosclerosis, which in turn increases the risk of coronary heart disease. The theory is therefore based on three statistical correlations. One is the correlation between the level of blood cholesterol and the amount of atherosclerosis in the arteries. which has been supported by autopsy studies. The second is the correlation between the amount of atherosclerosis in the arteries and coronary heart disease, which has also been supported by autopsy studies.[4]

The third correlation, between blood cholesterol levels and coronary heart disease rates, is an indirect relationship. According to statistical theory, indirect relationship always have weaker correlations than direct relationships. In this case, it is because atherosclerosis is produced by many factors besides blood cholesterol levels and coronary heart disease is produced by many factors besides atherosclerosis.

The relationship between blood cholesterol and coronary heart disease was examined in a number of prospective epidemiological studies that measured the blood cholesterol levels in a sample, followed the sample for a period of time, and compared the coronary heart disease rates of persons with different blood cholesterol levels. The pathbreaking and most rigorous study was the Framingham heart study. Based on thirty years of experience, the study found a statistical correlation between blood cholesterol and cardiovascular disease mortality rates for men who were ages 31–47 and women who were ages 40–47 at the study's inception. It found no correlation for men and women who were ages 48–65 and women who were ages 31–39 when the study began. These inconsistencies suggest that the correlations were fortuitous.[5]

Three larger studies used persons who were healthy enough to be employed or attend medical school, which reduced the number of unknown factors that could have caused any differences in outcomes. One study followed 9,902 male Israeli government employees ages 40 and over for 23 years. The sample had a mortality rate early in the study that was only 80% of the comparable Israeli Jewish population. The subgroups with cholesterol levels of less than 187 mg/dl and with levels of 188–216 mg/dl had similar coronary heart disease mortality rates, but the subgroup with levels above 216 mg/dl had higher rates. A study of 1,017 male students at the Johns Hopkins University medical school from 1949 to 1964 followed the members of the sample until 1991. The proportions in four subgroups with different blood cholesterol levels who developed angina pectoris or myocardial infarction were as follows: 118–172 mg/dl, 7%; 173–189 mg/dl, 12%; 190–208 mg/dl, 18%; 209–315 mg/dl, 35%. An English study followed 17,718 male civil servants ages 40–64 from 1967–69 to 1987 and found unusually high coronary heart disease mortality rates only in the subgroup with the highest serum cholesterol levels (227 mg/dl and above).[6]

The type of statistical correlation found in all three studies is a curvilinear relationship: groups with the highest blood cholesterol levels had the highest coronary heart disease rates, but groups with average and below average blood cholesterol levels had similar rates. The relationship between cholesterol level and coronary heart disease would be even weaker if it were possible to remove persons with the genetic disorder familial hypercholesterolemia from the high blood cholesterol group. By contrast, the relationships involving blood pressure or smoking are linear, with the highest levels having the highest coronary heart disease rates and the lowest levels having the lowest rates.

Drug Treatment of High Blood Cholesterol

As with essential hypertension, concern with blood cholesterol as a medical problem received its greatest stimulus from the development of drugs that

lowered blood cholesterol levels effectively. The earliest drugs, such as nia-
cin, were of limited benefit and had unpleasant side effects. The first modern cholesterol-lowering drug, clofibrate, was approved in 1967 after being
widely used in Europe. Clinical trials of clofibrate through the 1980s found
few statistically significant differences in coronary heart disease rates between treatment and placebo groups. Nevertheless, a 1985 consensus conference convened by the National, Heart, Lung and Blood Institute concluded that "reduction of blood cholesterol levels in people with relatively
high initial levels will reduce the rate of coronary heart disease," even though
"no study considered individually could be regarded as conclusive." In 1989,
the director of the Institute was less sanguine: "I do not think that the case
for cholesterol reduction has been proved to the degree we all would prefer." Nevertheless, billions of dollars worth of cholesterol lowering drugs
were sold in the 1970s and 1980s.[7]

In the 1990s a new class of statin drugs was examined in two major
clinical trials. One five-year study screened 80,000 Scottish male volunteers to obtain a sample of 6,595 men with an average age of 55 years and
extremely high blood cholesterol levels (an average of 272 mg/dl). Fifteen
percent of the sample had high blood pressure, 44% were smokers, and
34% were ex-smokers. The average blood cholesterol level of the treatment
group declined to 218 mg/dl after taking the drug while that of the placebo
group remained unchanged. The study divided the sample into a statin
drug group and a placebo group for five years and found that a myocardial
infarction or death from coronary heart disease occurred in 7.9% of the
placebo group (about 1.6% per year) compared to 5.5% of the treatment
group (about 1.1% per year). Thus the statin drugs lowered the risk of
severe coronary heart disease by about 0.5% per year in a group of men in
their late fifties who had extremely high blood cholesterol levels and a very
high rate of present or past cigarette smoking.[8]

The other major clinical trial screened 100,000 American volunteers
to obtain a sample of 6,605 men and women with an average age of 58
years and an average blood cholesterol of 221 mg/dl, which was normal for
the age group. Twenty percent were taking antihypertensive medication
and only 12% were current smokers. The average blood cholesterol level of
the treatment group declined to 184 mg/dl after one year while that of the
placebo group remained unchanged. After five years the study found that, per
100 patient-years, 1.1 of the placebo group compared to 0.7 of the treatment
group had a myocardial infarction, unstable angina, or sudden death. Thus
this trial reduced the risk of severe coronary heart disease in a group of volunteers in their late fifties with normal blood cholesterol levels by 0.4% per year.[9]

The unimpressive findings of these studies, which were financed by the pharmaceutical companies that manufactured the drugs, were exaggerated in the published reports. Instead of describing the arithmetic differences in event rates, they cited the percentage difference. One report described a 31% reduction in end points instead of a 0.5% annual difference between treatment and placebo groups, while the other claimed a 37% reduction instead of a 0.4% annual difference. In addition, the circumstances of the trials differed greatly from the standard practice of medicine. An observation by Allan Brett concerning clinical trials of earlier cholesterol-lowering drugs is appropriate: "The modest benefits . . . were achieved in a carefully orchestrated setting that included highly motivated patients and physicians, expert dietary counseling, and free care. It is unclear whether such programs can be duplicated in conventional practice settings." Regardless, lovastatin, the first statin drug, quickly became the most popular cholesterol-lowering drug despite its high cost and was prescribed to 2.8 million Americans in 1993.[10]

Cholesterol-lowering drugs produced the same public health issue that was so controversial in blood pressure: what was the minimum blood cholesterol level that benefited from medication? As with blood pressure, the blood cholesterol levels recommended for treatment were below those justified by the statistical evidence. In 1972, a joint committee of the American Medical Association and the Food and Nutrition Board of the National Academy of Sciences concluded that the risk of coronary heart disease was "relatively small" at levels less than 220 mg/dl. In 1982, the American Heart Association agreed and stated that the relationship between blood cholesterol and coronary heart disease "probably is curvilinear, so that above a certain 'threshold' region [of 200–220 mg/dl], risk accelerates with rising cholesterol levels." Despite the consensus of both recommendations, the AHA proposed an "ideal range of 130–190 mg/dl." By 1993, the National Cholesterol Education Program (NCEP) of the National Institutes of Health and the AHA both accepted the curvilinear relationship but recommended levels of "less than 200 mg/dl as desirable."[11]

These recommendations were designed to affect many millions of Americans. In 1990, blood cholesterol levels of 200 mg/dl or greater were found in close to one-half of all adults ages 35–44 and more than two-thirds of those ages 45 and over. Thus, according to the NCEP and the AHA, about 63 million adults in the United States in 1990 had undesirably high blood cholesterol levels. In 1985 a consensus conference of the National Institutes of Health defined "severe" high blood cholesterol as 240 mg/dl or higher, levels that occurred in 1990 in one-seventh of those

35–44, one-fourth of those 45–54, and one-third of those 55–64 and 65–74. Under this definition, 25 million Americans had severe high blood cholesterol.[12]

Health education programs for the 63 million adults with blood cholesterol levels of 200 mg/dl or higher would produce enormous demands on the American health care system. All of them would be urged to change their diets, which would often require professional counseling and monitoring. All 63 million would require annual or biennial blood tests to measure their blood cholesterol levels. Very few of these millions of persons would benefit from such a massive and costly program.

Physicians have become more concerned with blood cholesterol. In the early 1980s, a survey of 221 California physicians, mostly family physicians, found that only 34% felt that "raised blood cholesterol" had a "large effect on coronary heart disease," compared to about 80% who felt the same way about cigarette smoking and high blood pressure. In 1988 a survey of 633 midwest physicians found many more, 68%, who agreed that high blood cholesterol had a "substantial effect" on coronary heart disease, compared to 90% who agreed with regard to cigarette smoking and 80% for high blood pressure. Surveys of 1,277 internists, cardiologists, and family physicians in 1986 and 1,604 of them in 1990 found that the proportion who knew their own blood cholesterol level increased from 65% to 87%. The proportion who would institute drug treatment at blood cholesterol levels of 260 mg/dl or lower increased from less than one-third in 1986 to three-fourths in 1990. In 1990, according to the report, one-half of the physicians "thought that the current emphasis on high blood cholesterol was producing needless anxiety in their patients."[13]

Public attitudes changed in similar ways. Public opinion surveys of about two thousand adults found that the proportion who had heard of high blood cholesterol increased from 77% in 1983 to 93% in 1990, and the proportion who had their own level checked increased from 35% to 65%. Both the public and physicians considered blood cholesterol to have less impact on coronary heart disease than smoking and blood pressure.[14]

Dietary Cholesterol

Cholesterol in foods of animal origin is another key factor in the atherosclerosis theory of coronary heart disease. It adds an initial fourth step to the process: the consumption of foods with large amounts of cholesterol raises the blood cholesterol level, which increases atherosclerosis, which increases the risk of coronary heart disease. Because blood cholesterol, atherosclerosis, and coronary heart disease are all affected by factors in addition to dietary cholesterol, the statistical correlation between dietary cholesterol and coronary heart disease will be lower than any of the more direct correlations.

A finding that dietary cholesterol affects the development of atherosclerosis was first made in 1913 when rabbits fed cholesterol developed atheromas. The relevance of this finding to humans has been widely questioned. Cholesterol is found only in foods of animal origin, which rabbits are not biologically adapted to eat. The rabbits consumed enormous amounts of cholesterol. The deposits of cholesterol in the arteries of rabbits did not resemble human atherosclerosis and they also developed deposits of cholesterol in organs in which it has never been found in humans. Critics have called the cholesterol deposits in the rabbits a generalized lipid storage disease. Similar studies have used other animals, but no animal study has produced the sequence of events that occurs in humans.[15]

Most studies of humans have endeavored to establish a correlation between the consumption of foods containing cholesterol and blood cholesterol levels. The most thorough studies were conducted about mid-century by Ancel Keys. In one short-term experiment, twenty-seven men were fed either low or high cholesterol diets for four weeks and then switched to the other diet; trivial changes occurred in their blood cholesterol levels. As a long-term study, Keys examined groups of men in two towns on the island of Sardinia whose diets were practically identical except for egg consumption, which constitutes the single largest source of cholesterol in most human diets. He found no differences in blood cholesterol levels despite a two- and three-fold difference in cholesterol consumption. He did cross-sectional and longitudinal studies of men in Minnesota who consumed widely varying amounts of cholesterol and again found no relationship between the consumption of foods containing cholesterol and blood cholesterol levels. In 1956 he concluded: "the foregoing evidence is definitive, we think, in showing that variations in the intake of cholesterol over the whole range of natural diets do not influence the serum [cholesterol] level of physically active normal adult men so long as other elements in the diet are constant."[16]

Subsequent studies have confirmed Keys's findings. The Framingham heart study conducted an extremely thorough dietary study of 912 participants from 1957 to 1960 and found "no indication of a relationship between dietary cholesterol and serum cholesterol level," even when animal fat intake was considered. A review of a large number of studies also con-

cluded that variations in cholesterol consumption do not affect blood cholesterol, with one exception. In places where practically no animal food
(and therefore no cholesterol) is consumed, the consumption of animal
foods will raise blood cholesterol levels significantly. These and many other
studies led Keys to reiterate his position in 1991: "Many controlled experiments have shown that dietary cholesterol has a limited effect in humans.
Adding cholesterol to a cholesterol-free diet raises the blood [cholesterol] level
in humans, but when added to an unrestricted diet it has a minimal effect."[17]

Despite the lack of statistical correlations in studies relating dietary
cholesterol intake to blood cholesterol levels, private and government health
organizations have adopted the position that dietary cholesterol affects the
risk of coronary heart disease. This was not the case in 1956, when a joint
symposium of the National Heart Institute and the American Heart Association rejected concern with dietary cholesterol as "an insignificant atherogenic factor." In 1959, the American Heart Association was reported as
stating that "there is not enough cholesterol in eggs, compared with the
amount normally in the body, to make any difference." But beginning in
1973, the AHA, and later federal government agencies, recommended that
the daily consumption of dietary cholesterol be less than 300 milligrams,
which is between three-fourths and one-half of the daily consumption of
most people. In 1996, the American Heart Association conceded that "there
is considerable interindividual variation in response to dietary cholesterol,
which should be considered when making individual dietary recommendations." Frederick Stare and others observed in 1989 that the 300 milli-
gram amount "is arbitrary and more or less meaningless from a physiological standpoint. The figure does not represent any demonstrated change in
risk in any clinical study."[18]

Dietary Fats and Oils

The effect of diet on coronary heart disease was soon expanded beyond
dietary cholesterol to include fats and oils. Dietary fats and oils are components of animal and vegetable foods and an essential part of the human
diet: they are sources of fat-soluble vitamins like vitamin A, they are synthesized by the body into fatty acids that are a major source of energy, they
reduce gastric motility, and they make it possible to avoid bulky and unpalatable diets. Essential fatty acids, which are required in small quantities by
the body and are not synthesized internally, are obtained from animal and
vegetable fats.[19]

Vegetable oils, fish oils, and animal fats are often differentiated from each other by their melting temperatures. Some fats are solid at room temperature, such as butter, coconut oil, palm oil, and rendered animal fats like beef and chicken fat and lard. Others, including olive oil and fish oils, are naturally liquid at room temperature or, as in vegetable oils, are rendered liquid at room temperature by a complex industrial process. The melting temperature of a fat can be raised by partial hydrogenation, which also reduces its susceptibility to oxidation and rancidity.[20]

The melting temperatures of fats and oils are determined by the types of fatty acids that comprise them. All fats and oils are composed of varying proportions of saturated, monounsaturated, and polyunsaturated fatty acids, each subdivided into more specific kinds of fatty acids. Saturated fatty acids, which have the highest melting temperatures, predominate in butter and meat fats, monounsaturated fatty acids predominate in olive oil, and polyunsaturated fatty acids predominate in many vegetable oils. Partial hydrogenation of a vegetable oil increases the proportion of saturated fatty acids, usually by a small amount. Essential fatty acids are obtained from polyunsaturated fats in plant foods or herbivorous animals.[21]

The effect of fat and oil consumption on human blood cholesterol levels was first examined in the 1950s. E. H. Ahrens, Jr. and others used controlled laboratory feeding experiments with human subjects that varied the consumption of saturated and unsaturated fatty acids while keeping the total number of calories constant. Consumption of large amounts of fats with high concentrations of saturated fatty acids raised total blood cholesterol and LDL levels, while their replacement with fats with high concentrations of unsaturated fatty acids either lowered or did not raise the levels. The degree of saturation was shown to be a causal factor because increased saturation of vegetable oils by hydrogenation affected blood cholesterol levels in a manner similar to oils with the same levels of saturation naturally. Later feeding studies showed that specific kinds of fatty acids had different effects on blood cholesterol levels. Stearic acid, a saturated fatty acid that is a major component of the fats in beef, pork, butter, and chocolate, has little effect on blood cholesterol levels. Fats high in polyunsaturated fatty acids tend to lower blood cholesterol levels, while those high in monounsaturated fatty acids tend to be neutral in their effect on blood cholesterol levels.[22]

These laboratory findings led to studies to determine the relationship between dietary fat and coronary heart disease in natural environments. Some have been historical, others cross-cultural, and still others have examined groups of individuals within the same society.

The historical approach has investigated whether fat consumption in human diets increased contemporaneously with the onset of the coronary heart disease epidemic in America and Europe in the 1920s. Prehistoric hunter-gatherer societies subsisted largely on a diet of wild game, fruits, and nuts. Because the meat of wild game has much less fat but the same amount of cholesterol as that of domesticated animals, it is estimated that these people consumed much more protein, much less fat, and the same amount of cholesterol and carbohydrates as persons in modern western societies. Overhunting, climatic changes, and population growth more than 20,000 years ago led to agricultural societies that consumed more plant foods, fish, and shellfish. Their diets were lower in fat and protein, but with adverse effects on height, nutrition, and life expectancy. Most of the major dietary changes thereafter involved foods that were processed for longer storage. From the middle ages up to the mid-nineteenth century, European societies consumed fresh meats, fruits, and vegetables only in the summer and fall. During the rest of the year, they ate salted fish, pork, and other meats that were extremely fatty to make them palatable. They also consumed cereal grains, vegetables such as cabbage and potatoes that could be stored for long periods, and milk, butter, and cheese, which contain animal fats and cholesterol.[23]

The great transformation toward more varied and nutritious European and American diets began in the late nineteenth century. New modes of transportation brought fresh meat, fish, fruits, and vegetables to cities. Canneries used the new science of bacteriology to process vegetables, fruits, fish, and meats into canned foods that were inexpensive and available year round. Pasteurization increased the shelf life of milk and milk products. Cellophane and other types of improved packaging retarded spoilage and provided a greater variety of baked and other foods to consumers. People spent much of their steadily rising incomes on the growing number of reasonably priced and nutritious foods, so that per capita flour consumption declined from 226 pounds annually in the 1870s to 174 pounds in 1919. The new diet is considered to be a major factor in the improved health of the American population that occurred at this time.[24]

The most widely used statistics on American food consumption trends since 1909 have been foods available for consumption, which include domestic production and imports but do not subtract wastage during food preparation or at the table. Over the course of the century, animal fats available for consumption per person remained essentially unchanged while vegetable fats increased greatly. Specifically, beef, fresh fish, shellfish, and especially poultry available per person increased significantly, while pork products declined. Most of the butter was replaced by vegetable margarine, and most of the lard was replaced by vegetable shortening. Consumption of dairy products increased, despite less fluid milk consumption, because of more frozen dairy products and cheese (much of it in pizza). Egg consumption remained steady up to the Second World War, increased due to wartime shortages of other foods, and declined gradually thereafter. The amount of flour and cereal grains available for consumption per person declined by more than half. Consumption of vegetables rose to mid-century and levelled off thereafter. After mid-century consumption of fresh fruits declined while juice and other processed fruit consumption increased.[25]

Converted to nutrients, total calories available for consumption per person declined from 3,500 grams in 1909–13 to about 3,300 grams from mid-century through the 1970s, and rose to 3,800 grams in 1994. The proportion of total calories in the form of fats increased from 32% in 1909–13 to 42% in 1976, the proportion in the form of complex carbohydrates declined from 37% to 21%, and the proportion in the form of sugars rose from 12% to 18%. Protein available for consumption remained unchanged at about 100 grams, while carbohydrates and crude fiber available for consumption declined from about 500 grams early in the century to about 400 grams in the mid-1980s. Cholesterol consumption rose from about 500 milligrams in 1900–13 to 570 milligrams in 1947–49 and declined to just over 400 milligrams in the early 1990s, due primarily to changes in egg consumption. Fat consumption rose from about 125 grams to about 160 grams.[26]

Foods available for consumption are poor measures of actual consumption trends. They exclude home-grown foods, such as fruits, vegetables, eggs, chickens, and pigs, that were important early in the century when much of the population was rural. They cannot separate actual consumption from loss or wastage, even though only an estimated 70%–75% of foods available for consumption are actually consumed.[27] For example, early in the century many families saved meat fats, such as lard and chicken fat, for later use in frying and baking, while today they are discarded. The discarded animal fats are not subtracted from consumption, but the commercial vegetable oils and margarine that have replaced them are reported as additional fats available for consumption.

Historical statistics on actual food consumption are available from a few dietary surveys of college students and U.S. soldiers in the late nineteenth century. These found that about 40% of their calories were derived from fat, about the same proportion as in the late twentieth century. More recent food recall and diary studies have found that the proportion of calories from fat has remained constant at 38%–40% from the 1940s to the 1980s.[28]

Thus American diets have not changed during the nineteenth or twentieth centuries toward significantly greater consumption of the fats and cholesterol that are alleged to affect coronary heart disease rates. This was the conclusion of a committee of the American Heart Association in 1957: "The proposition that the character of the American diet has so changed during the past 50 years as to increase the incidence of coronary vascular disease cannot be supported."[29]

The relationship between dietary fat and coronary heart disease has also been examined cross-culturally, primarily by comparisons between modern hunter-gatherer societies and advanced western societies. The former consume little meat and fat, have very low blood cholesterol levels, and have practically no coronary heart disease, while the latter consume much more meat and fat and have high blood cholesterol levels and coronary heart disease rates. However, fat consumption is only one of many differences between the two types of societies and cannot be assumed to produce the differences in coronary heart disease rates. For example, coconut oil contains more saturated fat per gram than almost any other known food, but a study found that Polynesians on a remote atoll who consumed large amounts of coconut and saturated fats had lower blood cholesterol levels and rates of coronary heart disease than urbanized Polynesians who consumed less coconut and saturated fats.[30]

Western nations with different levels of fat consumption have also been compared to each other. Ancel Keys compared six technologically advanced countries in the 1950s and found that societies with greater amounts of fat consumption had higher coronary heart disease rates. Because of the nonrandom selection of the six countries, two researchers replicated the study for males ages 55–59 using the 22 countries for which all necessary data were then available. They also found that societies that consumed very little fat had low heart disease mortality rates. However, societies that consumed large amounts of fat varied so greatly in their heart disease mortality rates that no patterns were discernable.[31]

The most famous and influential cross-cultural study was the Seven Countries Study headed by Ancel Keys. According to the National Heart, Lung, and Blood Institute and the American Heart Association in 1989, the "Seven Countries Study provides the strongest evidence that diets high in saturated fatty acids increase the risk of coronary heart disease." About 1960 Keys selected 16 cohorts in a number of European countries, Japan, and the United States on the basis of convenience and cost factors rather than randomization. Most of the cohorts were agricultural or fishing villages with little contact with urban western cultures or diets, and the remainder consisted of workers in modern urban societies. The total sample included 12,763 men ages 40–59 (12,509 without coronary heart disease). The diets of the cohorts were determined by unstandardized dietary surveys varying in duration and methodology using 499 men, an average of 26 men per cohort. These dietary findings were used to represent the diets of all men in each cohort. Periodic medical examinations were performed on all men for ten years.[32]

The study found ecological statistical correlations between the average consumption of dietary fats and of saturated fats of the cohorts and their average blood cholesterol levels and coronary heart disease rates. They found that blood cholesterol levels above but not below 220 mg/dl were related to coronary heart disease rates; that smoking was not related to all-cause mortality and related only in some cohorts to coronary heart disease and lung cancer mortality; that relative weight (the average body mass index) was not related to coronary heart disease rates; and that blood pressure was related to coronary heart disease rates only for those in the top 20% of blood pressure levels.[33]

The Seven Countries Study was characterized by so many flaws in methodology and so many dubious findings that no generalizations are justified. The countries were not selected using any method of randomization. The individuals in each cohort were not selected using randomization, although a few of the cohorts included all of the men in the community. The dietary surveys were not conducted scientifically. The study never related the diets of each man to his development of coronary heart disease, but simply compared the average diet of each cohort to its coronary heart disease rate. These ecological correlations cannot be generalized to individuals with any confidence. The most striking findings were the nonexistent or weak relationships between coronary heart disease rates and smoking, obesity, and blood pressure. Any study that fails to find a relationship between these proven risk factors and coronary heart disease must be considered suspect.

A third type of study examined coronary heart disease rates in individuals in the same society who consumed different amounts and types of fat, a method that can provide much more trustworthy evidence concerning the health consequences of fat consumption. One of the most impressive was a 1957–60 dietary study of 912 participants in the Framingham Heart Study. The study used expert interviewers trained in nutrition to obtain detailed information on the diets of the participants on several occasions during the study. Blood cholesterol levels and the incidence of coronary heart disease were obtained from the periodic medical examinations, thereby assuring the accuracy of the data. The study found no relationships between total caloric, total fat, or animal fat consumption and either blood cholesterol levels or coronary heart disease rates.[34]

A methodologically sound study of individuals examined a random sample of 1,900 men ages 40–55 who were employed for two or more years at a large industrial firm in Chicago. Dietary information on fat and cholesterol consumption was obtained at the initial medical examination in 1957 and again one year later, but not thereafter (a major limitation). Death certificates of the sample members who died were acquired for the next nineteen years. Subgroups were constructed of the highest, middle, and lowest thirds for each of several characteristics measured at the initial medical examination. One characteristic was the percentage of calories from saturated fatty acids; after nineteen years 11.8%, 11.2%, and 10.9% of the three subgroups respectively died from coronary heart disease. Another characteristic was the percentage of calories from polyunsaturated fatty acids: after nineteen years 10.1%, 10.4%, and 13.5% of the three subgroups respectively died from coronary heart disease. The last characteristic was consumption of dietary cholesterol: after nineteen years 13.6%, 9.5%, and 10.9% of the three subgroups respectively died from coronary heart disease. When converted to annual mortality rates, these findings show no meaningful relationship between either dietary fat or cholesterol consumption and coronary heart disease.[35]

Despite the meaningless results of these and many other research studies, the diet-heart hypothesis attracted remarkable attention in the media, as shown by reports in the *New York Times*. In 1954 the World Congress of Cardiology was told that heart disease was most common where there was most fat in the diet. Ancel Keys was reported as informing the American Chemical Society that dietary fats were more important than the total number of calories in producing coronary heart disease. In 1956 an account of a national biology meeting stated that "evidence is mounting that diets rich in meat, milk and eggs—diets in which Americans take pride—are one of the major factors in the cause of . . . atherosclerosis" and it "may be possible to counter the presumed deleterious effects of animal fats by increasing the dietary consumption of vegetable fats." Another article in the same year compared research on smoking and diet and observed that "smoking has . . . attracted little attention among researchers as a possible factor in coronary disease" while "diet has been an object of much greater interest." In 1957 the differences between saturated and unsaturated fats were explained to readers. The newspaper reported occasional criticisms of the diet-heart hypothesis, but most articles stressed the importance of diet as a cause of coronary heart disease.[36]

About 1970, governments in the United States and elsewhere began funding clinical intervention trials that modified diet and other risk factors and measured their impact on coronary heart disease rates. Each trial selected a sample of volunteers and randomly divided it into an intervention and a usual care group, with the intervention group receiving periodic instruction and assistance in modifying risk factors. Both groups were followed for several years and their coronary heart disease rates compared.

Controlled clinical trials of behavioral changes of risk factors pose fundamental methodological problems. Measurements of many changes are based on patient statements that are questionable because of the natural desire of patients to please the investigators. Members of the control group may modify their behaviors in ways similar to the intervention group. The most serious problems occur in studies of highly motivated and health conscious volunteers, who probably already have adopted diets, exercise habits, and other lifestyles that are atypical of the general population.

The most famous trial was the Multiple Risk Factor Intervention Trial (MRFIT), which was also the first trial to deal with several risk factors simultaneously. Funding for the study, which cost $115 million over 10 years, was approved by Congress in 1972. Interested men were simply invited to appear at screening centers with no thought given to a sampling design, the foundation of every good epidemiological study. Volunteers flooded the 20 screening centers throughout the country seeking admission to the trial, and more than 350,000 men ages 35–57 were screened. Ultimately 12,000 volunteers were selected who were in the upper 10% of the population in terms of their risk of coronary heart disease based on their blood pressure, blood cholesterol, and smoking status. Although the sample was expected to have much higher than average mortality rates because of the risk factor levels, after six years its death rate was only two-thirds of the expected rate. Thus a study designed to lower mortality rates in a high-risk population used a sample with much lower-than-average mortality rates.[37]

The sample of 12,866 men was divided into two groups during the seven-year duration of the study. The members of the "usual care" group were referred to their regular source of care for treatment and invited to return annually for a medical check-up, with the results sent to their personal physicians. The members of the "special intervention" group were provided drug treatment for hypertension when appropriate and counseled at least every four months to change their diet to reduce saturated fat consumption and to stop smoking. Given the highly atypical volunteers, it is not surprising that the usual-care group changed its behavior almost as much as did the special-intervention group. After six years the 64% of both groups who were smokers declined to 32% for the special-intervention group and 45% for the usual-care group. The proportion receiving antihypertensive medication increased from 20% of both groups to 57% of the special-intervention group and 46% of the usual-care group. The average blood plasma cholesterol level dropped from 240 mg/dl for both groups to 228 mg/dl for the special-intervention group and 232 mg/dl for the usual-care group. Over ten years, the special-intervention group had 3.1 coronary heart disease deaths per 1,000 participants, while the usual-care group had 3.5, a difference in the rates of 0.004 deaths per 100 participants per year. The differences in the mortality rates from all cardiovascular diseases and in all-cause mortality rates were equally minuscule.[38]

Even if the study had produced meaningful findings, it was much too expensive to be applied to the general population. More than $2,000 per year was spent on each member of the intervention group solely for management of the three risk factors without treating any actual health problems. The failure to use cost-effective interventions has characterized almost all research studies designed to modify risk factors.

Numerous other trials have been undertaken to lower blood cholesterol levels by altering diets. Probably the most methodologically sophisticated was conducted about 1990 using a small sample of 58 men with an average age of 51 and 39 women with an average age of 57, both with higher-than-average cholesterol levels of 262 mg/dl. Every patient observed four regimens, each for a period of nine weeks: a high-fat diet plus a cholesterol-lowering statin drug; a high-fat diet plus a placebo; a low-fat diet plus the statin drug; and a low-fat diet plus the placebo. The high-fat diets contained about 2,250 calories, with 41% obtained from fat and 450 milligrams of cholesterol, a typical American diet; the low-fat diet, which was the more restrictive of two diets recommended by the National Cholesterol Education Program, contained about 1,570 calories, with 26% from fat and 145 milligrams of cholesterol. Extraordinary and very expensive efforts were made to ensure compliance with the diets, including careful selection of the participants, the use of expert dietitians as instructors, and about fifteen meetings with each participant before and during the thirty-six week trial.[39]

Both drugs and diet reduced blood cholesterol levels, but drugs had much the greater effect. When the placebo group switched from a high-fat to a low-fat diet, its average blood cholesterol level dropped from 274 mg/dl to 257 mg/dl. When the drug group switched from a high-fat to a low-fat diet, its average cholesterol level dropped from 219 mg/dl to 203 mg/dl. Thus the switch from high-fat to low-fat diets produced a drop of about 17 mg/dl in blood cholesterol levels. The switch from placebos to drugs produced a much greater drop of about 54 mg/dl. In order to be sure that the blood cholesterol levels had stopped declining at the end of the study, the levels of the placebo groups were examined after six weeks and found to be practically identical to their nine-week levels. Several human experiments in the 1950s also found that extreme dietary changes produced an initial rapid decline in blood cholesterol levels that leveled off after several weeks.[40]

The authors concluded that the 17–mg/dl decline in blood cholesterol levels produced by dietary changes was much greater than would occur under normal conditions. The study patients were carefully selected for willingness to comply, received detailed dietary guidance from experts, had frequent meetings with their physicians, and underwent each regimen for only nine weeks. Few patients could afford the extraordinarily expensive medical care provided at no cost to the participants and no society has the health manpower or resources to provide that level of care to the general population. Most people would not endure such severe dietary restrictions indefinitely.

The levels of cholesterol reduction that are possible with less restrictive diets have been examined using the more moderate diet recommended by the National Cholesterol Education Program. A review of multi-year trials of men with cholesterol levels of 210 to 270 mg/dl found that moderate dietary restriction produced an average cholesterol reduction of about 2%, or a meaningless drop of about 5 mg/dl for those with a cholesterol level of 260 mg/dl. More severe dietary restrictions produced greater reductions, but the authors concluded, "modification of diet can lower serum cholesterol concentrations substantially, but . . . the dietary treatment must be unpleasant to be effective."[41]

The authors of the review also observed that because the average decline in blood cholesterol levels was only 2%, some persons experienced declines of more than 2% and others actually raised their blood cholesterol levels due to increased internal synthesis. They concluded: "If reductions in cholesterol concentrations in individuals are regarded as real and not simply due to random variation, increases in concentration must also be considered real and potentially harmful. It is wrong to count as successes the responders and disregard those whose cholesterol concentration moved in the wrong direction."[42]

Supporters of the atherosclerosis theory have made highly misleading claims about the benefits of reducing blood cholesterol levels. The most frequent claim has been that a 1% reduction in blood cholesterol level produces a 2% reduction in the risk of serious coronary heart disease. This conclusion was based on the Lipid Research Clinics Coronary Primary Prevention Trial of the National Institutes of Health, which took ten years and cost $150 million. It was a seven-year placebo and drug trial of 3,806 men ages 35–59 with an extremely high average blood cholesterol level of 292 mg/dl, which declined to 279 mg/dl after the men were placed on a standard diet but before one-half of them began to receive drugs. After seven years, the drug group experienced an additional decline to an average blood cholesterol level of 257 mg/dl, while the placebo group remained practically unchanged at an average blood cholesterol level of 277 mg/dl. Over the seven years, 9.8% of the placebo group and 8.1% of the drug group experienced either definite coronary heart disease deaths or nonfatal myocardial infarctions.[43]

These statistical results can be described using either percentage or arithmetic differences. Using percentages, the 8% additional decline in blood cholesterol levels in the drug group produced a 19% drop in coronary heart disease deaths and nonfatal myocardial infarctions over seven years, or about a 2% decline in coronary heart disease rates for every 1% decline in cholesterol levels. Such statements say nothing about the actual number of persons who experienced adverse events. Using arithmetic differences, the additional 23 mg/dl drop in blood cholesterol levels in the drug group produced 32 fewer cases of severe coronary heart disease in 1,900 men over seven years, about 5 per year. The drug group therefore experienced 0.2 fewer events per hundred participants per year than the placebo group. Using a phrase offered in another context by Chalmers, the use of percentage rather than arithmetic differences can show that the mortality rate underwent an impressive decline while the funeral rate remained basically unchanged.[44]

Many other criticisms have been made about clinical trials concerning cholesterol reduction. In 1985, when the Lipid Research Clinics Coronary Primary Prevention Trial was published, a commentary complained that "the reported conclusions seem to go beyond what is reasonably justified on the basis of the actual results" and stated that "scientific presentations . . . should be free of such advocacy." Another study selected 22 cholesterol-lowering trials and examined references to them for six years in the *Science Citation Index,* a compilation of references to scientific journal articles. The 14 trials "regarded by their authors as supportive" were cited more than five times as often as those "considered unsupportive."[45]

Thus research concerning high blood cholesterol, like that involving high blood pressure, has been interpreted in ways that were not supported by the statistical findings. Recommendations have been made for population-wide changes in diet and the widespread use of cholesterol-lowering drugs. The commercial implications of the dietary recommendations were quickly recognized by food producers.

18

DIETARY RECOMMENDATIONS AND GUIDELINES

Stroll down a supermarket aisle these days. You could swear you're in a drug store. Cereal boxes proclaim that a bowl a day will help ward off cancer and heart disease. Vegetable oils vow to keep arteries free of unhealthy deposits. Orange juice with calcium aims to prevent brittle bones. . . . It's a brave new era in food marketing. The industry has discovered that promoting a product as helping to prevent disease is a surefire way to boost sales. And foodmakers are pursuing that strategy with a vengeance.[1]

It is surprising how difficult it has been to develop unequivocal data relating diet and chronic disease. In spite of epidemiologic and animal studies supporting many of these relationships, focused human clinical studies often have been negative or, at best, equivocal.[2]

Despite the absence of statistical correlations relating diet and coronary heart disease rates in studies of individuals in natural environments, public and private health organizations and food producers have actively promoted dietary changes for the entire population, not just those at high risk. The result has been a massive risk factor health education campaign that has placed greater emphasis on dietary fats and cholesterol than smoking, physical exercise, and overweight.

The Rise of Public Interest in the Diet-Heart Hypothesis

Throughout the twentieth century, Americans viewed food consumption as closely tied to other aspects of their lives. Early in the century, rising incomes and the greater availability of nutritious foods enabled many persons to reduce their caloric intake without experiencing nutritional deficiencies. Middle-class women, soon joined by men, began to value slenderness in lifestyles and clothing fashions. By 1910 people were speaking of dieting and diets and women's magazines and physicians were providing advice on losing weight. Interest in dieting waned during the depression of the 1930s, the Second World War, and the baby boom of the 1950s but revived thereafter.[3]

Healthy foods were a basic part of health education. In 1917 the U.S. Department of Agriculture began to recommend daily dietary intake levels of foods that supplied essential nutrients. The recommendations were revised periodically and widely promoted in school health curricula and the mass media. In the 1920s, the rising death toll from chronic diseases led to health education campaigns about food consumption, such as the relationship between obesity and diabetes. The American public was thus well prepared by mid-century for the claims relating foods to coronary heart disease.[4]

The American Heart Association (AHA) was the first major health organization to promote the diet-heart hypothesis, which holds that diets high in saturated (animal) fats and cholesterol are a major cause of coronary heart disease. In 1956, a symposium held jointly with the National Heart Institute stated the two cornerstones of the hypothesis: (1) human laboratory feeding experiments showed a relationship between fat consumption and serum cholesterol levels; and (2) tribal and agricultural societies with low fat diets had much lower coronary heart disease rates than industrial societies with high fat diets. In 1961, an AHA committee recommended "the reduction of fat consumption under medical supervision, with reasonable substitution of poly-unsaturated for saturated fats" as a "possible means of preventing atherosclerosis and decreasing the risk of heart attacks and strokes." The *New York Times* reported that the AHA's "highest scientific body has lent its stature to the view that reducing or altering the fat content of a person's diet may help to prevent heart disease." The article compared the high saturated fat content of dairy products and meat to the low saturated fat content of vegetable oils and fish.[5]

Food producers were divided about proposals to reduce fat consumption. In 1962, the American Medical Association advised physicians that patients with atherosclerosis should lower their dietary intake of saturated fats by eliminating or reducing their consumption of dairy products, eggs, fatty meats, and products with lard, shortening, or cocoa butter, plus all baked goods except bread. Even though the advice was represented as an "experimental therapeutic procedure" only for patients with existing atherosclerosis, it aroused a firestorm of criticism from the affected food industries. A few months later the AMA reversed itself and, according to the *New York Times,* issued a "warning both to 'do-it-yourself Americans' and food processors who have built advertising campaigns on cooking oils, margarine and other foods derived from vegetable oils." It now recommended that patients should reduce their serum cholesterol levels only under medical supervision and that all Americans should consume meat, milk, cheese, eggs, butter, fats, oils, and other foods. *Business Week* reported that the butter and cheese producers were "mollified" while the food producers that used unsaturated fats were "perplexed."[6]

Public interest in the diet-heart hypothesis was stimulated by the consumer movement of the 1960s, which responded to a series of crises involving the health and safety hazards of many products. A tragedy involving the drug thalidomide led to federal legislation in 1962 that transformed the testing and marketing of prescription and over-the-counter drugs. Also in 1962 Rachel Carson published *Silent Spring,* which mobilized concern about the dangers of pesticides and the abuse of the environment. In 1964, the Surgeon General's report on the health hazards of smoking was published. In 1966, descriptions of unsafe automobiles by Ralph Nader and others produced federal legislation establishing automobile safety standards. In 1967, publicity about unregulated and contaminated meat products led to the Wholesome Meat Act. The 1970 Occupational Safety and Health Act was enacted in response to the exposure of workers to industrial carcinogens and other hazards without their knowledge. Under the leadership of President Lyndon Johnson, fifteen consumer protection laws were enacted by Congress from 1966 to 1968 compared to two from 1962 to 1965, and others were enacted in the 1970s until the election of President Ronald Reagan in 1980.[7]

Public confidence in major corporations was greatly diminished by the disclosures. Senator Warren G. Magnuson observed in 1972 about the 1966 automobile safety legislation: "To a large extent that Act reflected a gnawing loss of consumer faith, both in the competence and in the social responsiveness of American business. . . . The automobile, which had come to symbolize the brilliance of American manufacturing genius, has progressively been revealed as a surface-styled, poorly-engineered, unsafe, primary polluter of the environment." He added: "The automobile does not stand alone as an object of consumer wrath; the cigarette—a 'consumer staple' . . . stands condemned by the medical and scientific community as a lethal health hazard."[8] Other critics, many associated with Ralph Nader, attacked pharmaceuticals, pesticides, processed foods, chemicals, and factory waste products released into the environment.

The public also lost confidence in federal government agencies, which were criticized as indifferent to the public welfare and subservient to the major corporations. The Food and Drug Administration permitted hundreds of food chemicals and additives, including older untested ones, to be added to foods without being identified on the labels. The sweetener cyclamate produced the greatest outcry because its risks to pregnant women were uncovered in the 1950s, yet it remained in widespread use as an unlabeled ingredient until publicity in 1969 led to its banning the following year. The Department of Agriculture was accused of serving the interests of farmers while failing to protect the environment and the health and safety of the public.[9]

Public opinion polls revealed the sharp drop in public confidence in many institutions. This is indicated by responses concerning two statements: "Government is run by a few big interests looking out for themselves," and "You can trust government in Washington to do what is right" either "some of the time," "just about always," or "most of the time." The proportions of respondents agreeing with the first and answering "some of the time" to the second increased from about 25% in 1964 to 70% or more in 1974 to 1980. Between 1966–67 and 1978–80, the proportion expressing a "great deal" of confidence in "major companies" dropped from 51% to 21%, in "medicine" from 66% to 41%, and in "education" from 59% to 34%.[10]

The consumer movement had two primary foci. Its supporters demanded that government do more to eliminate hazards to public health, safety, and the environment. They wanted an open government decision-making process that informed the public of the criteria and standards used to make the decisions. In addition, many supporters assumed greater personal responsibility for their lifestyles and exposure to health hazards. They especially wanted more useful and accurate information about the safety and health consequences of the foods that they consumed.[11]

Public and private health organizations and major food producers quickly realized the benefits of providing the public with more information about the health values of foods. Instead of being censured by consumer groups, they could become their allies. Government agencies recognized that providing information was much less controversial than regulating or banning business activities. Private health organizations knew that emphasizing the health values of foods could strengthen their ties with major corporations. Food producers realized that health information implied that they were committed to healthy products and diverted consumer attention from such issues as chemical additives, pesticide residues, and artificial ingredients.

In 1965, the American Heart Association gave its "top priority" to a "Risk Factor" program that emphasized lower serum cholesterol and blood pressure levels, "sound dietary practices," avoidance of obesity, and "regular activity," according to a history of the organization. Cigarette smoking, the most deadly risk factor, was not on the list. Some physician members of the AHA opposed the recommendations, citing lack of evidence, and the issue was bitterly debated at the association's annual conventions. In 1973, the AHA recommended specific changes in the diets of all Americans: the percentage of daily calories from fat should be reduced from the existing average of 40%–45% to less than 35%, equally divided among saturated, monounsaturated, and polyunsaturated fats; daily cholesterol consumption should be reduced from the existing average of 600–750 milligrams to 300 milligrams; and excessive consumption of salt should be avoided. Once again cigarette smoking was not mentioned, even though nine years had elapsed since the Surgeon General's report.[12]

Producers of vegetable oils and margarine were among the first to realize the potential advantages for their products of the advice to reduce saturated fat consumption. As early as the 1950s some margarine, vegetable oil, and vegetable shortening producers claimed that their products reduced serum cholesterol levels, which the Food and Drug Administration (FDA) called "false and misleading" in 1959. In 1971 the FDA permitted the producers of processed foods to advertise the types of fats contained in their products.[13]

The margarine industry became the primary early beneficiary of the saturated fat recommendations and demonstrated the enormous profits that could result from health claims for foods. Margarine was invented about 1870 in France with the encouragement of the French government as an inexpensive table spread for the poor to replace tallow and lard. It was manufactured by rendering the oils in the stearin or hard portion of beef fat and emulsifying them with milk and water. The first major American producers were national meat packing firms, which manufactured margarine as a byproduct of meat processing. Margarine soon became a commercial success, primarily in Europe, and has been widely recognized as one of the greatest modern innovations in foods.[14]

By 1900, technological innovations enabled most margarines to be made from coconut oil which, like beef fat, consisted primarily of saturated fatty acids and was solid at room temperature. From the 1920s to the 1940s producers gradually switched to cottonseed and soybean oils, which were unsaturated fatty acids rendered solid at room temperature by new methods of partial hydrogenation. Vegetable oil margarines were much more popular in America than in Europe and were manufactured primarily by local and regional firms. In the 1930s a few national food producers introduced more expensive brands of vegetable margarine and in the 1940s margarine producers added vitamins to replace those lost when vegetable oils replaced beef fat.[15]

Margarine was for many years the most controversial food product sold in America. Butter producers and dairy farmers bitterly opposed its sale, while other farmers had no interest in a product whose main ingredient was imported coconut oil. At least one state prohibited the sale of margarine and many others banned coloring the white margarine yellow to resemble butter or otherwise discouraged its sale. Nevertheless, the industry's difficulties were largely of its own making. American margarine producers refused to market margarine as a distinctive product but disguised it to resemble butter and advertised it as a cheap substitute. European producers differentiated margarine from butter and were much more successful, as were American producers of vegetable shortening, who advertised its greater resistance to spoilage and other advantages over butter and lard. Margarine also had an unappealing consistency and flavor and was tainted by frequent allegations of unhygienic manufacturing processes and low quality or unsafe ingredients. Even during the Great Depression when inexpensive products were very popular, a 1938 survey of 53,000 homes in sixteen cities found that 84% of the homes had butter, 92% had shortening or lard, but only 25% had margarine.[16]

Shortages of butter during the Second World War forced many families to consume margarine, so that production doubled between 1940 and 1944. After the war the domestic cotton and soybean industries, which supplied the vegetable oils, joined with public demand for an inexpensive alternative to butter to effect the repeal of the restrictive state laws. Once margarine could be sold in the same form in all states, national manufacturers became more prominent and placed greater emphasis on quality and taste.[17]

National margarine producers realized that the diet-heart hypothesis enabled them to contrast the vegetable oils in margarine with the animal fats in butter. They also had much more money to spend on advertising than the fragmented regional butter producers. In 1961 *Business Week* reported that "some of the margarine makers think they have discovered in recent medical findings a weapon that will enable them to lop off a fat slice of butter's share of the market." The magazine reported that advertisements for one brand "have become more medical in tone as favorable research evidence has piled up." The saturated fat content of margarine was further reduced by making a softer, less hydrogenated product sold in tubs rather than the solid sticks.[18]

The massive advertising of health claims for margarine transformed a generally disreputable product of inferior quality and flavor into a great commercial success. Between 1910 and 1940, consumption per person per year was about 2.5 pounds for margarine and 17 pounds for butter. By 1981, margarine consumption had increased to 11 pounds per person per year, while butter consumption dropped to 4 pounds. Margarine became popular during a period of economic prosperity when its health claims were a stronger selling point than its low cost. This is shown by the parallel success of the vegetable shortening industry, which contrasted its vegetable oils with the animal fats in lard and butter. Given the history of the American margarine industry, it is not surprising that in the 1970s the Federal Trade Commission demanded on two occasions that a margarine company stop advertising false claims about physician recommendations for Fleischmann's Margarine.[19]

Dietary Recommendations

In the years since 1950 the policies of federal government, quasi-government, and private health organizations have changed from ambivalence about the diet-heart hypothesis to almost total acceptance. In 1958 the Food and Nutrition Board of the National Academy of Sciences examined the hypothesis and observed that "in the United States, an average diet containing approximately 40 percent of the calories in the form of fat has been consistent with the attainment of one of the best health patterns in the world. A diet containing less than 25 percent of the calories as fat is not easily selected from foodstuffs commonly available in the United States and is not likely to be popular. There is as yet no proven nutritional or health reason for suggesting that its attainment is a desirable goal." The authors could personally recall the malnutrition that prevailed among the poor during the depression of the 1930s and were not prepared to recommend changes in the American diet without strong evidence. In a 1966 report, the Board reiterated its earlier concerns, but this time recommended a "moderate reduction in total fat intake and some substitution of polyunsaturated for saturated fat." This was to be decided on an individual basis without sacrificing a "varied, adequate, and not overly rich diet" that maintained "normal body weight."[20]

In 1970, a federal government commission of medical experts, the Intersociety Commission for Heart Disease Resources, recommended reduced intake of cholesterol, fat, and saturated fat with the objective of lowering blood cholesterol levels. The *New York Times* reported on its front page that the commission advised the public to eat less "egg yolks, butter fat, fatty meats, organ meats, shellfish, and fat-rich baked goods and candies." It cited high blood pressure and cigarette smoking as other major risk factors for coronary heart disease. The commission made the recommendation even though "definitive evidence linking dietary fats and cholesterol to human heart disease [was] not available." It did mention that the Framingham study found no statistical correlation between diet and serum cholesterol levels, but stated that the diets of the participants were not sufficiently varied.[21]

Within a year, a Task Force on Arteriosclerosis of the National Heart and Lung Institute of the National Institutes of Health took the opposite position. It concluded that the evidence relating diet and serum cholesterol levels was "scientifically not entirely convincing. Therefore, recommendations concerning diet are based on personal impressions and fragmentary evidence rather than on scientific proof."[22]

In 1972, a joint report entitled "Diet and Coronary Heart Disease" of the Food and Nutrition Board of the National Academy of Sciences and the American Medical Association Council on Foods and Nutrition concluded that "there is extensive evidence that the level of cholesterol in the plasma of most people can be lowered by appropriate dietary modification" consisting of less cholesterol and more unsaturated fats. They recommended that the blood cholesterol levels of adults should be measured periodically, but said that the risks associated with cholesterol levels below 220 mg/dl were "relatively small." Smoking was not considered an important risk factor (eight years after the Surgeon General's report) because the report listed only "heavy cigarette smoking" among a group of risk factors that included elevated serum cholesterol, high blood pressure, obesity, and physical inactivity.[23]

The debate escalated dramatically with the famous 1977 report of the U.S. Senate Select Committee on Nutrition and Human Needs chaired by Senator George McGovern, entitled *Dietary Goals for the United States.* This "revolutionary Senate committee report," according to a historian, was "written by a group of political activists with a nonprofessional interest and knowledge of nutrition." It became a "central document in the history of dietary guidelines" that influenced subsequent recommendations in the United States and throughout the world. It was especially significant as the first statement of its kind by an official United States government body.[24]

The testimony of witnesses at the committee hearings indicated the importance to many groups of dietary recommendations. Among food producers, the Salt Institute opposed limits on salt intake, citing lack of evidence that salt consumption contributed to hypertension. The International Sugar Research Foundation called sugar an "ideal energy source" when added to protein and other foods, because it consisted of "pure calories with no fat and no cholesterol." The foundation attributed obesity solely to lack of exercise. The National Dairy Council urged less concern with individual components of the diet and more with obesity produced by too many calories and too little exercise. The National Canners Association claimed that their foods were nutritious and inexpensive.[25]

The American Medical Association criticized government guidelines for food consumption as unwarranted government interference with the practice of medicine. Decisions should be based on "appropriate medical dietary counselling on an individual basis." The AMA did "not consider it appropriate for the government to adopt national goals that specify such matters as the amount and proportions of total fat, type of fat, sugar, cholesterol, or salt content in the diets of the general public as these national goals advocate." It reiterated this position in 1979.[26]

Many scientists testified that scientific evidence was lacking for the proposed dietary recommendations. One contrasted the "uncertain effects of diet alteration on total mortality" with the strong evidence concerning smoking and blood pressure. Another noted that "none of the [dietary] trials has been totally convincing, and they are not totally convincing in the aggregate. It is particularly noteworthy that none of the trials has demonstrated prolongation of life." A pathologist stated that "no animal models have been found which are sufficiently similar to human arteriosclerosis to permit etiological conclusions." A biochemist observed:

> The manufacturers of margarines, egg and meat substitutes, and other segments of the food industry have taken full advantage of the AHA [dietary

guidelines] and, in fact, have taken over the burden of indiscriminately weaning the public away from eggs, beef, pork, and dairy products containing butterfat. By constant repetition, in all advertising media they have made it appear as a truism that anyone who consumes animal products, including meat, eggs and dairy dishes, is in danger of [coronary heart disease], and that substitution of their products will prevent the disease. . . . The advertising campaigns have been so intense and so persistent that the word cholesterol has become almost synonymous with coronary heart disease in most people's minds, including not only the man in the street but many physicians and even nutritionists and other scientists. . . . It has been forgotten that the evidence is conflicting.[27]

The 1977 recommendations of the Select Committee on Nutrition and Human Needs were based on the rationale proposed by a witness: "The diet we eat today was not planned or developed for any particular purpose. It is a happenstance related to our affluence, the productivity of our farmers and the activities of our food industry. The risks associated with eating this diet are demonstrably large. The question to be asked, therefore, is not why should we change our diet but why not?" The committee's goal was greater consumption of fruits, vegetables, whole grains, poultry, fish, and nonfat milk products, and less of meat, eggs, cheese, butter, and foods containing large amounts of sugar, salt, or saturated fats, including baked goods, snacks, candy, and soft drinks. It recommended the following: complex carbohydrates in the diet increased from 28% to 48% of all calories; refined and processed sugars reduced from 18% to 10%; protein unchanged at 12%; overall fat reduced from 40% to 30%; cholesterol reduced to 300 milligrams per day; and salt reduced to 5000 milligrams per day. The report provided no recommendations concerning obesity and cigarette smoking, although each of them had a much greater impact on mortality than the dietary changes.[28]

In 1980, the National Institutes of Health asked the Food and Nutrition Board (FNB) of the National Academy of Sciences to evaluate the Select Committee's report. The FNB was chosen because it determined the recommended dietary intake used by the government for nutritional requirements. The board concluded that human laboratory feeding experiments found that fat consumption affected serum cholesterol levels. However, "intervention trials in which diet modification was employed to alter the incidence of coronary artery disease and mortality in middle aged men have been generally negative." It criticized the guidelines of the Select Committee and observed about public health policy, "if there is uncertainty about its effectiveness, there must be clear evidence that the proposed intervention will not be harmful or detrimental in other ways." The FNB did not believe that dietary fat and cholesterol recommendations met this criterion and instead focused on obesity, the "commonest form of malnutrition in the Western nations of the world." It recommended a "nutritionally adequate diet" from the several food groups and moderate salt consumption with no more "food and fat intake" than was necessary to maintain appropriate weight for height.[29]

The reactions to the FNB report were immediate, vociferous, and conflicting, despite general agreement that its conclusions were supported by the evidence. The *New York Times,* in several articles on its front page and elsewhere, reported that the FNB recommendations constituted "the first official dissent by a national scientific body on the subject." One article noted that in the last decade eighteen major organizations had recommended reduced consumption of fat, saturated fat, and cholesterol and that "government experts" criticized the FNB report as "inadequate and misleading." Another article reported that "the American Medical Association and food industry groups, including producers of eggs, meat and dairy products, were quick to express approval of the Food and Nutrition Board's rejection of fat and cholesterol warnings." A physician-columnist observed that most physicians considered blood pressure reduction and smoking cessation to be more beneficial than dietary modifications. An editorial stated that the FNB's "report can only increase the confusion of health-conscious eaters." A reporter for the *Wall Street Journal* wrote that the conclusions were "not exactly scientifically startling, let alone heretical." A subcommittee of the U.S. House of Representatives held hearings on the report, and, according to the *New York Times,* both sides "agreed that there was no scientific correlation between lowering of cholesterol and a reduction in coronary disease."[30]

Unfortunately, the substantive issues disappeared from view after the FNB was shown to have no credibility whatsoever. A reporter for *Science* observed, "The problem with the report lies not in its content—which has yet to be proved in error—but in its wrapping." Two members were food company executives and others, including the author of the report, were paid consultants to egg producers or other food companies. The board's only continuing source of funding, including all of the funding for the report, was food company contributions. An ex-member of the board reported that he was unable to locate a charter or mandate or to discover how committee members were selected. According to a reporter for *Science,* he claimed that the board's "range of expertise is too narrow, its ties with industry too close to avoid the suspicion of bias, its mandate is too ill-defined, and its mode of operation is too secret." Consumer groups had repeatedly attacked the board for its close ties to the food industry and disregarding or downplaying the hazards of food chemical additives. The report itself exhibited a profound ignorance of statistical and epidemiological methods and recommended reduced salt consumption using the same kind of evidence that it rejected for reduced fat consumption.[31]

The administration of President Ronald Reagan from 1981 to 1989 forced the Food and Drug Administration and the Federal Trade Commission to pay less attention to nutrition and health issues by significantly reducing their funding. Reagan also cut funding for practically every other government agency concerned with enforcing health and safety regulations and appointed administrators who shared his views. For example, in 1981 Reagan's Secretary of Agriculture, John R. Block, an Illinois hog farmer, told a congressional committee that hogs know what to eat without being told and "humans are as smart as a hog."[32]

The National Institutes of Health, which was shielded from these political machinations, continued to press for dietary changes. A major 1985 report by a consensus conference of the National, Heart, Lung and Blood Institute reached three major conclusions: (1) "elevated blood cholesterol is a major cause of coronary artery disease"; (2) "the blood cholesterol level of most Americans is undesirably high, in large part because of our high dietary intake of calories, saturated fat, and cholesterol"; and (3) "appropriate changes in our diet will reduce blood cholesterol levels." The consensus conference claimed that the first two conclusions were easily demonstrated but conceded that the third, the effect of dietary changes on coronary heart disease, "has been more challenging." It concluded that "an aggregate analysis" of the clinical trials considered as a whole indicated that "reduction of blood cholesterol level in people with relatively high initial levels will reduce the rate of coronary heart disease." Extrapolating far beyond its own conclusions, the conference proposed that the entire population reduce its blood cholesterol levels. It recommended that total fat intake be reduced to 30% of calories, roughly equally divided among saturated, monounsaturated, and polyunsaturated fats, and dietary cholesterol intake to less than 250–300 milligrams per day.[33]

Most of the controversy generated by the report concerned its population-wide recommendations. A reporter for *Science* magazine commented: "The question is not whether people at high risk for heart disease should be concerned about their cholesterol levels. It is about whether the data are strong enough to recommend that the entire population, including children, go on low-fat diets." The curvilinear relationship between serum cholesterol levels and coronary heart disease provided no justification for a population-wide program. Opponents were reported as saying that they "would like to see cholesterol-lowering programs tailored to the individual rather than presented as an edict to the population at large."[34]

In 1985, based on the consensus conference, the National Heart, Lung and Blood Institute of the NIH created the National Cholesterol Education Program (NCEP). It was modeled after the earlier National High Blood Pressure Education Program and was also a "partnership" with voluntary health and medical associations to develop educational programs for health professionals, patients, and the general public. In the minds of some, the NIH had moved far beyond the evidence. The American Academy of Pediatrics rejected the consensus conference recommendations as too stringent for children. The *New York Times* reported that "even a few of the world's leading cholesterol authorities, while calling for reasonable steps to reduce high cholesterol levels, have cautioned against exaggerating the likely benefits of such steps or the problem itself." Ancel Keys, the pioneer investigator of the subject, was quoted in 1987 as saying, "I've come to think that [blood] cholesterol is not as important as we used to think it was. . . . Let's reduce cholesterol by reasonable means . . . but let's not get too excited about it."[35]

Nevertheless, from this time forward, the diet-heart hypothesis was uncritically accepted by federal government reports, such as the *Surgeon General's Report on Nutrition and Health* of 1988. Although the report conceded that "only weak associations of dietary factors with plasma cholesterol levels or [coronary heart disease] have been shown" in studies of individuals, it claimed that these were due to methodological limitations. The report decided that the cumulative evidence somehow overrode the negative findings of the individual studies: "Taken together, these clinical trials provide compelling evidence that lowering plasma cholesterol reduces [coronary heart disease] morbidity and mortality." It did concede that "total mortality has generally not been reduced in these studies." It alleged, contrary to all of the evidence, that this finding was as valid for average and below-average serum cholesterol levels as for above-average ones. It recommended that population serum cholesterol levels be reduced to below 200 mg/dl, a level also proposed by an expert panel of the NCEP in the same year.[36]

In 1989 the National Academy of Sciences published a report by a chastened and reorganized Food and Nutrition Board. This report concluded that "highest priority is given to reducing fat intake, because the scientific evidence concerning dietary fats and other lipids and human health is strongest and the likely impact on human health is greatest." Its recommendations were similar to those of the NCEP and other groups. The FNB added, without evidence, that further reductions in saturated fat and dietary cholesterol "may confer even greater health benefits."[37]

The FNB report was practically alone in attempting to provide a scientific rationale for its conclusions. It conceded that statistical correlations between individual fat consumption and coronary heart disease rates produced "somewhat inconsistent and inconclusive" findings, but blamed these on unidentified methodological problems. Lacking evidence from studies of individuals, the FNB resorted to ecological correlations: "There are many examples of diet-disease correlations that are strong when based on population means (e.g. dietary and serum cholesterol levels) but weak or nonexistent when based on values for individuals. Prominent examples are the strong ecological correlations found between dietary fats and [coronary heart disease] . . . and the weak or absent individual correlations for the same pair of variables." Ecological correlations had the advantages of greater variations in diets among the groups in the study and less "random variability" than studies of individuals. However, the dietary variations in the studies of individuals were typical of the American population and more than adequate to demonstrate the benefits of the recommended dietary changes. Furthermore, reducing random variability meant disregarding individual differences within the groups and focusing on group averages, but differences in group averages can never be generalized directly to individuals.[38]

The American Heart Association and the National Heart, Lung, and Blood Institutes added their support in 1989, according to the *New York Times,* when they "issued a joint statement . . . that the evidence that reducing [serum] cholesterol helps save lives is overwhelming" and that dietary changes can reduce serum cholesterol levels. They conceded that the evidence was based exclusively on studies of highly atypical individuals: "Even though these and many other studies were conducted on people at the highest risk of heart trouble, the doctors contended that sensible eating and lower cholesterol are good for everyone." Thus the "overwhelming" evidence consisted solely of extrapolations from persons at very high risk, many with a genetic disorder, to those at average and low risk.[39]

The NCEP's most important policy decision was to codify many of the recommendations into guidelines for physicians in 1988. An expert panel defined high blood cholesterol as 240 mg/dl or higher and "borderline-high blood cholesterol" as 200–239 mg/dl. These two groups together included the majority of the adult population of the United States. Cholesterol-lowering drugs were to be given based on LDL levels, other risk factors, and the presence of coronary heart disease. Those at the borderline-high level without evidence of coronary heart disease and fewer than two other risk factors were to be given dietary advice and annual blood tests. The risk factors included male sex, cigarette smoking, hypertension, "severe obesity" (even though indisputable evidence existed for the health risks of all levels of obesity), diabetes, a family history of premature coronary heart disease, and low HDL levels. The panel did not estimate the cost of its recommendations.[40]

The NCEP recommendations were sufficiently important to warrant hearings by the Subcommittee on Health and the Environment of the Committee on Energy and Commerce of the U.S. House of Representatives in 1989. All those testifying agreed that sufficient evidence existed for the benefits of cholesterol reduction in middle-aged men with serum cholesterol levels of 240 mg/dl or higher *plus* other risk factors or preexisting coronary heart disease. They disagreed about the benefits of a population-wide program. One physician testified that "many physicians question the value of aggressively treating high cholesterol in older men, women of any age, or mildly hypercholesterolemic middle-aged men who do not have symptoms of heart disease. The effectiveness of treating such people has never been established and there are good reasons to doubt that they will gain as much from treatment as the middle-aged, high-risk men who participated in the major studies of the health consequences of cholesterol reduction." Another observed that serum cholesterol "is not nearly as important a risk factor for coronary heart disease as several others, such as smoking, high blood pressure, obesity, diabetes, lack of adequate physical activity, and probably stress." A representative of the Office of Technology Assessment reported that the recommendations were "resource intensive" and that 60 million Americans (36% of the adult population) would receive diet or drug therapy and require frequent blood tests and visits to physicians.[41]

The reactions of corporations indicated the great commercial significance of the NCEP's recommendations. Two of its most controversial guidelines called for periodic blood tests of the serum cholesterol levels of many millions of adults and drug therapy for relatively low cholesterol levels, regardless of age, gender, and other factors that affect risk. In 1996 the American College of Physicians disagreed and proposed routine serum cholesterol screening only for men ages 35–64 and women 45–64, as well those at high risk because of smoking, obesity, or a family history of coronary heart disease. The *Wall Street Journal* reported:

[This alternative] recommendation predictably drew fire from pharmaceutical giants Merck and Co. and Bristol-Myers Squibb Co., leading makers of a class of hot-selling cholesterol-lowering medicines. Known as statin drugs, they are widely prescribed for patients who have had heart attacks or other symptoms of heart disease, but the companies are expected to try to expand the market to otherwise healthy patients with high cholesterol levels. Aggressive screening programs would be critical to the success of such a strategy.[42]

In the 1990s some proponents of the diet-heart hypothesis began to modify their positions, as indicated by the periodic "diet-heart" statements of the American Heart Association. The 1993 statement acknowledged the curvilinear relationship between serum cholesterol and coronary heart disease and admitted that the risk was "most marked" at serum cholesterol levels above 240 mg/dl. It conceded that the problem was largely limited to a group of genetically abnormal persons by admitting that "most" of the highest 25 percent of persons in terms of their serum cholesterol levels "probably also have genetic forms of hypercholesterolemia." The statement also acknowledged that the AHA emphasized serum cholesterol at the expense of risk factors like blood pressure and smoking, but claimed that the other risk factors "appear to play an atherogenic role against a background of high cholesterol levels." No research study has ever supported this conclusion.[43]

The next set of AHA "dietary guidelines" in 1996 questioned other basic premises of the diet-heart hypothesis. It took the astounding position (for the AHA) of recommending a minimum level of fat in the diet: "The AHA endorses the recommendations of the World Health Organization for a lower limit of 15 percent of calories as total fat." Its rationale was the risk of "potential nutrient deficiencies in certain subgroups such as children, pregnant women, and the elderly." The report also reiterated the importance of "underlying genetic influences" and stated that "individualized dietary and lifestyle recommendations may provide more effective approaches to prevention of" coronary heart disease. These statements implicitly questioned the need for dietary changes in the entire population.[44]

The Diet-Heart Hypothesis and the Food Industry

Food producers considered the diet-heart hypothesis to be only one of several health issues of concern to consumers. A 1993 national survey of 17,000 women ages 18–34 found that they gave the following reasons for the times when they were careful about what they ate: 60% mentioned a desire to lose weight, 57% cited proper nutrition, and only 37% referred to lowering the risk of disease. Other concerns included the health risks of chemical food additives, pesticides, and food contamination. Food producers therefore inundated consumers with as many health claims for each product as they could muster. New food products in 1993 made 847 claims for reduced or low fat, 609 claims for reduced or low calorie, 543 for no additives or preservatives, 473 for reduced or low sugar, 449 for all natural ingredients, 385 for organic ingredients, 287 for reduced or low cholesterol, and 242 for reduced or low salt.[45] The complexity of the situation has produced varied reactions to the recommendations to reduce consumption of animal fats and cholesterol, as shown by the dairy, meat, fast-food restaurant, and vegetable oil industries.

The dairy industry was ill prepared for the recommendations to reduce consumption of animal fats. For many years milk was priced by its fat content, which encouraged the use of cow breeds that produced high-fat milk. Dairy producers believed that their products were sacrosanct because of their favorable treatment by state and federal governments, including price supports and the purchase of dairy products for school lunch programs. By 1962, however, the *New York Times* reported that "whereas people once thought of dairy products in terms of health and vitality, many now associate them with cholesterol and heart ailments." Between 1970 and 1997 consumption of fluid whole milk declined from 214 to 73 pounds per person while that of low-fat and skim milk increased from 41 to 124 pounds, a net decline of 58 pounds per person. The industry responded by introducing non-fat and low-fat dairy products, which comprised more than one-half of the 800 dairy products introduced in 1988. On the other hand, consumption trends for some popular high-fat dairy products indicated little consumer concern with animal fats. From 1970 to 1995 cheese consumption per person (much of it in pizza) increased from 11 to 27 pounds and ice cream and butter consumption declined only slightly.[46]

The meat industry experienced similar problems. Traditionally, cattlemen and hog farmers were paid for the entire carcass, and beef that was heavily marbled with fat received the highest prices and government ratings. Consequently, producers had no interest in leaner meat. Nevertheless, between 1970 and 1995 red meat consumption, including beef, veal, lamb, mutton, and pork, declined from 132 to 115 pounds per person, while poultry consumption increased from 34 to 63 pounds. Most agricultural economists believe that poultry's lower cost was more responsible for the trends than concern over fats and cholesterol.[47]

Fast-food restaurants found that consumers had little interest in low fat and low cholesterol foods. Responding to pressures from nutritionists and consumer groups, the restaurants changed their methods of food preparation and introduced new foods. They replaced fried chicken with broiled, grilled, or baked chicken, even though the fat and caloric content was practically the same. McDonald's, a leading franchiser, switched the oil used to fry its french fried potatoes from one containing primarily beef fat to a vegetable oil. The chains added salad bars with low-fat dressings, lower-fat hamburgers, low-fat Mexican food, and one even added cottage cheese and pineapple. Sales were disappointing and most of the products were soon discontinued.[48]

The vegetable oil industry experienced different problems because most of its production was sold to food producers, not consumers. The various types of vegetable oils were readily interchangeable for most products, so the food producers could easily switch to those that they thought appealed to consumers at the moment. As a result, vegetable oils high in saturated fatty acids lost sales. Others that were high in unsaturated fatty acids and were once used exclusively for products like paints and linoleum suddenly became popular ingredients in baked and fried foods, margarines, and salad dressings. When the NCEP began a mass media campaign in 1987 to stress the significance of serum cholesterol levels, the American Soybean Association immediately attacked imported palm and coconut oils, which were less expensive but had more saturated fatty acids, "with advertisements raising the specter of cholesterol," according to the *Wall Street Journal.* Major food producers removed the tropical oils from some of their most popular products. Shortly thereafter, rapeseed oil appeared on the American market with a new name, canola oil. The genetically engineered rape plant was a major crop in Europe and Canada and its oil had less saturated fat than soybean oil. Food producers thereupon replaced soybean oils with canola oil in some products.[49]

A major problem for food producers was the need for external verification of their health claims. In 1988, the American Heart Association announced a program to award a seal of approval on selected foods for a fee of $40,000 (later reduced to $10,000) for testing the product and an annual endorsement fee of $5,000 to $1 million (later reduced to $600,000), depending on the size of the company. The AHA refused to divulge its criteria, but it did approve foods consisting largely or wholly of fats and oils. The Food and Drug Administration and the Department of Agriculture claimed that the program could be misleading and confusing to consumers. Shortly after its introduction in 1990, the *New York Times* reported that the AHA, which was "besieged by stinging criticism and threats of strong Government action" and especially the defection of most of the companies, cancelled the program. In 1992, the AHA revived the idea as the "heart-check certification program," this time adopting FDA labeling guidelines and charging a nominal fee. It entered into other arrangements with the same food producers, some for millions of dollars, to promote foods such as lean cuts of beef and citrus products and to develop television programs. The American Cancer Society and the Arthritis Foundation later entered into multimillion dollar agreements to place their names on foods and/or drugs.[50]

In 1987 the administration of President Ronald Reagan adopted a policy that "officially permitted disease prevention claims" on products, according to the *New York Times*. The newspaper reported in 1990 that "over the past three years, a product could make virtually any claim without evidence." The policy produced a free-for-all of exaggerations, deceptions, and outright fabrications in violation of federal law. When the FDA took a small company to court in 1989 for claiming that its product could treat heart disease, the court ruled that the agency could not enforce its rules against small companies because it did not enforce them against large companies. The Reagan administration policy of refusing to regulate food producers was an extension of a 1986 policy that essentially gave the biotechnology industry "control . . . over its own regulatory destiny," according to the *New York Times*. That policy adopted or eliminated regulations according to the preferences of the biotechnology industry and restricted the actions of the Environmental Protection Agency, the Department of Agriculture, and the Food and Drug Administration.[51]

By 1990 about one-third of all food advertisements, which totaled $3.6 billion, contained health or disease prevention claims. A food company executive conceded that "it's really a mixed bag because the consumer is so foolable." Another added, "I think you mislead more people than you educate." Companies listed smaller serving sizes on their packages to make it appear that their products had fewer calories and less fat and salt. Some producers claimed that a product prevented heart disease because it had little of one allegedly harmful ingredient, such as fat, even though it had enormous quantities of some other ingredient, such as salt. The only force for moderation was that fat reduction affected the taste of the products. Convinced that consumers believed that health foods were not tasty, food producers were unwilling to advertise many foods as health foods.[52]

Disagreements soon developed within the food industry about the desirability of unregulated health claims. On the one hand, a 1991 article in the *Wall Street Journal* claimed that "health claims in food marketing have brought nutritional issues to the forefront of consumer attention rather than leaving them to languish in medical journals and obscure advice columns." It maintained that "the ability to focus on health provides manufacturers with the incentive to improve foods in ways that nutritionists have advocated for years." On the other hand, three major food companies did not object when the Food and Drug Administration accused them in 1991 of false advertising by putting "no cholesterol" claims on vegetable oils, which cannot contain cholesterol because vegetables have no cholesterol. The claim could seem plausible because a public opinion survey found that one-half of the respondents did not know the foods that did or did not contain cholesterol. Proctor and Gamble, one of the companies accused by the FDA, stated that it was "quite willing to help defuse these claims from our packages" and removed the claims. One of the other companies stated that "we support what the FDA is doing in clarifying food labels."[53]

The issue came to a head because of oat bran, which was found to reduce serum cholesterol levels. Public interest was quickly aroused to such an extent that the *New York Times* reported in 1989 that "throwing in a spoonful of oat bran into literally anything seems to guarantee a torrent of cash." Oat bran did not have an appealing flavor, so very small quantities were added to the foods. As a result, according to the newspaper, "you would need to eat staggering quantities before you did your cholesterol count any good."[54]

The oat bran mania was used to greatest effect by breakfast cereals. Cheerios, an oat cereal with a very small amount of oat bran, quickly became the country's most popular cereal, and other manufacturers brought out similar products. One reporter noted that cereal manufacturers were making "their section of the supermarket sound more like a drugstore." Meanwhile, the W. K. Kellogg and General Mills companies introduced cereals called Heartwise and Benefit respectively that contained both oat bran and the outer husk of psyllium, a grain grown in India that reduced cholesterol. Psyllium was also used in commercial laxatives, so the laxative manufacturers insisted that they should be able to claim that their products reduced cholesterol levels. Because psyllium is considered a drug, the question arose as to whether the cereals should require approval as drugs.[55]

At this point, government officials in several states decided they would no longer condone the false and deceptive food health claims being tolerated by President George Bush, Reagan's successor. In 1989, the attorney general of Texas, joined by eight other states, sued the Quaker Oats Company, claiming that its advertisements "falsely claim that eating the cereal reduces cholesterol and the risk of heart attack." The company, which saw sales of the product jump after the oat claims, replied that it was "extremely disheartening to see the attorney general obstructing . . . the goal of nutrition education." In 1989 and 1990, the state banned the two breakfast cereals with psyllium, accusing their manufacturers of deceptive labeling. Late in 1990 the state of Iowa and five others accused the Kellogg company of "deceptive and misleading" advertising for several of its cereals.[56]

The suits raised the frightening prospect for the industry that every food label and every food advertisement would have to be approved separately by each of the fifty states. In 1989, *Business Week* reported that

> food companies . . . want to use health claims to gain a competitive edge. But marketeers know that an escalating war of aggressive health claims could bring an even harsher regulatory backlash than what's unfolding now. That fear is why so many are calling for the feds to step in. Claims "should be controlled by federal guidelines and not state by state," says . . . Kellogg's vice-president for public affairs. "That would be financial havoc."[57]

Although President George Bush had ignored complaints from consumer groups about fraudulent nutrition claims for foods, he reversed his position after the major food producers demanded federal government regulations. In 1990, according to the *New York Times,* his administration announced "broad and strict regulations intended to halt the proliferation of disease-prevention claims on food packages."[58] The regulations were enacted as part of the Nutrition Labeling and Education Act of 1990, which preempted most state regulations at the insistence of the food industry. The new regulations, based on federal government dietary recommendations, proved to be much more favorable to food producers than to the public.

Federal Government Dietary Guidelines

The federal government has developed two types of dietary recommendations. The U.S. Department of Agriculture adopted the first type, now termed recommended dietary intake, in 1917 as a list of nutrients that had been scientifically determined to prevent nutritional deficiencies and so are essential for life. The original list included five food groups, based on existing American food preferences, that met the need for carbohydrates, fats, and proteins in the diet. The discovery of the need for vitamins and minerals led to new sets of recommendations in the 1920s and 1930s that added these and other nutrients. In 1941 the concept of Recommended Dietary Allowances (later Recommended Dietary Intake) was adopted to quantify the amounts of nutrients that should be consumed daily by healthy persons. In the 1950s the recommendations increased the emphasis on the nutrients in the foods rather than the food classes.[59]

The second type of dietary recommendation, dietary guidelines, was designed to reduce the possibility of developing chronic diseases and recommended modifications of existing consumption patterns. According to A. Stewart Truswell, "although most [recommended dietary intakes] are well-established scientifically, [dietary] guidelines are more provisional, being based on indirect evidence about the complex role of food components in the cause of multifactorial diseases with long incubation periods." The first American dietary guidelines were proposed by the American Heart Association in the 1960s and the first government guidelines were those of the U.S. Senate Select Committee in 1977. In 1980 the Department of Agriculture and the Department of Health and Human Services jointly published *Nutrition and Your Health: Dietary Guidelines for Americans,* which has been revised periodically. It has become, according to one description, "the key Federal policy document on nutrition that serves as the basis for all Federal nutrition programs. It represents the Federal Government's best advice for persons 2 years of age and older about what to eat to stay healthy." Federal law requires the guidelines to be based on the best available medical and scientific knowledge and to be used by "any Federal food, nutrition, or health program."[60]

Similar dietary guidelines have been adopted by many other countries, but the American guidelines go beyond most of them in some important respects. The great majority of national dietary guidelines recommend a nutritionally adequate diet with a variety of foods; less fat, particularly saturated fat; food intake sufficient to maintain proper weight; greater consumption of foods with complex carbohydrates and fiber; reduced salt consumption; and moderate alcohol use. The United States is one of very few countries that specifies dietary cholesterol levels and one of a minority that refers to polyunsaturated fats.[61]

The Nutrition Labeling and Education Act of 1990 required practically all processed foods to contain a label with specific nutrition information about the food. The law exempted most bulk and raw foods, including fresh fruits, vegetables, meats, and poultry. Previously, food producers had listed nutritional information on food packages but, with a few exceptions, the information was voluntary and the manufacturer could choose the nutrients. Under the new legislation, the nutritional information was mandatory and the Food and Drug Administration determined the nutrients to be listed. The label listed the amount of each nutrient present in the food for a specified serving size and the appropriate minimum or maximum daily consumption of the ingredient based on the recommended dietary intake or the dietary guidelines. Descriptive advertising terms like *light, lean, good source of, reduced, fewer,* and *more* were defined, almost always to the advantage of the food industry and the confusion of the consumer. The most controversial issues were the size of the servings and the specific nutrients to be listed.[62]

One of the most significant concessions to the food industry in the legislation was the authorization of health claims for foods based on language specified by the Food and Drug Administration. Seven claims were authorized, three of which involved coronary heart disease: (1) low sodium foods may reduce the risk of high blood pressure; (2) foods low in saturated fats and cholesterol may reduce the risk of coronary heart disease; and (3) fiber contained in fruits, vegetables, and grains (e.g., breakfast cereals) may reduce the risk of coronary heart disease. Three other authorized claims were permitted for foods that were thought to lower the risk of cancer: dietary fats; fiber-containing grain products; and fruits and vegetables. Last, products containing certain levels of calcium were permitted to claim that they reduced the risk of osteoporosis. With the exception of the calcium health claim, which also called for regular exercise, food producers using a specific claim were not required to mention other risk factors associated with the listed diseases.[63]

The FDA's most egregious capitulation to the food industry was the omission of any reference to total caloric intake. Michael Fumento has described this approach as the "calories-don't-count, only-fat-does thesis." The FDA and other agencies have recommended that individuals consume a maximum of 30% of their total calories from fat, but "the government doesn't say *how many* calories the fat should be 30% of." Media health coverage has followed the lead of the government. The Center for Media and Public Affairs monitored news coverage from 37 different media outlets for three months and found, according to Fumento, that "fat consumption occupied twice as much coverage as any other nutritional topic. . . . The media warned against fat consumption four times as often as the overconsumption of calories." A 1996 public opinion survey found that 72% of the respondents used the fat content on the label in making food choices compared to 9% who used total calories.[64]

The information on the nutrition label and the authorized health claims are especially important because consumers receive most of their nutritional advice from commercial sources with close ties to the food industry. One 1993 survey of 17,000 women found that 86% obtained nutritional advice from magazines, many of which receive a significant part of their revenue from food advertisements. In addition, 53% of the women used food labels and advertising and 52% used books, but only 8% used government publications.[65]

Health professionals and the media receive much of their information about foods from nutritionists and dietitians. Marion Nestle has observed that for food companies, "coopting experts—especially academic experts—is an explicit corporate strategy." It involves consulting and lecture fees and research grants for individual scholars, and funding for academic departments, conferences, journals, and professional societies. Food companies fund large amounts of research that can be published in scholarly journals only with their explicit permission. The American Dietetic Association (ADA), which enrolls 70,000 registered dietitians, received 15% of its budget in 1995 from the food industry. According to Nestle, "The association apparently is willing to enter into partnerships with any food company or trade organization, regardless of the nutritional quality of its products." Each of the ADA's approximately seventy fact sheets is sponsored by a corporation, usually a manufacturer of the product being described. The *New York Times* noted that "nothing negative is ever included in materials produced by the [ADA], a fact that critics attribute to its link to industry."[66]

It is not surprising that public opinion surveys have indicated widespread consumer confusion. The most serious problem has been the inability of the public to differentiate more serious risk factors from less serious ones. One poll in the 1980s found that the public ranked "not smoking" tenth "among the nation's health and safety priorities" while health professionals rated it first. With regard to dietary fat, a survey in 1988 found that 55% of the respondents thought that dietary fat was a risk factor for coronary heart disease, but 35% thought that it was a risk factor for high blood pressure and 70% could not differentiate the kinds of fats that did and did not contain cholesterol.[67]

Exercise and Obesity As Risk Factors

The focus of the health education programs of federal government agencies and national health organizations on dietary fat and cholesterol has diverted attention from other lifestyle risk factors that are universally recognized as much greater risks. Besides cigarette smoking, two other risk factors that have received insufficient attention in health education programs are physical exercise and overweight.

Although interest in physical exercise has a long history, perceptions of its benefits for healthy persons have undergone periodic shifts. Throughout the nineteenth century physical exercise was believed to instill moral values and counterbalance the evils of urban life. During the early twentieth century, exercise was recognized as an aid in weight control, but was considered less important than caloric intake. After mid-century, the decline in strenuous physical exercise due to workplace changes and the automobile has led to the recognition of the health benefits of physical exercise for cardiovascular functioning, circulation, muscle tone, joint mobility, and weight control.[68]

Research on the relationship between physical activity and coronary heart disease was first undertaken about mid-century and became a component of risk-factor research. A 1990 analysis of a number of studies found a dose-response relationship: persons with the highest physical activity levels had the lowest coronary heart disease rates, persons with the lowest activity levels had the highest rates, and persons with moderate activity levels had rates between the two extremes. The review also found that the relationship was stronger in the studies judged to be methodologically superior. However, the findings of practically all studies of physical activity are affected by the tendency of persons in poorer health to select sedentary occupations and avoid vigorous exercise. Given the small number of cases of coronary heart disease in most studies, even a few such persons in a sample can affect the findings. At least part of the statistical correlation between physical activity and coronary heart disease results from the self-selection of persons into high and low physical activity groups based on their preexisting health status.[69]

Overweight became one of the most rapidly growing health problems toward the end of the twentieth century. Between 1960–62 and 1988–94, the age-adjusted proportion of all Americans ages 20–74 who were significantly overweight rose from 24% to 35%, with increases occurring for both sexes and all age groups. Significant overweight was defined as a body mass index in the top 15% of the population using a distribution based on a sample of men and women ages 20–29 in a 1976–80 national survey. Among children, the age adjusted proportion of boys and girls who were defined as overweight increased from 5% in 1963–70 to 14% in 1988–94 of those ages 6–11 and from 5% to 12% of those ages 12–17, using a more restricted definition of overweight.[70]

The adverse health consequences of obesity have been most convincingly demonstrated by many life insurance longitudinal studies. These are among the most impressive studies of risk factors ever conducted: they have very large samples, long time durations, and statistically valid methods of selecting representative samples from the population of life insurance policyholders. The policyholders were given medical examinations and found to be in good health when they purchased insurance and therefore were less likely to have unrelated illnesses that affected their mortality rates. They were more homogeneous than the general population with regard to socio-economic status, which reduced differences in that important determinant of mortality. Policyholders are rarely lost to follow-up over the course of the study because of the need to present evidence of death. The life insurance mortality studies before mid-century are especially valuable because few treatments were available to extend the lifespans of policyholders who died of causes related to obesity.

A study of 25,998 overweight men and 24,901 overweight women who purchased ordinary life insurance policies from the Metropolitan Life Insurance Company between 1925 and 1934 followed them until 1950, an average duration of twenty years. During the period 3,713 deaths occurred among the men and 2,687 among the women. The policyholders were sufficiently overweight to be sold substandard insurance policies but had no other impairments with regard to physical condition, medical history, or occupation. This is an extremely important condition because it reduces the probability that preexisting illnesses could have raised their mortality rates. Using age at issuance, the mortality rates of the overweight policyholders compared to policyholders who purchased standard policies were as follows: 80% higher for men ages 20–29; 69% higher for men ages 30–39; 52% higher for men ages 40–49; and 31% higher for men ages 50–59. Among women the overweight groups had mortality rates that were 34 to 52% higher, but no age trends were evident. The higher death rates from some specific diseases for men and women respectively were as follows: diabetes mellitus 3.8 and 3.7 times standard risks; coronary and organic heart disease 1.4 and 1.8 times standard risks; stroke 1.6 and 1.6 time standard risks; and chronic nephritis 1.9 and 2.1 times standard risks. The overweight policyholders were at no greater risk of dying from cancer or pneumonia. A 1997 review of more recent studies not conducted by the life insurance industry also found a strong relationship between obesity and total and cardiovascular disease mortality rates.[71]

Many studies have found a strong dose-response relationship between body weight and mortality rates. The 1959 Build and Blood Pressure Study of the Society of Actuaries examined several million men and women who purchased ordinary life insurance policies from 26 large life insurance companies from 1935 to 1953 and followed them to the anniversary of their policies in 1954. Mortality rates of overweight policyholders with no other known impairments that affected their insurability were compared to the mortality rates of all standard risk policyholders. By age at policy issuance, men 10% above average weight had a 3% higher mortality rate at ages 15–39 and an 8% higher at ages 40–69. Men 20% above average weight had a 15% higher mortality rate at all ages. Those 30% above average weight had a 30% higher mortality rate at all ages. Women 10% above average weight had no higher mortality rate, those 20% above average weight had a 6% higher mortality rate for those ages 15–39 and 15% higher for those ages 40–69, and those 30% above average weight had a 12% higher mortality rate for those ages 15–39 and 25% higher for those ages 40–69. The mortality rates for the most overweight policyholders are greatly understated, because many persons in this category will not be approved for life insurance.[72]

The 1959 Build and Blood Pressure Study also showed that the presence of additional risk factors in men exacerbated the adverse health effects of overweight, even though the levels of the other risk factors were low enough to qualify for standard insurance. Moderate elevation of blood pressure increased mortality rates of overweight men by nearly 60% and a family history of early cardiovascular-renal disease increased the mortality rate by 35%. Higher mortality rates also occurred for overweight men who had elevated blood sugar, asthma, albuminuria, and other conditions.[73]

Overweight heightens the risk of chronic diseases such as high blood pressure and diabetes. A study of the home office employees of the Metropolitan Life Insurance Company about 1950 found that, among those ages 45–54 with diastolic blood pressure of 90 mm/Hg or higher, 45% had a "heavy build" while only 20% had a "light build." Another study of thousands of patients at a diabetes clinic found that 85% of those who contracted diabetes at ages 40 or over were overweight, 60% of them "markedly overweight."[74]

Obesity is a highly salient public health issue because its adverse health effects are reversible. The 1959 Build and Blood Pressure Study studied excessively overweight policyholders who purchased substandard life insurance and then lost weight and qualified for standard rate insurance. Of the male policyholders who initially were about 25% overweight, those who lost weight and qualified for standard rates had a mortality rate that was 9% above standard risks while all those who were 25% overweight originally had a mortality rate 28% higher than standard risks. Of those who were initially 35–40% overweight, the weight losers had a mortality rate 4% less than standard risks, while the mortality rates of all those who were 35–40% overweight originally was 51% greater than standard risks.[75]

Even though the adverse health effects of obesity have been recognized for decades, the leading government agency concerned with blood cholesterol levels has repeated minimized their importance, a position it shares with many other public health organizations. The 2001 report of the National Cholesterol Education Program Expert Panel on Detection, Evaluation, and Treatment of High Blood Cholesterol in Adults adopted a new emphasis on persons with multiple risk factors. The "major, independent risk factors" considered in addition to LDL blood cholesterol level were cigarette smoking, high blood pressure, a family history of premature coronary heart disease, and age. Overweight and a sedentary lifestyle were excluded, even though they can be reversed while age and family history cannot.[76]

Weight reduction of the overweight and smoking cessation are two public health programs that can produce many times the health benefits of lowering blood cholesterol levels. Both have strong statistical correlations with a number of life-threatening diseases, whereas high serum cholesterol levels have only a moderate association with coronary heart disease. Both can be managed with little or no medical intervention. Yet the FDA nutrition labels and authorized health claims for processed foods make no mention of adjusting food intake to maintain appropriate weight. The National Institutes of Health has no programs to help individuals reduce weight or stop smoking comparable to the National Cholesterol Education Program and the National High Blood Pressure Education Program. Most major voluntary health organizations have shown little interest in weight control.

The growing prevalence of overweight poses particular problems for public health programs because it has resulted from broad social changes. Sedentary occupations of men have distorted the traditional balance between caloric intake and physical activity. The employment of more women in the labor force has produced greater consumption of prepared foods, which usually have more calories than home-made foods. Rising incomes have reduced the economic necessity of preparing and consuming inexpensive labor-intensive foods based on traditional recipes with fewer calories than processed foods.

The greatest barrier to effective public health education programs concerning overweight is the economic interests of food producers. Food producers and national retail food franchises and chains are among the nation's largest corporations and have great economic and political influence. Their widespread advertising in the mass media discourages such important sources of health information as television and women's magazines from addressing the problem in all its ramifications. Food producers also exert great influence through the content of their advertising. By the year 2000, food processors and retail food establishments were spending $11 billion annually on direct media advertising, primarily for highly processed fast foods, snacks, beverages, and convenience foods. Much of the advertising claimed health benefits for the foods.[77]

Health education campaigns to reduce overweight will succeed only if they describe in detail the major classes of high-calorie foods and vigorously discourage their consumption. They must also educate the public about a low-calorie diet, teach individuals to recognize overweight in themselves, and inform them of methods of losing weight safely. Appropriate actions could involve expanding food nutrition labels to include desirable height/weight tables and requiring all food health claims on packages and advertisements to contain warnings about overweight similar to those used for cigarettes. Such a program requires a direct confrontation with major corporate food producers, which public and private organizations concerned with public health have assiduously avoided.

19

THE SECULAR DECLINE IN THE CORONARY HEART DISEASE EPIDEMIC

The announcement for this reversal in the long-term upward trend [of coronary heart disease mortality] was received with great astonishment, both in the United States and in other countries.[1]

No one has yet established a convincing fit of trends for any risk factor with cardiovascular mortality trends.[2]

The Secular Decline In The Coronary Heart Disease Pandemic

The great twentieth-century coronary heart disease pandemic, which killed millions of persons in westernized countries, abated after 1960 and continued to wane for the remainder of the century. Its rise and fall has usually been explained by population-wide changes in personal risk factors, which include excessive animal fats and cholesterol in the diet, obesity, smoking, sedentary living, lack of physical exercise, and stress. According to this theory, a meaningful decline in coronary heart disease rates occurred after the risk factors were modified in large numbers of persons.

From one perspective, it is inconceivable that an international pandemic of any disease could be caused or eliminated by changes in personal behaviors. The millions of persons affected by the coronary heart disease pandemic lived in two dozen countries with different social and economic structures, customs, traditions, diets, and work and recreational activities. Such diversity could never produce identical patterns of personal behavior that materialized and diminished simultaneously in all of the countries. Furthermore, personal behaviors have never been considered responsible for the great pandemics of the past, such as the nineteenth and early twentieth centuries pandemics of cholera, tuberculosis, and influenza. All great pandemics have been explained by singular combinations of social, economic, and technological changes, usually including new patterns of transportation that permitted the spread of the disease across countries and continents.

From another perspective, the factors that produced great pandemics were never the same as those that produced different rates of the disease in specific groups. For example, before, during, and after the coronary heart disease pandemic, the disease was more prevalent in men, lower socio-economic groups, and hypertensive persons. Thus these factors could not have caused the pandemic to develop or diminish.

To demonstrate a correlation between risk factor changes and the decline in coronary heart disease mortality rates, it is necessary to compare the date of onset of the decline in coronary heart disease rates to trends in the prevalence of risk factors. This analysis will employ statistics from a variety of sources and use death rates of persons under age 65 because of more accurate reporting of cause of death.

United States vital statistics show that coronary heart disease became a much less important cause of death for both men and women in the last three decades of the twentieth century. Between 1970 and 1993, the coronary heart disease mortality rates among men ages 45–54 and 55–64 dropped by more than 60% (see Table 19.1). This greatly exceeded the decline in overall mortality rates, with coronary heart disease producing about 37% of all deaths in 1970 but only 20% in 1993. Women experienced a similar 60% decline in coronary heart disease mortality rates even though their rates were only about 25% of those of men at ages 45–54 and about 35% at ages 55–65 throughout the period. The proportion of all deaths among women that resulted from coronary heart disease dropped by about half from 1970 to 1993.

The declining proportion of deaths due to coronary heart disease has reversed the trend toward greater longevity of women than men, because

Table 19.1: Major Causes of Death at Ages 45–64 by Sex, 1970–1996

	(per 1,000 persons) *Age 45–54* *Male*		*Female*	
	1970	1996	1970	1996
All causes	9.6	5.7	5.2	3.2
Coronary heart disease	3.4	1.0	0.8	0.3
All heart disease	3.8	1.6	1.1	0.6
Cancer	1.8	1.4*	1.8	1.4*
Stroke	0.4	0.2*	0.4	0.2*

	Age 55–64 *Male*		*Female*	
	1970	1996	1970	1996
All causes	22.8	13.9	11.0	8.3
Coronary heart disease	9.0	3.0	3.0	1.1
All heart disease	9.9	4.5	3.5	1.9
Cancer	5.1	4.8*	3.4	3.6*
Stroke	1.4	0.5*	1.0	0.4*

*1995

Sources: U.S. Bureau of the Census, *Statistical Abstract of the United States: 1985* (Washington, DC: 1984), 71, 77; U.S. Bureau of the Census, *Statistical Abstract of the United States: 1999* (Washington, DC: 1999), 95, 104–5; National Center for Health Statistics, *Health, United States, 1996–97* (Hyattsville, MD: 1997), 133.

other causes of death with no meaningful gender differences have become relatively more important (see Table 19.2). The number of additional years of life expectancy at age 40 for white women compared to white men increased steadily from about 1920 to about 1970, when it reached 6.2 years. The decline in coronary heart disease mortality rates stabilized the difference in the 1970s and lessened it subsequently, to 4.5 years in 1997.

As coronary heart disease mortality rates declined, the condition became predominantly a disease of the very old (see Table 19.3). In 1970, 38% of all coronary heart disease deaths among men and 51% of those among women occurred in persons ages 75 and over. By 1997, the proportions had increased to 57% for men and 77% for women, with 24% of male deaths and 45% of female deaths occurring in persons ages 85 and over. Coronary heart disease has increasingly become a disease of senescence, as it was perceived by physicians before the epidemic began in the 1920s.

The trend toward older ages of death for coronary heart disease victims indicates that the actual decline was greater than reported in vital

Table 19.2: Life Expectancy at Age 40 for White Men and Women, 1919–1997

	Men	Women	Number of extra years for women
1919–21	29.9	30.9	1.0
1939–41	30.0	33.3	3.3
1959–61	31.7	37.1	6.0
1969–71	31.9	38.1	6.2
1979–81	34.0	40.2	6.2
1990	35.6	41.0	5.4
1997	36.6	41.1	4.5

Sources: U.S. Bureau of the Census, *Statistical Abstract of the United States: 1970* (Washington, DC: 1970), 53; U.S. Bureau of the Census, *Statistical Abstract of the United States: 1999* (Washington, DC: 1999), 93.

statistics. Among the very old, coronary heart disease is frequently overreported because it is a diagnosis of convenience to comply with legal regulations. Robert R. Kohn has observed that "an old person usually dies with a variety of diagnoses. It may not be clear, either clinically or from post-mortem examination, which process was an important cause of death. Indeed, no cause of death may be obvious, particularly in very old people. A cause of death chosen from a standard list must, however, go on the death certificate." Coronary heart disease is an obvious and medically acceptable choice because it is associated with many serious diseases. For example, decreased lung or kidney function places greater demands on the pumping action of the heart and can produce or aggravate coronary heart disease. As was shown in earlier chapters, postmortem examinations have found that coronary heart disease is erroneously listed as the cause of death much more often in elderly persons. As the average age of death from coro-

Table 19.3: Age Distribution of Coronary Heart Disease Deaths, by Sex, 1970–1997

Age	Men		Women	
	1970	1997	1970	1997
0–54	13%	9	5	3
55–64	21	13	10	5
65–74	29	25	24	15
75–84	27	33	37	32
85+	11	24	24	45
Total	100	100	100	100

Source: 1970: U.S. Public Health Service, *Vital Statistics of the United States, 1970,* Vol. IIA (Rockville, MD, 1974), 216–17; 1997: unpublished U. S. government vital statistics.

nary heart disease increase, so does the amount of overreporting, which slows down the apparent rate of decline.[3]

The date when the coronary heart disease epidemic began to abate is crucial to establishing correlations between coronary heart disease mortality trends and risk factor trends. Fortunately, classification problems are reduced because the decline began during a single revision of the International Classification of Diseases. Each revision changed some of the specific conditions included within the ischemic (coronary) heart disease category and so is not precisely comparable with the others. The sixth revision spanned 1949–1957, the seventh revision 1958–1967, and the eighth revision 1968–1978.[4]

According to United States vital statistics, the onset of the decline in coronary heart disease mortality rates occurred in the late 1960s. Table 19.4 lists mortality rates from coronary heart disease and for all causes for selected years from 1950 to 1994 for white men and women ages 45–54 and 55–64 (rates for nonwhite groups were not available for all years listed). The epidemic peaked from the mid-1950s to the late 1960s in both men and women. Consistent rates of decline began for men in the late 1960s and in the early 1970s for women. Trends in the epidemic were unrelated to total mortality trends, because total mortality rates declined steadily throughout the period.

The onset of the decline occurred earlier in the vital statistics of urban than rural states. Thirteen states, most with large urban populations, experienced the onset for white males ages 55–64 before 1961: California, Florida, New York, Pennsylvania, New Jersey, Maryland, Massachusetts, Connecticut, Rhode Island, New Hampshire, Washington, Idaho, and Wyoming. All other highly urbanized states experienced the onset of their declines in the early 1960s. States with large urban populations had much more accurate diagnostic capabilities at that time because of their better-trained physicians and superior medical facilities.[5]

Coronary heart disease mortality rates based on vital statistics include the total population, both sick and healthy. Healthy persons will benefit sooner and to a greater degree from a secular decline than will persons with a previous history of heart disease or other serious diseases. Persons with a previous myocardial infarction, some other form of coronary heart disease, diabetes, or left ventricular hypertrophy have irreversible conditions that produce much higher mortality rates from coronary heart disease than healthy persons.

Healthy men experienced the onset of the decline in coronary heart disease mortality rates about 1960. One source of evidence is the ordinary

Table 19.4: Coronary Heart Disease and Total Mortality Rates by Age and Sex,
1950–1994

	(rates per 1,000 white persons)							
	Coronary Heart Disease Age				Total Mortality Age			
Year	45–54		55–64		45–54		55–64	
	M	F	M	F	M	F	M	F
Sixth revision								
1950	3.2	0.7	8.1	2.7	9.8	5.5	23.0	12.9
1957	3.4	0.6	8.9	2.8				
Seventh revision								
1958	3.4	0.6	8.9	2.7				
1959	3.5	0.6	8.9	2.7				
1960	3.5	0.6	9.0	2.8	9.3	4.6	22.3	10.8
1961	3.5	0.6	8.9	2.6				
1962	3.5	0.7	8.9	2.7				
1963	3.5	0.7	9.1	2.7				
1964	3.5	0.7	9.0	2.6				
1965	3.5	0.7	9.0	2.6				
1966	3.5	0.7	9.1	2.6				
1967	3.4	0.7	8.9	2.5				
Eighth revision								
1968	3.5	0.7	9.5	2.8				
1969	3.4	0.7	9.2	2.7				
1970	3.3	0.7	9.0	2.7	8.8	4.6	22.0	10.1
1972	3.2	0.7	8.8	2.6				
1978	2.6	0.5	6.9	2.1				
Ninth revision								
1979	2.2	0.5	6.0	1.8	7.0	3.7	17.3	8.8
1984	1.8	0.4	5.0	1.6				
1990*	1.3	0.3	3.8	1.4	5.5	3.1	14.7	8.2
1996*	1.0	0.3	3.0	1.1	5.2	2.9	13.1	7.8

*All races for coronary heart disease only

Source: Millicent W. Higgins and Russell V. Luepker, eds., *Trends in Coronary Heart Disease Mortality: The Influence of Medical Care* (New York: Oxford University Press, 1988), 284–85; U.S. Bureau of the Census, *Statistical Abstract of the United States, 1999* (Washington, DC; U.S. GPO, 1999), 95, 104; National Center for Health Statistics, *Health, United States, 1999* (Hyattsville, MD: 1999), 160–62.

policyholders of the Metropolitan Life Insurance Company, who were required to pass a medical examination to qualify for life insurance policies
and also had above-average socio-economic levels (see Table 19.5). During
the 1960s Metropolitan ordinary policyholders ages 35–64 had significantly
lower coronary heart disease mortality rates than the U.S. white population, the most comparable national group. The male policyholders experi-

Table 19.5: Coronary Heart Disease Mortality Rates by Age and Sex: Standard Risk Ordinary Policyholders, Metropolitan Life Insurance Company, 1962–1973

	(rates per 1,000 policies)									
	1962		*1967*		*1969*		*1973*		*1977*	
	M	F	M	F	M	F	M	F	M	F
45–49	2.3	0.3	2.0	0.3	1.8	0.3	1.6	0.3	1.4	0.2
50–54	4.3	0.6	3.9	0.7	3.8	0.7	3.0	0.6	2.4	0.6
55–59	6.9	1.4	6.8	1.4	6.1	1.4	5.1	1.5	4.1	1.1
60–64	10.9	2.9	10.8	3.2	10.3	2.8	8.4	2.6	6.8	2.3
65–69	16.3	7.6	15.9	7.0	15.1	7.3	12.3	5.7	10.9	4.9

Ages 35–64 age–adjusted coronary heart disease mortality rates

Policyholders	3.5	0.7	3.4	0.7	3.1	0.7	2.6	0.7	—	—
U.S. white Population	3.8	1.0	3.8	0.9	3.7	1.0	3.4	0.9	—	—

Sources: "Recent Trends in Mortality from Heart Disease," *Statistical Bulletin* 56 (June, 1975): 3–6; "Recent Trends in Mortality from Cardiovascular Diseases," *Statistical Bulletin* 60 (April–June, 1979: 7.

enced steady and significant declines in their coronary heart disease mortality rates from 1962 to 1977 and the report stated that the onset of the decline antedated 1962. The decline occurred for all age groups from 45–49 to 65–69 but the rate of decline in the early part of the period was greatest for the youngest groups, as would be expected by their generally better health. The onset of the decline for female policyholders occurred in the 1970s, as it did for the U.S. female population. The decline proceeded at a faster rate between 1962 and 1973 for ordinary policyholders ages 35–64 than for the U.S. white population, again indicating that persons in better health benefited more from the decline.

A 1960 date for onset of the decline in healthy men was also found in a longitudinal study of 294,000 holders of government life insurance policies, almost all issued to white men who passed a medical examination and served in the U.S. Armed Forces between 1917 and 1940. The sample was much healthier than the general population because its overall mortality rate was only 73% of that of white men of comparable ages in the U.S. population. Cause of death was obtained for 97% of the deceased because of the need to file claims to receive death benefits. The sample consisted of the 84% of the policyholders who returned questionnaires in 1954 or 1957 that included a question about their smoking status. Considering the period from 1954 to 1980, nonsmoking veterans ages 55–69 experienced the onset of the decline in coronary heart disease mortality rates between 1954 and 1960. The rates for smokers rose from 1954 to 1960 and declined after 1960 among those ages 55–64 and after 1965 among those ages 65–69.[6]

Evidence of a 1960 date for the decline is also found in studies of coronary heart disease morbidity and mortality. A nationwide study examined 75,000 to 94,000 male employees of the E. I. DuPont de Nemours and Company from 1957 to 1983. About 95% were covered by health insurance, which suggests generally accurate diagnoses. The age-adjusted rates of first myocardial infarctions and sudden deaths attributed to coronary heart disease per 1,000 employees declined from 3.2 in 1957–59 to 3.1 in 1960–62, 2.9 in 1963–65, and 3.0 in 1966–68. A steeper rate of decline then occurred to 2.7 in 1969–71 and 2.3 in 1981–83. Rates for the higher-paid salaried workers declined earlier and to a greater extent than for the lower-paid wage workers. Another study of the incidence of initial myocardial infarctions, angina pectoris, and sudden unexpected deaths in residents of Rochester, Minnesota, from 1950 through 1982 found that the rate peaked for men in the 1950s and declined steadily thereafter. The decline occurred primarily among those ages 30–69. The trends were much weaker among women, whose rates were about one-fourth those of men at ages 30–49 and one-half at older age groups.[7]

Other evidence that healthy persons were the primary beneficiaries of the decline consists of a downward trend in mortality rates of persons without preexisting heart disease, while no such trend occurred in persons with preexisting disease up to the late 1980s. A community-wide study examined 793 validated coronary heart disease deaths among white males ages 35–44 in the Pittsburgh, Pennsylvania, area between 1970 and 1981. The age group was chosen because of its high autopsy rate and the infrequency of previous coronary heart disease. From 1970–72 to 1979–81 the group experienced a 50% decline in coronary heart disease mortality rates, primarily due to fewer new cases of the disease. The greatest decline occurred for sudden coronary heart disease deaths without a previous history of coronary heart disease. In addition, out-of-hospital deaths and cases who were dead on arrival declined by 62%, while in-hospital deaths declined by only 33%.[8]

Studies elsewhere produced similar findings. Sixteen hospitals in the Worcester, Massachusetts, metropolitan area experienced a steady decrease in death rates from initial acute myocardial infarction and in out-of-hospital deaths from coronary heart disease for both men and women between 1975 and 1988. No changes occurred for in-hospital death rates or survival rates of patients discharged from the hospitals after acute myocardial infarctions. A study of one million subscribers to the Kaiser-Permanente health plan in northern California from 1971 to 1977 found that the downward trend in coronary heart disease mortality rates was due to fewer new cases rather than higher survival rates of those with the disease. A New York City study of first myocardial infarctions compared the 4.5 year post-hospitalization survival rates of 436 men ages 35–64 in 1961–70 to 697 men in 1971–80. Although this was a period of steadily declining coronary heart disease mortality rates, no differences in survival rates occurred between the two groups or between subgroups that had infarctions of the same degree of severity.[9]

These studies provide convincing evidence that about 1960 rates of first myocardial infarctions and coronary heart disease mortality began to decline steadily in healthy men. The study samples varied widely in composition and geographic locations. The onset of the decline occurred during a single revision of the International Classification of Diseases, thereby eliminated classification changes as a possible explanation. Coronary heart disease mortality rates for women declined later than those for men, but the pandemic was much milder for women.

The coronary heart disease pandemic occurred during the same time period in North America, western and northern Europe, Australia, and other advanced westernized countries. These countries experienced steadily increasing coronary heart disease mortality rates for men from the 1920s through the 1960s. After about 1970, practically all of them experienced steadily declining rates for both men and women. The gender patterns of the pandemic were very similar in all of the countries.[10]

Trends in Risk Factors and Coronary Heart Disease Rates

Coronary heart disease is produced by a combination of factors that interact and operate in the human body over years or decades. Changes in the causal factors must therefore occur long before the onset of the decline. If the decline in coronary heart disease rates in healthy men began about 1960, their risk factors must have begun changing no later than the early 1950s. Proponents of the risk factor theory describe three types of changes: (1) new treatments for persons who experienced coronary heart disease; (2) modifications of risk factors in persons at high risk of the disease; and (3) modifications of risk factors in the general population.

Improvements in the treatment of coronary heart disease made no contribution to the decline in mortality rates until long after 1960. Most innovations in treatment became widely used in the 1970s or 1980s, including prehospital resuscitation, coronary artery bypass graft surgery, angioplasty, thrombolytic therapy, and drugs such as beta-blockers. Another widely cited intervention, the coronary care unit, was developed in the early 1960s to treat potentially fatal heart arrhythmias in patients with recent myocardial infarctions. By 1966, 350 units were in operation and thousands more were established in the next decade. These units were generally ineffective during the 1960s and 1970s: many patients in them were misdiagnosed, the staffs were untrained and often lacked authority to treat patients immediately, and resuscitation was soon found to be less useful than prevention of arrhythmias. Studies in England found little benefit of the units for patients with mild or moderate myocardial infarctions.[11] Furthermore, therapeutic innovations were implemented at different times and to widely varying degrees in the countries that experienced similar declines in coronary heart disease mortality. More generally, no major epidemic has ever been halted by therapeutic innovations, but only by preventive measures and changes in social and environmental conditions.

Modification of risk factors in high risk persons did not contribute to the secular decline that began about 1960. The benefits of declines in smoking rates can be measured by mortality rates from lung cancer, which began to decline after 1970 in men ages 35–44 and after 1980 in men ages 45–54 and women ages 35–54. Diabetes mellitus showed little change, with age-adjusted death rates per 1,000 population remaining level at 0.14 in 1950, 1960, and 1970, declining to 0.10 in 1980, and rising to 0.13 in 1995.[12]

Trends in high blood pressure, high blood cholesterol, and overweight were measured in physical examinations of samples of the American population in 1960–62, 1971–74, 1976–80, and 1988–94. The 45–54 year-old age group is described here, but the same trends occurred in all other age groups. Essential hypertension was defined as a blood pressure of at least 140 mm/Hg systolic or 90 mm/Hg diastolic or being on antihypertensive medication. The rates of any one of those conditions in the four surveys were 48%, 55%, 54%, and 34% for men and 43%, 44%, 47%, and 25% for women. No decline occurred until the 1988–94 survey. A high serum cholesterol level was defined as 240 mg/dl or higher. The rates of those levels in the four surveys were 39%, 38%, 37%, and 27% for men and 47%, 39%, 41%, and 27% for women. No decline occurred for men until the 1988–94 study. Overweight was defined as being in the top 15% of the body-mass index scores of persons 20–29 in the 1976–80 survey. In the four surveys 28%, 28%, 31%, and 38% of men were overweight, as were 31%, 32%, 33%, and 45% of women. Overweight rates increased over the time period.[13]

Modifications of risk factors in the general population also were not responsible for the secular trend. Jeremiah Stamler stated in 1992 that there are four "established major risk factors"—'rich' diet, diet-related optimal levels of serum total cholesterol and blood pressure, and cigarette smoking. . . . [T]he population-wide eating pattern is the key in three of these four established major risk factors."[14]

The impact of diet on persons at average risk can be measured by changes in the average blood cholesterol levels for the American population as measured in the national surveys in 1960–62, 1971–74, 1976–80, and 1988–94. The average serum cholesterol levels for men ages 35–44 were 227, 221, 217, and 206 mg/dl, those for men ages 45–54 were 231, 229, 227, and 216 mg/dl, those for women ages 35–44 were 214, 207, 207, and 195 mg/dl, and those for women ages 45–54 were 237, 232, 232, and 217 mg/dl. The only meaningful changes in blood cholesterol levels occurred after 1976–80, long after the onset of the decline in coronary heart disease rates.[15]

These data demonstrate conclusively that changes in personal risk factors were not responsible for the secular decline in coronary heart disease mortality and morbidity rates.

Social and Economic Factors Related To Coronary Heart Disease

The emphasis on personal risk factors for coronary heart disease has been accompanied by a disregard of social risk factors. For this reason it is important to establish that a variety of social characteristics have had a significant impact on coronary heart disease rates.

The strongest evidence comes from the disparities in the coronary heart disease rates of workers with different job titles in the same organizations, which are among the most methodologically rigorous studies of their kind. Studies of workers exclude persons too ill to work, who are atypical in many respects. Job titles in individual large organizations are much more internally consistent with regard to education, earnings, and work responsibilities than census occupational categories or occupations reported on death certificates. Workers employed by the same organization were hired using the same health standards, had the same health insurance benefits, and shared many aspects of their working conditions. Information on coronary heart disease was obtained from reliable sources and the deaths occurred at ages where reporting of cause of death is most accurate.

The nationwide study of 73,573 male employees ages 17–64 of E.I. DuPont de Nemours and Company found that 1331 were "stricken with a myocardial infarction" in the years from 1956 to 1961. Myocardial infarctions were measured by annual medical examinations of all employees ages 30 and over and information provided by the company's group life and health insurance plans. The workers were placed in five groups of 1,143 to 46,050 employees each, which included one for hourly wage employees and four for different types of salaried employees. Myocardial infarction rates were based on the average number of workers in each group over the period. The lowest age-adjusted annual myocardial infarction rates per 1,000 employees were 2.2 for high level managers and 2.5 for the group consisting of professionals, salesmen, and middle-level managers. The highest rates were 4.0 for first-level supervisors, most of whom started their careers as hourly wage workers, 3.7 for clerical workers and laboratory technicians, and 3.5 for hourly wage skilled, semiskilled, and unskilled workers. Blood pressure, serum cholesterol levels, smoking, and weight were examined in a sample of workers in different occupations and the differences among occupational groups were found to be small.[16]

The Whitehall study conducted medical examinations of 17,530 English male civil servants between 1967 and 1969 and followed them for an average of 7.5 years. Most of the men were employed in physically undemanding occupations, so that self-selection into occupations by health status did not occur to any meaningful degree. Using men ages 50–59 as an example, during the course of the study 2.9% of those in administrative and professional grades died of coronary heart disease compared to 4.5% of those in the clerical and similar grades. Only 40% of the difference was explained by dissimilarities in serum cholesterol levels, systolic blood pressure, smoking status, body mass index, physical activity outside of work, blood glucose levels, or presence of coronary heart disease at entry into the study. The study concluded that "a man's grade of employment was a stronger predictor of his subsequent risk of [coronary heart disease] death than any of the other major risk factors."[17]

A study that followed 85,000 white male U.S. Army veterans from their discharge in 1946 to 1969 found lower coronary heart disease mortality rates among those who held higher level positions while in the army. The average age at discharge was 24 years and the average age at the study's termination was 47 years. The total mortality rate of the veterans was 84% of the rate of the general population of similar ages. Compared to white males in the general population with the same age distributions, the commissioned officers had only 50% as many coronary heart disease deaths, the noncommissioned officers had 88%, and the privates had 98%. The comparable proportions for all causes of death were 59%, 77%, and 100%

respectively. Within each rank, veterans with more education had lower total mortality rates than those with less education.[18]

These studies found significant differences in coronary heart disease rates by occupational grade that were independent of personal risk factors. The same conclusion was reached in a report approved by the Science Advisory Committee of the American Heart Association in 1993. It stated that socio-economic status "is an important factor in the etiology and progression of cardiovascular disease" and "the relation between measures of [socio-economic status] and cardiovascular events remain substantial when accepted cardiovascular risk factors are considered simultaneously."[19]

These conclusions are consistent with the finding that overall mortality rates are greatest at the lowest socio-economic levels and least at the highest levels. Differential access to health care is not the primary explanation for the gradient, which occurs for diseases that are treatable and untreatable and in countries with and without universal health insurance. Differences in diet cannot explain the gradient. Department of Agriculture surveys examined the self-reported diets of high, medium, and low socio-economic status groups in 1965, 1977–78, and 1989–91. In all three surveys the three groups were very similar in the percentage of their calories from fat, saturated fat, and intake of dietary cholesterol and sodium. All three groups reduced their consumption of these nutrients from the first to the third surveys, which provides additional evidence of the similarities in their choices of foods.[20]

Place of birth and ethnicity, two social factors that were related to mortality in the early twentieth century, affect coronary heart disease rates. The Framingham Heart Study found in the 1950s that the foreign-born participants had lower rates of coronary heart disease than the native-born. A later study examined coronary heart disease mortality rates in New York City for 1988–92 for blacks born in the South, blacks born in the Northeast, blacks born in the Caribbean, and whites born in the Northeast. Because all of the deaths occurred in New York City, the standards of diagnosis and treatment were reasonably similar for all groups. As predicted by the westernized lifestyle theory, the lowest rates occurred for blacks born in the Caribbean, whose coronary heart disease mortality rates per 1,000 persons ages 45–64 were 1.7 for men and 1.1 for women. Although the theory would also predict low rates for blacks born in the then rural South, southern–born blacks had the highest rates with 4.1 deaths for men and 2.2 for women. Blacks born in the highly urbanized Northeast were between the two extremes, with 3.2 coronary heart disease deaths for men and 1.5 for women. These rates were practically identical to those for whites born in the Northeast, which were 3.4 for men and 1.3 for women.[21]

Table 19.6: Mortality Rates by Cause of Death: Selected Countries, 1992–1994

(rates per 1,000 population)
Age Standardized

Country	Coronary Heart Disease Rate	Stroke Rate	Lung Cancer Rate*	Crude Death Rate
Japan	0.4	0.8	0.3	7.9
France	0.6	0.5	0.4	9.0
Spain	0.7	0.8	0.3	8.9
Italy	0.9	0.9	0.4	9.9
Netherlands	1.2	0.7	0.5	8.7
Sweden	1.7	0.7	0.2	11.3
Canada	1.5	0.5	0.5	7.2
Germany	1.5	0.8	0.4	11.1
Australia	1.6	0.6	0.4	6.9
United States	1.6	0.5	0.6	8.8
Switzerland	1.0	0.7	0.3	9.6
England/Wales	2.0	0.8	0.5	11.2**

*1997

**United Kingdom

Source: U.S. Bureau of the Census, *Statistical Abstract of the United States 1997* (Washington, DC: U.S. GPO, 1997), 832–34.

Evidence of cultural determinants of coronary heart disease is shown in the differences in coronary heart disease rates among westernized countries. Although all technologically advanced nations experienced significant declines in their coronary heart disease mortality rates after 1970, their relative rankings have remained largely unchanged since before 1950. Table 19.6 lists crude death rates and age-standardized mortality rates for coronary heart disease, stroke, and lung cancer for selected westernized countries in the early 1990s. Coronary heart disease rates varied widely among the countries and showed a low statistical correlation with their overall mortality rates or stroke or cancer mortality rates. The disparities among the countries are also much greater for coronary heart disease than for stroke, lung cancer, or total mortality.

Racial differences in coronary heart disease mortality rates indicate that coronary heart disease has been disproportionately a disease of white males. Before 1950 white males had much higher coronary heart disease mortality rates than black males, the opposite of practically all other diseases. In 1979 and 1997 black males had somewhat higher coronary heart disease rates than white males and black females had much higher rates than white females (see Table 19.7). However, in every age group, a smaller

Table 19.7: Coronary Heart Disease Mortality Rates by Age, Sex and Race, 1979–1997

(rates per 1,000 population)

1979

	Male		Female	
	White	Black	White	Black
35–44	0.5	0.7	0.1	0.3
45–54	2.2	2.6	0.5	1.1
55–64	6.0	6.0	1.8	3.0
65–74	13.9	11.3	5.9	7.1

1997

	Male		Female	
	White	Black	White	Black
35–44	0.2	0.3	0.1	0.1
45–54	1.0	1.4	0.2	0.6
55–64	2.8	3.7	1.0	1.9
65–74	7.2	7.4	3.3	4.9

Proportion of All Deaths from Coronary Heart Disease, 1979–1997

1979

	Male		Female	
	White	Black	White	Black
35–44	19.0	9.4	6.4	8.5
45–54	31.5	17.2	12.6	14.7
55–64	34.8	21.6	20.8	20.3
65–74	34.8	23.1	29.4	24.2

1997

	Male		Female	
	White	Black	White	Black
35–44	9.5	6.0	4.5	4.8
45–54	19.2	12.2	8.7	9.6
55–64	22.5	16.1	13.2	14.0
65–74	23.0	17.2	17.1	17.9

Source: Unpublished data, Mortality Statistics Branch, National Center for Health Statistics.

proportion of the total mortality of black males compared to white males resulted from coronary heart disease. In 1979, 32% of all deaths of white males ages 45–54 were caused by coronary heart disease compared to 17% of deaths among black males. In 1997, the proportions were 19% and 12% respectively. Similar differences occurred for the 55–64 and the 65–

74 year-old groups. White and black women, however, had practically identical proportions of their deaths caused by coronary heart disease.

Thus convincing evidence exists that a downward secular trend in the great coronary heart disease pandemic began about 1960 and that changes in personal risk factors were not responsible for the decline. There is also clear-cut evidence that social factors have a strong impact on coronary heart disease rates.

20

EPILOGUE

> The most vital contribution to the "risk epidemic" . . . has come from
> the development of scientific thinking itself. Within this thinking there
> has been a movement from a paradigm of monocausal determinism
> towards a paradigm of multiple causes and effects, accepting uncer-
> tainty as a vital factor.[1]

Risk factors have not been completely accepted in public health and clinical medicine, largely because of ambivalence about inferential statistics.
Their prominent role in the health education movement has raised several
fundamental issues, including individual versus social responsibility for disease and population-wide- versus high-risk strategies.

Risk factors have brought public health and clinical medicine closer
together than ever before. The role of public health is to identify risk factors, educate the public about prevention and treatment, and promote
changes in individuals and public and private organizations. The role of
clinical medicine is to diagnose risk factors in individual patients and treat
them through lifestyle changes or medications.

The identification and treatment of risk factors rely on inferential
statistics, which has become the standard method of finding relationships
in samples of persons and generalizing the findings to populations of interest. Inferential statistics has had a long record of achievements in the social

sciences, agriculture, education, and business, where it produced a fundamental reorientation of their conceptual frameworks. Probabilistic modes of analysis replaced deterministic ones, multifactorial etiology replaced the analysis of one causal factor at a time, and correlations replaced cause-and-effect relationships as the objectives of research investigations.

In public health and medicine, inferential statistics has had to compete with older methodologies: clinical observation, pathology, laboratory investigation, and vital and other descriptive statistics. These methodologies produced revolutionary and profound discoveries in disease etiology, prognosis, and therapy. Their successes have made them the criteria by which all new methodologies are judged. They dominate the philosophical and methodological bases of professional education; they are pervasive in journals and conferences; they serve as the evidence of last resort in controversies.

Inferential statistics was brought into public health and medicine partly because of the limitations of the dominant methodologies when applied to chronic and degenerative diseases. Clinical observation, pathology, and laboratory investigation could not explicate the etiology of diseases with extremely long latency periods. This was most strikingly shown by their failure to recognize that smoking was one of the greatest public health problems of the twentieth century. Neither could the traditional methods explain the multiple etiological factors in coronary heart disease.

Inferential statistics also entered medicine because of public concern over the many new preventive and therapeutic interventions. The public demanded that the risks of these measures be quantified, promulgated, and debated, and that public officials balance safety, efficacy, and cost in their decisions. Once again inferential statistics became the methodology of choice, such as the 1970 decision of the Food and Drug Administration to use controlled clinical trials to evaluate drugs for safety and efficacy.[2]

Critics of medical procedures also used inferential statistics to scrutinize and evaluate the dominant methodologies. An example is a 1971 criticism of surgical research by David H. Spodick, a proponent of statistics: "It is therefore urgent to . . . objectively establish the merits of direct coronary operations before they become more or less 'accepted' as was the case with certain formerly and still popular procedures, some of which inspired second thoughts only after large numbers of patients had received their dubious benefits." Spodick noted that physicians applied "heroic measures in ominous circumstances, but it is the patient who has been, willy nilly, the hero." He criticized surgeons for drawing unwarranted inferences from animal experiments, for poorly designed clinical trials, and for basing conclusions on impressionistic rather than statistical evidence. One surgeon defended surgery by claiming that quantitative clinical trials are inappropriate for surgical procedures. By the time the results are published, the procedures have often been modified: "Techniques are refined; mortality and morbidity fall, often precipitously, and the results obtained by other surgeons commonly surpass those of the initiator." Surgery also has a "system of intrinsic controls" involving "the referral of patients for surgical therapy by primary physicians, who are not surgeons and are rewarded only by good results."[3]

Reservations about inferential statistics have led to the accusation that risk factors are an alien approach imposed on public health and medicine. The distinguished physician-statistician, Alvan Feinstein, acknowledged that in risk factor research "the reported evidence is almost always a statistical analysis of epidemiologic data, and the scientific tactics that produced the evidence are almost always difficult to understand and evaluate." Another physician, Robert Aronowitz, called risk factors an "unquestioned, implicit, ill-defined, and largely invisible framework for understanding disease," in contrast to the observable pathological and laboratory investigations and the "shared values or insights from the clinical care of individual patients."[4]

Aronowitz also stated that risk factor methodology has not been subjected "to much explicit debate or analysis." This is in striking contrast to the almost identical concept of carcinogens, which has been more closely associated with the physical than the biomedical sciences. Carcinogenesis has been subjected to intensive conceptual and methodological scrutiny. The lack of such analysis for risk factors also explains why they have been so unevenly applied.[5]

Risk factors also entered public health and medicine for reasons unrelated to statistics; they meshed closely with the growing popular attention to the concept of risk. The public has demanded to know more about the risks associated with public health, medicine, foods, science, and technology. Academe, government, and the professions have responded accordingly. Risk, risk analysis, risk assessment, and risk management have become important subjects in scholarly and professional disciplines and journals. Risk has been a central theme in reports of the National Academy of Sciences and other prestigious organizations. The growing concern with risk in public health and medicine is shown by analyses of Medline, the most complete index of health-related periodicals. The proportion of articles with the word "risk" in the title increased from 0.1% in 1967 to 5% in 1991 for all journals and to an average of about 10% for the leading medical journals in the United States, England, and Scandinavia.[6]

This qualitative approach to risk often manifests little concern with quantitative measures and defines risk simply as the possibility of some kind of adverse event. It has greatly broadened the notion of risk and has produced greater receptivity to risk factors or levels of risk factors that pose relatively little danger or are only weakly supported by statistical evidence. It has become popular in the mass media because it is more easily understood by laypersons.

The greater receptivity to risk factors not supported by convincing statistical evidence jeopardizes the hard-earned popular trust in public health recommendations. For most of history, health recommendations were vague and ineffectual and usually disregarded by the public. In the late nineteenth century, bacteriology produced a new type of health recommendation based on conclusive research evidence. It slowly and laboriously acquired a reputation for scrupulous accuracy and trustworthiness. Public health recommendations became the standard of the best that government could offer its citizens. Today many recommendations concerning risks derive from inconclusive research and are later revised or reversed. For example, the recommendations made by organizations such as the American Cancer Society and the National Cancer Institute for mammography for asymptomatic women in their forties changed at least six times in the years prior to 1997, and in that year an NIH consensus conference was unable to agree on any recommendation. These frequent changes reduce the credibility of recommendations of proven benefit. The confusion also extends to the mass media, which often lack the expertise to present findings in context or with the necessary qualifications.[7]

The Health Education Movement

One of the basic issues involving risk factors for chronic diseases concerns individual versus social responsibility for health and disease. Practically all modifiable risk factors must be altered in each individual separately, which has led supporters of the individual-responsibility position to conclude that personal lifestyles are the major determinant of health status. Those who prefer the social-responsibility position assert that individual behavior is constrained by social and economic institutions and that government plays a key role in fostering and regulating them. An example is the many years when the federal government subsidized the tobacco industry and state governments refused to enforce laws banning the sale of tobacco products to minors while enforcing similar laws regarding alcoholic beverages. The social-responsibility approach assigns a primary role to government to enhance health and reduce the risk of disease.

The social-responsibility theory was dominant from the late 1940s through the 1960s because of major advances in medicine and public health, such as antibiotics, new surgical procedures, and the polio vaccine. Health was believed to depend primarily on the availability and quality of health services, so federal and state governments increased the number of hospital beds, the supply of health care professionals, funding for medical research, and health insurance for the elderly and indigent. A 1976 task force report of the John E. Fogarty International Center of the National Institutes of Health stated that "the individual's role in his or her health maintenance has been largely presented in terms of adequate health insurance coverage, access to a physician or hospital, and, in the view of a minority, an annual physical checkup." Faith in this approach waned in the late 1960s due to the difficulties of preventing and treating chronic and degenerative diseases and to risk factor research concerning individual behaviors like cigarette smoking. Modifying individual behavior to prevent disease appeared to be a more useful and less expensive strategy for improving health.[8]

In 1971 President Richard Nixon sent a health message to Congress that advocated the individual-responsibility approach.

> In the final analysis, each individual bears the major responsibility for his own health. Unfortunately, too many of us fail to meet that responsibility. . . . These are personal questions, to be sure, but they are also public questions. For the whole society has a stake in the health of the individual. . . . Through tax payments and through insurance premiums, the careful subsidize the careless; the non-smokers subsidize those who smoke; the physically fit subsidize the run-down and the overweight; the knowledgeable subsidize the ignorant and the vulnerable. . . . It is in the interest of our entire country, therefore, to educate and encourage each of our citizens to develop sensible health practices. Yet we have given remarkably little attention to the health education of our people.[9]

If individuals are responsible for their own health, improved health require the health education of the public. The health education movement originated as a popular social movement of interested laypersons. Many of them conceived of health not merely as freedom from disease, but a continuous process of physical and mental self-enhancement. The movement overlapped with other social movements such as those concerned with the environment, women's rights, and the elderly. It was also supported by providers of alternative forms of medical care, including holistic medicine and nutritional therapies.[10]

In 1973 President Nixon appointed a Committee on Health Education, which concluded: "We are convinced that the results of any changes or improvements in the delivery and financing of health care will be virtually nullified unless there is, at the same time, an improvement in health education." In 1976 Congress enacted the National Consumer Health Information and Health Promotion Act, which created the office of Health Information and Health Promotion in the Department of Health, Education, and Welfare (HEW). The health education movement developed in other countries as well, and in 1984 the World Health Organization established a similar program in its regional office for Europe.[11]

In 1979 the Surgeon General of the Public Health Service issued a report, *Healthy People,* which stated that the public was receptive to health education. "The American people are deeply interested in improving their health. The increased attention now being paid to exercise, nutrition, environmental health and occupational safety testify to their interest and concern with health promotion and disease prevention." It concluded that "with the growing understanding of causes and risk factors for chronic diseases, . . . prevention is an idea whose time has come. We have the scientific knowledge to begin to formulate recommendations for improved health." While social factors were important determinants of disease, "it is the controllability of many risks—and, often the significance of controlling even only a few—that lies at the heart of disease prevention and health promotion."[12]

Health education was defined by President Nixon's Committee on Health Education as "a process that bridges the gap between health information and health practices. Health education motivates the person to take the information and do something with it" by "persuading people to change their lifestyles." The major "problem areas" for health education were stated in 1980 in *Promoting Health/Preventing Disease: Objectives for the Nation,* a report of the Department of Health and Human Services, the successor to HEW. They were (1) "preventive health services," including control of high blood pressure, family planning, prenatal care, infant health, and immunization; (2) "health promotion," including smoking cessation, nutrition, alcohol and drug use, physical fitness, and control of stress and violent behavior; and (3) "health protection," including occupational safety, accident prevention, fluoridation, and toxic agent and infectious disease control.[13]

A basic issue for health education is whether programs for chronic diseases should be directed at the total population or only at high-risk groups. The rationale for a population-wide approach has been that persons not at high risk generate most cases of chronic disease. It was the original strategy of the modern public health movement in protecting the public against bacterial diseases using programs such as water purification, milk pasteurization, smallpox vaccination, and mass screening for tuberculosis. These programs shared several characteristics: they were directed at the total population regardless of level of risk; they involved extensive activities by public health departments and government agencies that regulated private businesses; and they required no or infrequent participation by the public and physicians in private practice.

Population-wide health education programs for risk factors, on the other hand, place great demands on the public. They expect the great majority of persons to make significant changes in their lifestyles and be screened regularly for asymptomatic risk factors. The public must continuously learn about new risk factors, change their lifestyles accordingly, and discard obsolete risk factors. Most persons are not willing to learn, keep informed about, and make the many lifestyle changes expected of them. They emphasize a few changes, often based on personal convenience. Even more important, most persons do not know which lifestyle changes provide the greatest benefits or are supported by the most convincing evidence.

Population-wide programs also place heavy demands on physicians. Physicians are well prepared by training and experience to administer and monitor medication regimens in selected groups, such as patients with high blood pressure. They lack the training and the time to provide dietary therapy, assist smokers to stop smoking, motivate the overweight to lose weight, and arouse the sedentary to become physically active. They lack the staffs to monitor and continually re-educate patients and their families. Aronowitz has observed that it is not clear that "statistical risks and lifestyle issues" are the "proper domain of physicians or other sorts of professionals, and whether such tasks make the best use of their training and interests." Most physicians have recognized this and have focused on those risk factors that they are best qualified to treat.[14]

Population-wide programs do have strong appeal to certain organizations. Government agencies and voluntary health associations use them to demonstrate their contribution to the public's health. Food companies use health claims to promote the sale of their products. Pharmaceutical companies develop drugs in order to sell them to millions of persons who are at moderate as well as high risk from specific risk factors.

The alternative to a population-wide strategy is a selective approach targeted at high-risk groups. The advantages of the selective strategy are lower costs, fewer demands on the health care system, and less need for the involvement of the general public. The key issues in this approach are the level of risk that warrants modification, the benefits and cost-effectiveness of alternative strategies to reduce the risks, methods for screening the population to identify those at high risk, and the capabilities of the health care system to provide the necessary services.[15] These issues require a level of knowledge and expertise that is seldom available.

To be effective, health education must be provided to the healthy as well as the sick. The 1976 NIH report warned that consumer health education "cannot succeed in an environment where national health policy and the allocation of national health resources are keyed almost exclusively to health care (the diagnosis and treatment of illness and disability)."[16] The American medical care system has consistently emphasized acute diseases and acute episodes of chronic conditions, such as myocardial infarctions in coronary heart disease. This is clearly shown by the types of medical conditions covered by public and private health insurance plans and the resources available in hospitals and clinics.

Acute care is also the major focus of medical research, as indicated by the priorities of the National Institutes of Health, which funds most research on health and disease. In 1996 the NIH provided $1.4 billion in research funding for HIV/AIDS, an acute disease, but only $62 million for chronic obstructive pulmonary diseases (primarily bronchitis and emphysema), which killed 2.3 times as many people annually as AIDS and constitute a growing chronic health problem in children and adults. The agency also provided research funding of $300 million for diabetes mellitus and $269 million for coronary heart disease, two chronic diseases that affect millions more persons than HIV and AIDS. The emphasis of the NIH on acute conditions is indicated by the weak statistical correlations between its funding for specific diseases and number of existing cases of the diseases, number of new cases per year, or days in acute care hospitals. Moderately low correlations (about 0.4) were found between the amount of funding and both mortality rates and years of life lost.[17]

The application of the risk factor concept has also suffered from the confusion between scientific evidence and conclusions drawn from the evidence. Clinical trials always cite statistical significance, the probability that chance variations explain the differences between experimental and control groups, as the key factor in demonstrating a relationship. Yet experts in statistics have repeatedly warned against such an oversimplified analysis. Statistical tests are designed to attach great weight to the size of the samples, so that very large samples make trivial differences statistically significant. The user must decide whether the differences are meaningful. Thomas

Dawber, a physician who served as the first director of the Framingham Heart Study, cautioned:

> One distinction . . . of great consequence to practicing physicians is that between statistical significance and clinical importance. . . . Observations on differences in many characteristics . . . if made on very large numbers of subjects, may find small differences, which because of the size of the population are highly significant statistically. The physician may find that regardless of the significance level, the findings have no clinical importance; they do not warrant action. Public health officials will not find them administratively significant.[18]

For this reason policy decisions about risk factors that are based on statistical evidence require judgments. A committee of the National Academy of Sciences has observed: "Science alone can never be an adequate basis for a risk decision. . . . Risk decisions are, ultimately, public policy choices because the levels of risk that are considered acceptable and the risks that should be considered as important require decisions that involve societal values."[19]

The history of the use and misuse of the risk factor and its statistical methodology has followed a familiar path in the annals of public health and medicine. Every revolution has posed fundamental challenges to accepted practices and produced an initial period of confusion and conflict followed by greater comprehension and consensus. The unique challenge for the risk factor concept is its influence on billions of dollars of consumer and health care expenditures, and therefore on private corporations and providers of health services and products. In this environment health policies are no longer based on the expertise of disinterested public health and medical professionals, but are strongly influenced by those with direct economic interests in the outcomes. As an example, the Dietary Supplement Health and Education Act of 1994 enabled manufacturers of dietary supplements and botanical products to limit government regulation of the safety of their products and make extraordinary health claims for their products without evidence.[20] If risk factors are to serve the objectives for which they were created, health professionals and laypersons must have greater understanding of the methodological and substantive issues involved.

NOTES

Notes to Preface

1. See Gary Taubes, "Looking for the Evidence in Medicine," *Science* 272 (1996): 22–24; Alvan R. Feinstein, "Meta-Analysis: Statistical Alchemy for the 21st Century," *Journal of Clinical Epidemiology* 48 (1995): 71–79.

2. Audrey B. Davis, "Life Insurance and the Physical Examination: A Chapter in the Rise of American Medical Technology," *Bulletin of the History of Medicine* 55 (1981): 392–406.

Notes to Chapter 1

1. Ellen K. Silbergeld, "Risk Assessment and Risk Management: An Uneasy Divorce," in *Acceptable Evidence: Science and Values in Risk Management,* ed. Deborah G. Mayo and Rachelle D. Hollander (New York: Oxford University Press, 1991), 101.

2. See John D. Graham, Laura C. Green, and Marc J. Roberts, *In Search of Safety: Chemicals and Cancer Risk* (Cambridge, MA: Harvard University Press, 1988).

Notes to Chapter 2

1. L. E. Maistrov, *Probability Theory: A Historical Sketch* (New York: Academic Press, 1974), 41–55. A history of numerical methods applied to medicine and public health is Kerr L. White, *Healing the Schism: Epidemiology, Medicine, and the Public's Health* (New York: Springer-Verlag, 1991), 27–120.

2. The two kinds of data are often called a priori and a posteriori data respectively. For a history of early probability and statistics, see Stephen M. Stigler, *The History of Statistics: The Measurement of Uncertainty before 1900* (Cambridge, MA: Harvard University Press, 1986), 62–63.

3. See Maistrov, *Probability Theory;* Stigler, *The History of Statistics.*

4. Ian Hacking, *The Taming of Chance* (Cambridge: Cambridge University Press, 1990), 1; Loren R. Graham, *Between Science and Values* (New York: Columbia University Press, 1981), 35–36, 48, 52–53.

5. Ian Hacking, *The Emergence of Probability: A Philosophical Study of Early Ideas about Probability, Induction, and Statistical Inference* (London: Cambridge University Press, 1975), 28, passim.

6. Walter F. Willcox, *Studies in American Demography* (1940; New York: Russell and Russell, 1971), 491–520. Willcox lists about 150 definitions of statistics written between 1749 and 1934.

7. Lorraine Daston, *Classical Probability in the Enlightenment* (Princeton, NJ: Princeton University Press, 1988), pp. 126–27; James H. Cassedy, *Demography in Early America: Beginnings of the Statistical Mind, 1600–1800* (Cambridge, MA: Harvard University Press, 1969), 7–8, 118; Andrea A. Rusnock, "The Quantification of Things Human: Medicine and Political Arithmetic in Enlightenment England and France" (Ph.D. dissertation, Princeton University, 1990), 27–36.

8. M. J. Cullen, *The Statistical Movement in Early Victorian Britain: The Foundations of Empirical Social Research* (New York: Barnes and Noble, 1975), 8; John M. Eyler, *Victorian Social Medicine: the Ideas and Methods of William Farr* (Baltimore: Johns Hopkins University Press, 1979), 43; Rusnock, "Quantification of Things Human," 169.

9. The authorship of the book has been a contentious topic. See Cullen, *The Statistical Movement in Early Victorian Britain,* 2–5.

10. John Graunt, *Natural and Political Observations Mentioned in a Following Index and Made Upon the Bills of Mortality* (1662; New York: Arno Press, 1975), 43, 28–29, 51.

11. Maistrov, *Probability Theory,* 54.

12. George Rosen, "Problems in the Application of Statistical Analysis to Questions of Health: 1700–1880," *Bulletin of the History of Medicine* 29 (1955): 28.

13. Eyler, *Victorian Social Medicine,* 73; Anders Hald, *A History of Probability and Statistics and Their Applications Before 1750* (New York: Wiley, 1990), 134–41; Rosen, "Problems in the Application of Statistical Analysis to Questions of Health: 1700–1880," 29.

14. Daston, *Classical Probability in the Enlightenment,* 141–50, 169; Hald, *A History of Probability and Statistics and Their Applications Before 1750,* 7, 509–13.

15. Genevieve Miller, *The Adoption of Inoculation for Smallpox in England and France* (Philadelphia: University of Pennsylvania Press, 1957), 29–34.

16. Ibid., 41–44, 49–51, 273.

17. Ibid., 80–87, 96.

18. Rusnock, "The Quantification of Things Human: Medicine and Political Arithmetic in Enlightenment England and France," 75–97; Patricia Cline Cohen, *A Calculating People: The Spread of Numeracy in Early America* (Chicago: University of Chicago Press, 1982), 96–103.

19. Miller, *The Adoption of Inoculation for Smallpox in England and France,* 111–22.

20. Ibid., 156, 170; John Duffy, *Epidemics in Colonial America* (Baton Rouge: Louisiana State University Press, 1953), 27, 35, 40.

21. Miller, *The Adoption of Inoculation for Smallpox in England and France,* 180–94, 197, 229–39; Rusnock, "The Quantification of Things Human: Medicine and Political Arithmetic in Enlightenment England and France," 132–58.

22. Pierre Charles A. Louis, *Researches on the Effects of Bloodletting in some Inflammatory Diseases,* trans. C. G. Putnam (Boston: Hilliard, Gray, 1836), 64–69.

23. Ibid., 56–60.

24. Ibid., 9; J. Rosser Matthews, *Quantification and the Quest for Medical Certainty* (Princeton: Princeton University Press, 1995), 14–20.

25. George Weisz, "Academic Debate and Therapeutic Reasoning in Mid-19th Century France," in *Medicine and Change: Historical and Sociological Studies of Medical Innovation,* ed. Ilana Lowy (Paris: John Libby Eurotext, 1993), 287–315; William Coleman, *Death is a Social Disease: Public Health and Political Economy in Early Industrial France* (Madison: University of Wisconsin Press, 1982), 124–25.

26. Claude Bernard, *An Introduction to the Study of Experimental Medicine* (1865; reprint, New York: Schuman, 1949), 139, 1–2.

Notes to Chapter 3

1. Ian Hacking, *The Taming of Chance* (Cambridge: Cambridge University Press, 1990), 15.

2. Lambert A. J. Quetelet, *A Treatise on Man and the Development of his Faculties* (Gainesville, FL: Scholars' Facsimiles and Reprints, 1969), 80.

3. Ibid., 6, 83.

4. Theodore M. Porter, *The Rise of Statistical Thinking: 1820–1900* (Princeton, NJ: Princeton University Press, 1986), 111–12.

5. Stuart J. Woolf, "Towards the History of the Origins of Statistics: France 1789–1815," in Jean-Claude Perrot and Stuart J. Woolf, *State and Statistics in France, 1789–1815* (Chur, Switzerland: Harwood Academic Publishers, 1984), 99.

6. Edvard Arosenius, "The History and Organization of Swedish Official Statistics," 542–43; Fernand Faure, "The Development and Progress of Statistics in France," 255–56, in *The History of Statistics: Their Development and Progress in Many Countries,* ed. John Koren (1918; New York: Burt Franklin, 1970).

7. George Rosen, "Problems in the Application of Statistical Analysis to Questions of Health: 1700–1880," *Bulletin of the History of Medicine* 29 (1955): 34.

8. Faure, "The Development and Progress of Statistics in France," 250–57; Arosenius, "The History and Organization of Swedish Official Statistics," 540–42; A.N. Kiaer, "The History and Development of Statistics in Norway," 447, in *The History of Statistics: Their Development and Progress in Many Countries.*

9. U.S. Bureau of the Census, *A Century of Population Growth: From the First Census of the United States to the Twelfth, 1790–1900* (Washington: GPO, 1909), 3–15.

10. Carroll D. Wright, *The History and Growth of the United States Census* (1900; New York: Johnson Reprint Corp., 1966), 132, 926. This volume contains the complete text of every census schedule, the names of all census publications, all legislation pertaining to the census in the nineteenth century, and an analysis by Wright.

11. W. Stull Holt, *The Bureau of the Census: Its History, Activities, and Organization* (Washington: Brookings Institution, 1929), 4–35.

12. Faure, "The Development and Progress of Statistics in France," 287–88; William Coleman, *Death is a Social Disease: Public Health and Political Economy in Early Industrial France* (Madison: University of Wisconsin Press, 1982), 142–47.

13. D. V. Glass, *Numbering the People: The Eighteenth Century Population Controversy*

and the Development of Census and Vital Statistics in Britain (Farnbourough, Eng.: Saxon House, 1973), 91–94; M. J. Cullen, *The Statistical Movement in Early Victorian Britain: The Foundations of Empirical Social Research* (New York: Barnes and Noble, 1975), 13, 38, 96.

14. Frank H. Hankins, *Adolphe Quetelet as Statistician* (New York: 1908), 28–29, 42; Walter F. Willcox, *Studies in American Demography* (1940; New York: Russell and Russell, 1971), 86.

15. See George C. Alter and Ann G. Carmichael, "Classifying the Dead: Toward a History of the Registration of Causes of Death," *Journal of the History of Medicine* 54 (1999): 114–32.

16. John M. Eyler, *Victorian Social Medicine: The Ideas and Methods of William Farr* (Baltimore: Johns Hopkins University Press, 1979), 37–38; William Coleman, *Death is a Social Disease: Public Health and Political Economy in Early Industrial France* (Madison: University of Wisconsin Press, 1982), 139; Faure, "The Development and Progress of Statistics in France," 242, 262–64.

17. Coleman, *Death is a Social Disease,* 140, 147.

18. Glass, *Numbering the People,* 119; Cullen, *The Statistical Movement in Early Victorian Britain,* 29–33; F. B. Smith, *The People's Health: 1830–1910* (New York: Holmes and Meier, 1979), 67–68. John M. Eyler, *Sir Arthur Newsholme and State Medicine, 1885–1935* (Cambridge: Cambridge University Press, 1997), 30–31.

19. Willcox, *Studies in American Demography,* 200.

20. S. N. D. North, "Seventy-Five Years of Progress in Statistics," in *The History of Statistics: Their Development and Progress in Many Countries,* 31–32.

21. U.S. Children's Bureau, *Birth Registration: An Aid in Protecting the Lives and Rights of Children; Necessity for Extending the Registration Area* Monograph No. 1 (Washington: U.S. GPO, 1913), 6, 6n; James H. Cassedy, *American Medicine and Statistical Thinking, 1800–1860* (Cambridge, MA: Harvard University Press, 1984), 203–4; Robert Gutman, *Birth and Death Registration in Massachusetts, 1639–1900* (New York: Milbank Memorial Fund, 1959), 25, 40, 50–1, 102.

22. James H. Cassedy, "The Registration Area and American Vital Statistics," *Bulletin of the History of Medicine* 39 (1965): 225–26.

23. Wright, *The History and Growth of the United States Census,* 98, 229–33.

24. Ibid., 63, 71; Cassedy, "The Registration Area and American Vital Statistics," 221–23.

25. U.S. Bureau of the Census, *Mortality Statistics, 1907,* 8th Annual Report (Washington, DC: U.S. GPO, 1909), 12–14; U.S. Bureau of the Census, *Mortality Statistics, 1908,* 9th Annual Report (Washington, DC: U.S. GPO, 1910), 11.

26. Association of Life Insurance Presidents, *Birth and Death Bookkeeping: Need for Better Vital Statistics* (New York: 1912), 6.

27. Gary W. Shannon and Gerald F. Pyle, *Disease and Medical Care in the United States: A Medical Atlas of the Twentieth Century* (New York: Macmillan, 1993), 4; Willcox, *Studies in American Demography,* 210, 232; Grace L. Meigs, *Maternal Mortality from all Conditions Connected with Childbirth,* U.S. Children's Bureau Publication No. 19 (Washington, DC: US GPO, 1917), in *The Health of Women and Children* (New York: Arno Press, 1977), 37.

28. Sam Shapiro, Edward R. Schlesinger, and Robert E. Nesbitt, Jr., *Infant, Perinatal, Maternal, and Childhood Mortality in the United States* (Cambridge, MA: Harvard University Press, 1968), 4; Willcox, *Studies in American Demography,* 211.

Notes to Chapter 4

1. Lambert A.J. Quetelet, *A Treatise on Man and the Development of his Faculties* (Gainesville, FL: Scholars' Facsimiles and Reprints, 1969), 6.

2. James H. Cassedy, *American Medicine and Statistical Thinking, 1800–1860* (Cambridge, MA: Harvard University Press, 1984), 166–72, 163–65.

3. Gerald N. Grob, *Edward Jarvis and the Medical World of Nineteenth Century America* (Knoxville: University of Tennessee Press, 1978), 113–14.

4. Kenneth Allen de Ville, *Medical Malpractice in Nineteenth Century America: Origins and Legacy* (New York: New York University Press, 1990), 25–26, 104–6; Frank H. Hamilton, "Report on Deformities after Fractures: Part Third," *Transactions of the American Medical Association* 10 (1857): 299–307.

5. Ibid., 242.

6. Ibid., 298–99; de Ville, *Medical Malpractice in Nineteenth Century America*, 106–8, 215–17.

7. Grob, *Edward Jarvis and the Medical World of Nineteenth Century America*, 120–33.

8. M. J. Cullen, *The Statistical Movement in Early Victorian Britain: The Foundations of Empirical Social Research* (New York: Barnes and Noble, 1975), 77–133; Philip Abrams, *The Origins of British Sociology: 1834–1914* (Chicago: University of Chicago Press, 1968), 13n, 16.

9. Cullen, *The Statistical Movement in Early Victorian Britain*, 112–14, 135, 146. See also Martin Bulmer, Kevin Bales, and Kathryn K. Sklar, eds., *The Social Survey in Historical Perspective: 1880–1940* (Cambridge: Cambridge University Press, 1991).

10. Cullen, *The Statistical Movement in Early Victorian Britain*, 100–1.

11. B. W. Richardson, "John Snow, M.D.," in John Snow, *Snow on Cholera* (New York: Commonwealth Fund, 1936), xxxii, xlii, xlvii; Reinhard S. Speck, "Cholera," in *The Cambridge World History of Human Disease*, ed. Kenneth F. Kiple (Cambridge: Cambridge University Press, 1993), 642–49; Snow, *Snow on Cholera*, 2, 9.

12. Snow, *Snow on Cholera*, 11–12, 15–16.

13. Richardson, "John Snow, M.D.," xxxvi.

14. Snow, *Snow on Cholera*, 45, 112–13.

15. John M. Eyler, *Victorian Social Medicine: the Ideas and Methods of William Farr* (Baltimore: Johns Hopkins University Press, 1979), 117–22.

16. Lindsay Granshaw, "'Upon This Principle I have Based a Practice': The Development and Reception of Antisepsis in Britain, 1867–90," in *Medical Innovations in Historical Perspective*, ed. John V. Pickstone (New York: St. Martin's Press, 1992), 26.

17. Biographies of Quetelet are in Frank H. Hankins, *Adolphe Quetelet as Statistician* (New York: 1908), 9–35; and Solomon Diamond, "Introduction," in Quetelet, *A Treatise on Man and the Development of his Faculties* v–xii. This account relies on Stephen M. Stigler, *The History of Statistics: The Measurement of Uncertainty before 1900* (Cambridge, MA: Harvard University Press, 1986), 161–220.

18. Quetelet, *A Treatise on Man and the Development of his Faculties*, 7–10; Hankins, *Adolphe Quetelet as Statistician*, 62–82.

19. Quetelet, *A Treatise on Man and the Development of his Faculties*, 99.

20. Modern social scientists would deal with interactions among the variables using multiple regression, but this method was not available to Quetelet.

21. Stigler, *The History of Statistics*, 180–81.

22. Ibid., 213, 144–45; Theodore M. Porter, *The Rise of Statistical Thinking: 1820–1900* (Princeton, NJ: Princeton University Press, 1986), 6–7, 13, 91–100.

23. Porter, *The Rise of Statistical Thinking,* 106–7; Stigler, *The History of Statistics,* 203–15.

Notes to Chapter 5

1. Arthur M. Master, Charles I. Garfield, and Max B. Walters, *Normal Blood Pressure and Hypertension: New Definitions* (Philadelphia: Lea and Febiger, 1952), 7.

2. Samuel C. Robinson and Marshall Brucer, "Range of Normal Blood Pressure," *Archives of Internal Medicine* 64 (1939): 412.

3. Frank H. Hankins, *Adolphe Quetelet as Statistician* (New York: 1908), 53; Lorraine J. Daston, "The Domestication of Risk: Mathematical Probability and Insurance 1650–1830," in Lorenz Krüger, Lorraine J. Daston, and Michael Heidelberger, *The Probabilistic Revolution Vol. 1: Ideas in History* (Cambridge, MA: MIT Press, 1987).

4. William G. Rothstein, *American Medical Schools and the Practice of Medicine: A History* (New York: Oxford University Press, 1987), 105–7, 155–56.

5. Audrey B. Davis, "Life Insurance and the Physical Examination: A Chapter in the Rise of American Medical Technology," *Bulletin of the History of Medicine* 55 (1981): 397; U.S. Bureau of the Census, *Historical Statistics of the United States: Colonial Times to 1970* (Washington, DC, 1975), I:76.

6. Lorraine Daston, *Classical Probability in the Enlightenment* (Princeton, NJ: Princeton University Press, 1988), 165–66, 175.

7. Ian Hacking, *The Taming of Chance* (Cambridge: Cambridge University Press, 1990), 48; John H. Magee, *Life Insurance,* 3rd ed. (Homewood, IL: Irwin, 1958), 104–5.

8. Theodore M. Porter, *The Rise of Statistical Thinking: 1820–1900* (Princeton, NJ: Princeton University Press, 1986), 12–13; Louis I. Dublin, *A Family of Thirty Million: The Story of the Metropolitan Life Insurance Company* (New York: 1943), 313.

9. Daston, *Classical Probability in the Enlightenment,* 176–77.

10. Morton Keller, *The Life Insurance Enterprise, 1885–1910: A Study in the Limits of Corporate Power* (Cambridge, MA: Harvard University Press, 1963), 6–8: U.S. Bureau of the Census, *Historical Statistics of the United States, Colonial Times to 1970* (Washington, DC: 1975), II:1057–58.

11. James M. Hudnot, *History of the New-York Life Insurance Company: 1895–1905* (New York: 1906), 8–9; Joseph B. Maclean, *Life Insurance* 9th ed. (New York: McGraw-Hill, 1962), 173–75; Haley Fiske, "A Mother's Beauty in Metropolitan Business," *Addresses Delivered at the Triennial Conventions and Mangers' Annual Banquets of the Metropolitan Life Insurance Company* Vol. I (New York: 1923), 300–2.

12. See H. Roger Grant, *Insurance Reform: Consumer Action in the Progressive Era* (Ames: Iowa State University Press, 1979).

13. Joseph B. Maclean, *Life Insurance* (New York: McGraw-Hill, 1929), 182–88; Shepard B. Clough, *A Century of American Life Insurance: A History of the Mutual Life Insurance Company of New York 1843–1943* (1946: reprint ed.: Westport, CT: Greenwood Press, 1970), 79–84, 170.

14. S. Josephine Baker, *Fighting for Life* (1939; New York: Arno Press, 1974), 54.

15. Clough, *A Century of American Life Insurance,* 78, 174–75.

16. Ibid., 78–79; Maclean, *Life Insurance,* 78.

17. Marquis James, *The Metropolitan Life: A Study in Business Growth* (New York: Viking, 1947), 42–43.

18. Theodore M. Porter, *Trust in Numbers: The Pursuit of Objectivity in Science and Public Policy* (Princeton, NJ: Princeton University Press, 1995), 102–13; Robert B. Mitchell, *From Actuarius to Actuary: The Growth of a Dynamic Profession in the Canada and the United States* (n.p.: Society of Actuaries, 1974), 3–7, 12, 15, 17.

19. Malvin E. Davis, *Industrial Life Insurance in the United States* (New York: McGraw-Hill, 1944), 4–5; Magee, *Life Insurance,* 105–6.

20. Davis, *Industrial Life Insurance in the United States,* 6; S. B. Ackerman, *Industrial Life Insurance: Its History, Statistics and Plans,* 2nd ed. (Chicago: Spectator Co., 1926), 50–67; *The Metropolitan Life Insurance Company: Its History, Its Present Position in the Insurance World, Its Home Office Building and its Work Carried on Therein* (New York: Metropolitan Life Insurance Company, 1914), 11.

21. Robert C. Chapin, *The Standard of Living among Workingmen's Families in New York City* (New York: Russell Sage Foundation, 1909), 191–97; Baker, *Fighting for Life,* 58–59.

22. Comment of Edna L. Foley in *Addresses Delivered at the Triennial Conventions and Mangers' Annual Banquets of the Metropolitan Life Insurance Company* Vol. I (New York: 1923), 486–87.

23. Michael M. Davis, Jr., *Immigrant Health and the Community* (1921; Montclair, NJ: Patterson Smith, 1971), 92–111; William I. Thomas, *Old World Traits Transplanted* (1921; Montclair, NJ: Patterson Smith, 1971), 125–26; Peter Roberts, *The New Immigration* (1912; New York: Arno Press, 1970), 187–99. See also David T. Beito, *From Mutual Aid to the Welfare State: Fraternal Societies and Social Services, 1890–1967* (Chapel Hill: University of North Carolina Press, 2000).

24. Olivier Zunz, *Making America Corporate 1870–1920* (Chicago: University of Chicago Press, 1990), 97–99.

25. James, *The Metropolitan Life,* 168, 172; *The Metropolitan Life Insurance Company…,* 145–48.

26. Dublin, *A Family of Thirty Million,* 40–1, 44, 125, 261; James, *The Metropolitan Life,* 77–79.

27. Zunz, *Making America Corporate,* 98; U.S. Bureau of the Census, *Historical Statistics of the United States,* I:166–67.

28. James, *The Metropolitan Life,* 86, 180, 270.

29. Ibid., 120–22, 159.

30. Ibid., 95–96, 178, 180, 200; Metropolitan Life Insurance Company, *An Epoch in Life Insurance: A Third of a Century of Achievement,* 2nd ed. (New York: Metropolitan Life Insurance Company, 1924), 32.

31. Zunz, *Making America Corporate,* 98–100.

32. James M. Hudnot, *History of the New-York Life Insurance Company: 1895–1905* (New York: 1906), 25–26, 28; Arthur Hunter, "Selection of Risks from the Actuarial Standpoint," *Transactions of the Actuarial Society of America* 12 (1911): 5–7.

33. Franklin B. Mead, "Substandard Insurance: Its Evolution and a Review of Some of its Principles," *Record of the American Institute of Actuaries* 11 (1922): 158–86; Robert Henderson, "Insurance of Substandard Lives," *Annals of the American Academy of Political and Social Science* 130 (March 1927), 16–17; Hudnot, *History of the New-York Life Insur-*

ance Company, 26–29; Haley Fiske, "A Mother's Beauty in Metropolitan Business," *Addresses Delivered at the Triennial Conventions,* 306–8.

34. Harold M. Frost, "History and Philosophy of Life Insurance Medicine," in *Life Insurance and Medicine: The Prognosis and Underwriting of Disease,* ed. Harry E. Ungerleider and Richard S. Gubner (Springfield, IL: Thomas, 1958), 207.

35. Davis, "Life Insurance and the Physical Examination: A Chapter," 401–2; Frost, "History and Philosophy of Life Insurance Medicine," 204; "The Slowness with Which Important Medical Discoveries are Generally Put to Practical Use," *JAMA* 276 (1996): 1932 [originally in *Journal of the American Medical Association* 27 (1896): 1210–11]; Robert L. Martensen, "The Effect of Medical Conservatism on the Acceptance of Important Medical Discoveries," *JAMA* 276 (1996): 1933; Hudnot, *History of the New-York Life Insurance Company* (New York: 1906), 95.

36. Mitchell, *From Actuarius to Actuary,* 33–34; Frost, "History and Philosophy of Life Insurance Medicine," 207–10.

37. Clough, *A Century of American Life Insurance,* 237–38; "Historical Highlights of ALIMD, 1889–1964," *Transactions of the Association of Life Insurance Medical Directors of America* 73th Annual Meeting (New York: 1965), 281; R. D. C. Brackenridge, *Medical Selection of Life Risks: A Comprehensive Guide to Life Expectancy for Underwriters and Clinicians,* 2nd ed. (New York: Nature Press, 1985), 34.

38. Louis I. Dublin, Alfred J. Lotka, and Mortimer Spiegelman, *Length of Life: A Study of the Life Table,* revised ed. (New York: Ronald, 1949), 193; Brackenridge, *Medical Selection of Life Risks,* 97–102.

39. David L. Ellison, *Healing Tuberculosis in the Woods: Medicine and Science at the End of the Nineteenth Century* (Westport, CT: Greenwood, 1994), 82.

40. Louis Dublin, *After Eighty Years: The Impact of Life Insurance on the Public Health* (Gainesville, FL: University of Florida Press, 1966), 39–40, 45.

41. Arthur Hunter, "Selection of Risks from the Actuarial Standpoint," *Transactions of the Actuarial Society of America* 12 (1911): 5, 11–12.

42. See Maclean, *Life Insurance,* 207–24.

43. Theodore C. Janeway, *The Clinical Study of Blood-Pressure: A Guide to the Use of the Sphygmomanometer* (New York: Appleton, 1904), 44 and passim; Master, Garfield, Walters, *Normal Blood Pressure and Hypertension,* 11–36; Hughes Evans, "Losing Touch: The Controversy over the Introduction of Blood Pressure Instruments into Medicine," *Technology and Culture* 34 (1993): 784–807. See Arthur Ruskin, ed., *Classics in Arterial Hypertension* (Springfield, IL: Thomas, 1956).

44. See George W. Pickering, *High Blood Pressure* (New York: Grune and Stratton, 1955).

45. Master, Garfield, and Walters, *Normal Blood Pressure and Hypertension,* 27–29; Theodore Janeway, *The Clinical Study of Blood-Pressure: A Guide to the Use of the Sphygmomanometer* (New York: Appleton, 1910), vii. Riva Rocci originally used a narrow cuff, but a wider cuff was soon found to be more accurate, and all blood pressure readings cited use the wide cuff.

46. Harold N. Segall, "Quest for Korotkoff," *Journal of Hypertension* 3 (1985): 317–26; Yury L. Shevchenko and Joshua E. Tsitlik, "90th Anniversary of the Development By Nikolai S. Korotkoff of the Auscultatory Method of Measuring Blood Pressure," *Circulation* 94 (1996): 116–18; Francis A. Faught, *Blood-Pressure: From the Clinical Standpoint* (Philadelphia: Saunders, 1913), 47–56.

47. Peter C. English, *Shock, Physiological Surgery, and George Washington Crile: Medi-*

cal Innovation in the Progressive Era (Westport, CT: Greenwood Press, 1980), 96–113; Harvey Cushing, "On Routine Determinations of Arterial Tension in Operating Room and Clinic," *Boston Medical and Surgical Journal* 148 (1903): 254, 250–56.

48. Janeway, *The Clinical Study of Blood-Pressure* (1910); Arthur M. Fishberg, *Hypertension and Nephritis* (Philadelphia: Lea and Febiger, 1930), 137; Emanuel Goldberger, *Heart Disease: Its Diagnosis and Treatment* (Philadelphia: Lea and Febiger, 1951), 26.

49. W. H. Cowing, *Blood Pressure: Technique Simplified* (Rochester, NY: Taylor Instrument Companies, 1912), 3d. ed. 27; Francis A. Faught, "The Status of the Blood Pressure Observation in Life Insurance Examinations," *New York Medical Journal* 92 (1910): 168–71.

50. C. H. Willitts, "Discussion," *Proceedings of the Association of Life Insurance Medical Directors of American from the Twenty-third to and Including the Twenty-fifth Annual Meeting* (New York: 1915), 266.

51. H. W. Cook, "Report of Blood Pressure Committee," in *Abstract of the Proceedings of the Thirty-Second Annual Meeting of the Association of Life Insurance Medical Directors of America* (New York: 1922), 38–42.

52. "Discussion," *Abstract of the Proceedings of the Association of Life Insurance Medical Directors of America from the Twenty-third to and Including the Twenty-fifth Annual Meeting, 1913–1915* (New York: 1915), 104, 258; "Discussion," *Abstract of the Proceedings of the Association of Life Insurance Medical Directors of America from the Seventeenth to the Twenty-second Annual Meeting, 1907–12* (New York: 1912), 433.

53. Brackenridge, *Medical Selection of Life Risks*, 9–10.

54. "Report of Committee on Blood Pressure," *Abstract of the Proceedings of the Thirty-First Annual Meeting of the Association of Life Insurance Medical Directors of America* (New York: 1921), 26: *Abstract of the Proceedings ... to and Including the Twenty-fifth Annual Meeting*, 106–7.

55. George W. Norris, *Blood-Pressure: Its Clinical Applications* (Philadelphia: Lea and Febiger, 1914), 124–25.

56. J. W. Fisher, "The Diagnostic Value of the Sphygmomanometer in Examinations for Life Insurance," *Journal of the American Medical Association* 63 (1914): 1752–54.

57. Robinson and Brucer, "Range of Normal Blood Pressure," 413; Brandreth Symonds, "The Blood Pressure of Healthy Men and Women," *Journal of the American Medical Association* 80 (1923): 236.

58. Edgar V. Allen and Edgar A. Hines, Jr., "Normal Blood Pressure and its Physiologic Variations," in *The Diagnosis and Treatment of Cardiovascular Disease*, ed. William D. Stroud, 4th ed. (Philadelphia: Davis, 1950) I:838.

59. Master, Garfield, and Walters, *Normal Blood Pressure and Hypertension*, 45–46; Robinson and Brucer, "Range of Normal Blood Pressure," 412–13.

60. Janeway, *The Clinical Study of Blood-Pressure*, 1st ed. 135; Master, Garfield, and Walters, *Normal Blood Pressure and Hypertension*, 81–83.

61. Robert M. Daley, Harry E. Ungerleider, and Richard S. Gubner, "Prognosis in Hypertension," *Journal of the American Medical Association* 121 (1943): 384.

62. Pickering, *High Blood Pressure*, 122–26, 226–40.

63. Edward K. Root, "The Decreasing Mortality from Tuberculosis," *Proceedings of the Association ...from the Twenty-third to and Including the Twenty-fifth Annual Meeting*, 361.

64. Ibid., 359–60.

65. Hunter, "Selection of Risks from the Actuarial Standpoint," 1–2.

66. Clough, *A Century of American Life Insurance,* 289; "Historical Highlights of ALIMD, 1889–1964," 282–84.

Notes to Chapter 6

1. Antonio Stella, "The Effects of Urban Congestion on Italian Women and Children," *Medical Record* 73 (1908): 724.

2. Charles Loring Brace, *The Dangerous Classes of New York, and Twenty Years' Work among Them* (1872; Washington, DC: NASW Classics, 1973), 35–36; Hutchins Hapgood, *The Spirit of the Ghetto* (Cambridge, MA: Harvard University Press, 1967), 5.

3. Leslie Moch, "The History of Migration and Fertility Decline: The View from the Road," in *The European Experience of Declining Fertility, 1850–1970: The Quiet Revolution,* ed. John R. Gillis, Louise A. Tilly, and David Levine, (Cambridge, MA: Blackwell, 1992), 175–92.; Leslie Moch, *Moving Europeans: Migration in Western Europe Since 1650* (Bloomington: Indiana University Press, 1992), 23–59.

4. Moch, "The History of Migration and Fertility Decline," 185; Philip Taylor, *The Distant Magnet: European Emigration to the U.S.A.* (New York: Harper and Row, 1971), 7, 16–18; John Burnett, *Plenty and Want: A Social History of Diet in England from 1815 to the Present Day,* rev. ed. (London: Scolar Press, 1979), 133–37.

5. Dino Cinel, *The National Integration of Italian Return Migration, 1870–1929* (Cambridge: Cambridge University Press, 1991), 96–115; Mark Wyman, *Round-Trip to America: The Immigrants Return to Europe, 1880–1930* (Ithaca: Cornell University Press, 1993), 25–32.

6. Suzanne W. Model, "Work and Family: Blacks and Immigrants from South and East Europe," in *Immigration Reconsidered: History, Sociology, and Politics,* ed. Virginia Yans-McLaughlin (New York: Oxford University Press, 1990), 132–33.

7. Taylor, *The Distant Magnet,* 48; Gianfausto Rosoli, "Italian Migration to European Countries from Political Unification to World War I," in *Labor Migration in the Atlantic Economies: The European and North American Working Classes During the Period of Industrialization,* ed. Dirk Hoerder (Westport, Ct: Greenwood, 1985), 100–6; Dino Cinel, *From Italy to San Francisco: The Immigrant Experience* (Stanford, CA: Stanford University Press, 1982), 1–2; Cinel, *The National Integration of Italian Return Migration, 1870–1929,* 101–8.

8. Charles Tilly, "Transplanted Networks," in *Immigration Reconsidered: History, Sociology, and Politics,* 84–85; Wyman, *Round-Trip to America,* 83.

9. Dirk Hoerder, "An Introduction to Labor Migration in the Atlantic Economies, 1815—1914," in *Labor Migration in the Atlantic Economies,* 9; Wyman, *Round-Trip to America,* 63–66, 53; Jeremiah W. Jenks, W. Jett Lauck, and Rufus D. Smith, *The Immigration Problem: A Study of American Immigration Conditions and Needs,* 6th ed. (New York: Funk & Wagnalls, 1926), 35, 102.

10. U.S. Bureau of the Census, *Statistical Abstract of the United States, 1921* (Washington, DC: U.S. GPO, 1922), 55–60; Niles Carpenter, *Immigrants and their Children* (1927; New York: Arno Press, 1969), 29.

11. U.S. Bureau of the Census, *Statistical Abstract of the United States, 1921,* 64, 74.

12. Carpenter, *Immigrants and their Children*, 379.

13. Peter Roberts, *The New Immigration* (1912; New York: Arno Press, 1970), 5, 364–66; Jenks, Lauck, and Smith, *The Immigration Problem*, 138.

14. George Rosen, "Urbanization, Occupation and Disease in the United States, 1870—1920: The Case of New York City," *Journal of the History of Medicine* 43 (1988): 395, 407–8; Model, "Work and Family: Blacks and Immigrants from South and East Europe," 132–34; Roberts, *The New Immigration*, 75.

15. Henry Fairchild, *Immigration: A World Movement and its American Significance*, rev. ed. (New York: Macmillan, 1925), 195–96; Jenks, Lauck, and Smith, *The Immigration Problem*, 37–39.

16. Roberts, *The New Immigration*, 367–69.

17. U.S. Bureau of the Census, *Historical Statistics of the United States, Colonial Times to 1970* (Washington, DC: U.S. GPO, 1975), I:105–7.

18. Walter F. Willcox, *Studies in American Demography* (1940; New York: Russell and Russell, 1971), 391, 412; Jenks, Lauck, and Smith, *The Immigration Problem*, 44–45.

19. Jenks, Lauck, and Smith, *The Immigration Problem*, 140–46.

20. Walter Laidlaw, *Population of the City of New York, 1890–1930* (New York: 1932), 243; Robert W. DeForest, "Tenement Reform in New York Since 1901," xvii–xviii, and Robert W. DeForest and Lawrence Veiller, "The Tenement House Problem," 3, 7–9, in *The Tenement House Problem*, ed. Robert W. DeForest and Lawrence Veiller, (1903; New York: Arno Press, 1970); Michael M. Davis, Jr., *Immigrant Health and the Community* (1921; Montclair, NJ: Patterson Smith, 1971), 76–77.

21. Davis, *Immigrant Health and the Community*, 124; W. Gilman Thompson, *The Occupational Diseases: Their Causation, Symptoms, Treatment, and Prevention* (New York: Appleton, 1914), 48, 77–79, 58.

22. Charles Bolduan, "Some Statistics on Pneumonia," in New York City Department of Health, *Annual Report of the Board of Health for the Year Ending Dec. 31, 1906* (New York: 1907), II:715.

23. Louis I. Dublin, Alfred J. Lotka, and Mortimer Spiegelman, *Length of Life: A Study of the Life Table*, rev. ed. (New York: Ronald Press, 1949), 213.

24. The percentages were quite similar for cities of 100,000–250,000 and 25,000–100,000. Carpenter, *Immigrants and their Children*, 405–6.

25. See Alan M. Kraut, *Silent Travelers: Germs, Genes, and the "Immigrant Menace"* (New York: Basic Books, 1994).

26. Wyman, *Round-Trip to America*, 85.

27. Lee K. Frankel and Louis I. Dublin, *Heights and Weights of New York City Children: A Study of Measurements of Boys and Girls Granted Employment Certificates* (New York: Metropolitan Life Insurance Company, 1916), 1–2. See Roderick Floud, Kenneth Wachter, and Annabel Gregory, *Height, Health and History: Nutritional Status in the United Kingdom, 1750–1980* (Cambridge: Cambridge University Press, 1990).

28. Frankel and Dublin, *Heights and Weights of New York City Children*, 24–25.

29. "Mortality in the First Month of Life According to Nativity of Mother" *Statistical Bulletin of the Metropolitan Life Insurance Company* 4 (Dec. 1923): 7–8; Henry H. Hibbs, Jr., *Infant Mortality: Its Relation to Social and Industrial Conditions* (New York: Russell Sage, 1916), 77–79.

30. Richard A. Meckel, *Save the Babies: American Public Health Reform and the Prevention of Infant Mortality, 1850–1929* (Baltimore: Johns Hopkins University Press, 1990),

178–85; Robert M. Woodbury, *Causal Factors in Infant Mortality: A Statistical Investigation Based on Investigations in Eight Cities,* U.S. Children's Bureau Publication No. 142 (Washington: U.S. GPO: 1925), 10, 21, 174, 178–81.

31. Woodbury, *Causal Factors in Infant Mortality,* 110–13.

32. Carpenter, *Immigrants and Their Children,* 207; Patricia Thornton and Sherry Olson, "Infant Vulnerability in Three Cultural Settings in Montreal, 1880," in *Infant and Child Mortality in the Past,* ed. Alain Bideau, Bertrand Desjardins, and Hector Brignoli (Oxford: Clarendon Press, 1997), 216–22.

33. Gretchen A. Condran and Ellen A. Kramarow, "Child Mortality among Jewish Immigrants to the United States," *Journal of Interdisciplinary History* 22 (1991): 224–27.

34. Carpenter, *Immigrants and Their Children,* 185.

35. Jenks, Lauck, and Smith, *The Immigration Problem,* 137; S. Josephine Baker, *Fighting for Life* (New York: Macmillan, 1939), 70–71.

36. See Condran and Kramarow, "Child Mortality Among Jewish Immigrants to the United States."

Notes to Chapter 7

1. John E. Gordon, "Evolution of an Epidemiology of Health," in *The Epidemiology of Health,* ed. Iago Galdston (New York: Health Education Council, 1953), 27.

2. C.-E. A. Winslow, *The Life of Hermann M. Biggs: Physician and Statesman of the Public Health* (Philadelphia: Lea and Febiger, 1929), 139.

3. Jon C. Teaford, *The Unheralded Triumph: City Government in America, 1870–1900* (Baltimore: Johns Hopkins University Press, 1984), 122–26.

4. Ibid., 84.

5. Ibid., 201, 219–27; John Duffy, *A History of Public Health in New York City: 1866–1966* (New York: Russell Sage, 1974), 105–6, passim.

6. Alan M. Kraut, *Silent Travelers: Germs, Genes, and the "Immigrant Menace"* (New York: Basic Books, 1994).

7. George C. Whipple, "Fifty Years of Water Purification," 161–80; and Frederic P. Gorham, "The History of Bacteriology and its Contribution to Public Health Work," 79–83, both in *A Half Century of Public Health,* ed. Mazyck P. Ravenel (1921; New York: Arno Press, 1970).

8. Duffy, *A History of Public Health in New York City: 1866–1966,* 630–32. See New York City Department of Health, *Annual Report for the Calendar Year 1920* (New York: 1921).

9. Walter Laidlaw, *Population of the City of New York City, 1890–1930* (New York: 1932), 299; New York City Department of Health, *Annual Report of the Board of Health for the Year Ending Dec. 31, 1900* (New York: 1901), 8.

10. William H. Park, and Charles Bolduan, "The Value of Diphtheria Antitoxin in the Treatment of Diphtheria as Established by Ten Years of Trial," in New York City Department of Health, *Annual Report of the Board of Health for the Year Ending Dec. 31, 1905* (New York: 1906), II:515–61. See Evelynn M. Hammonds, *Childhood's Deadly Scourge: The Campaign to Control Diphtheria in New York City, 1880–1930* (Baltimore, MD: Johns Hopkins University Press, 1999).

11. Winslow, *The Life of Hermann M. Biggs*, 97, 103–5; William H. Park, and Alfred L. Beebe, "Diphtheria and Pseudo-Diphtheria," *Medical Record* 46 (1894): 386–87; Duffy, *A History of Public Health in New York City: 1866–1966*, 92, 95, 97.

12. Winslow, *The Life of Hermann M. Biggs*, 112–16.

13. Ibid., 116; J. H. McCollum, "Section on Medicine" *Medical News* 63 (1896): 81; J. E. Winters, "Comment," in John W. Brannon, "Observations of Antitoxine in Diphtheria" *New York Medical Journal* 63 (1896): 224.

14. Winters, "Comment," 224.

15. Brannon, "Observations of Antitoxine in Diphtheria," 220–22, 225–26; L. Emmett Holt, et al., "The Report of the American Pediatric Society's Collective Investigation into the Use of Antitoxin in the Treatment of Diphtheria in Private Practice," *Medical News* 69 (1896): 2.

16. Brannon, "Observations of Antitoxine in Diphtheria," 221; Winslow, *The Life of Hermann M. Biggs*, 117.

17. William H. Park, "The History of Diphtheria in New York City," *American Journal of Diseases of Children* 42 (1931): 1443.

18. T. Madsen and Sten Madsen, "Diphtheria in Denmark: I. Serum Therapy," *Danish Medical Journal* 3 (1956): 114–15.

19. Ibid., 115.

20. Holt, et al., "Report of the American Pediatric Society's Collective Investigation," 1–2.

21. Ibid., 1–12.

22. William T. Watson, "Personal Experience with Laryngeal Diphtheria," *Maryland Medical Journal* 36 (1897): 246–47.

23. Holt, et al, "Report of the American Pediatric Society's Collective Investigation," 11; New York City Department of Health, *Annual Report of the Board of Health for the Year Ending Dec. 31, 1902* (New York: 1904), 246–48; Abram S. Berenson, ed., *Control of Communicable Diseases in Man*, 15th ed. (Washington, DC: American Public Health Association, 1990), 141.

24. New York City Department of Health, *Annual Report of the Board of Health for the Year Ending Dec. 31, 1904* (New York: n.d.), I:13, 296.

25. "Regulations of the Department of Health Relating to the Attending Physician in Cases of Diphtheria," New York City Department of Health, *Annual Report of the Board of Health for the Year Ending December 31, 1908* (New York: 1909). 1:190–93; New York City Department of Health, *Annual Report of the Board of Health for the Year Ending December 31, 1909* (New York: 1911), 115.

26. John M. Grange, "Tuberculosis," in Topley and Wilson's *Principles of Bacteriology, Virology and Immunology*, 7th ed., ed. G. R. Smith (Baltimore: Williams and Wilkens, 1983–84), III:33; H.O. Lancaster, *Expectations of Life: A Study of the Demography, Statistics, and History of World Mortality* (New York: Springer-Verlag, 1990), 81–88; Lydia B. Edwards, and Carroll E. Palmer, *Tuberculosis* (Cambridge, MA: Harvard University Press, 1969), 7–8, 15–16.

27. The Metropolitan mortality statistics assumed that each person held only one policy and so used the number of policies as the population. Louis I. Dublin, *Mortality Statistics of Insured Wage-Earners and Their Families* (New York: Metropolitan Life Insurance Company, 1919), 1–4, 23.

28. Dublin, *A 40 Year Campaign Against Tuberculosis*, 57; Dublin, *Mortality Statistics of Insured Wage-Earners and Their Families*, 2, 23, 44, 52.

29. Robert Koch, *Essays of Robert Koch,* trans. K. Codell Carter (Westport, CT: Greenwood Press, 1987), 94–95, 143–45, 149.

30. Thomas M. Daniel, *Captain of Death: The Story of Tuberculosis* (Rochester, NY: University of Rochester Press, 1997), 115–17; Dublin, *A Forty Year Campaign against Tuberculosis,* 88–89; Henry D. Chadwick, and David Zacks, "The Incidence of Tuberculous Infection in School Children," *New England Journal of Medicine* 200 (1929): 332–37.

31. Karl Pearson, *The Fight Against Tuberculosis and the Death-rate from Phthisis* (London: Cambridge University Press, 1911), 20–27; Rene and Jean Dubos, *The White Plague: Tuberculosis, Man and Society* (Boston: Little, Brown, 1952), 122–23.

32. Louis I. Dublin, *Health and Wealth: A Survey of the Economics of World Health* (New York: Harper, 1928), 108.

33. Chadwick and Zacks, "The Incidence of Tuberculous Infection in School Children," 333–35; Alan M. Kraut, "Plagues and Prejudice: Nativism's Construction of Disease in Nineteenth- and Twentieth-Century New York City," in *Hives of Sickness: Public Health and Epidemics in New York City,* ed. David Rosner (New Brunswick, NJ: Rutgers University Press, 1995), 77.

34. U.S. Bureau of the Census, *Historical Statistics of the United States, Colonial Times to 1970* (Washington, DC: 1975), I:58–59, 63.

35. Louis I. Dublin and Robert J. Vane, Jr., *Causes of Death by Occupation,* U.S. Bureau of Labor Statistics Bulletin No. 507 (Washington, DC; U.S. GPO, 1930), 102.

36. U.S. Bureau of the Census, *Historical Statistics of the United States, Colonial Times to 1970,* I:58; New York City Department of Health, *Health for 7,500,000 People: Annual Report of the Department of Health for 1937* (New York: n.d.), 335, 338.

37. "Causes of the Recent Decline in Tuberculosis and Outlook for the Future," *Statistical Bulletin* 4 (June, 1923): 1–4.

38. New York City Department of Health, *Annual Report for the Calendar Year 1913* (New York: 1914), 189.

39. New York City Department of Health, *Annual Report of the Board of Health for the Year Ending Dec. 31, 1902* (New York: 1904), 9–10.

40. Winslow, *The Life of Hermann M. Biggs,* 131, 134–45, 143–44, 149–52; Daniel M. Fox, "Social Policy and City Politics: Tuberculosis Reporting in New York, 1889–1900," *Bulletin of the History of Medicine* 49 (1975): 169–95; New York City Department of Health, *Annual Report for the Calendar Year 1922* (New York: 1923), 75.

41. New York City Department of Health, *Annual Report of the Board of Health for the Year Ending Dec. 31, 1902,* 10; New York City Department of Health, *Annual Report of the Board of Health for the Year Ending Dec. 31, 1904* (New York: n.d.), 173–76; New York City Department of Health, *Annual Report for the Calendar Year 1920* (New York: 1921), 91–93.

42. New York City Department of Health, *Annual Report of the Board of Health for 1910–11* (New York: 1912), 71; New York City Department of Health, *Annual Report for the Calendar Year 1919,* 62; New York City Department of Health, *Annual Report 1926* (NY: n.d.), 52; New York City Department of Health, *Guarding the Health of Seven Million People: Annual Report 1930–31* (New York: n.d.), 58.

43. Michael R. Albert, Kristen G. Ostheimer, and Joel G. Breman, "The Last Smallpox Epidemic in Boston and the Vaccination Controversy, 1901–1903," *New England Journal of Medicine* 344 (2001): 375–79; S. Josephine Baker, *Fighting for Life* (1939; New York: Arno Press, 1974), 67–68, 72–77; New York City Department of Health, *Health for New*

York City's Millions: An Account of Activities of the Department of Health of the City of New York for 1938 (New York: n.d.), 155; Judith Leavitt, *Typhoid Mary: Captive to the Public's Health* (Boston: Beacon Press, 1996).

44. New York City Department of Health, *Annual Report of the Board of Health for the Year Ending Dec. 31, 1902*, 10; New York City Department of Health, *Annual Report of the Board of Health for the Year Ending Dec. 31, 1906,* (New York: 1907), 59–61; New York City Department of Health, *Annual Report of the Board of Health for the Years 1910 and 1911* (New York: 1912), 101–3. See Barbara Bates, *Bargaining for Life: A Social History of Tuberculosis, 1876–1938* (Philadelphia: University of Pennsylvania Press, 1992).

45. Louis I. Dublin, Alfred J. Lotka, and Mortimer Spiegelman, *Length of Life: A Study of the Life Table*, rev. ed. (New York: Ronald, 1949), 204–5; Michael E. Teller, *The Tuberculosis Movement: A Public Health Campaign in the Progressive Era* (New York: Greenwood, 1988), 89. See also Louis I. Dublin, *A Forty Year Campaign against Tuberculosis* (New York: Metropolitan Life Insurance Company, 1952), 37–50.

46. New York City Department of Health, *Annual Report of the Board of Health for the Year Ending Dec. 31, 1900* (New York: 1901), 35; New York City Department of Health, *Annual Report of the Board of Health for the Year Ending Dec. 31, 1907* (New York: 1908), 302.

47. New York City Department of Health, *Annual Report of the Board of Health for the Year Ending December 31, 1908* (New York: 1909), I:528, 539, 547; New York City Department of Health, *Annual Report of the Board of Health for the Years 1910 and 1911* (New York: 1912), 65; Hermann M. Biggs, "A Brief History of the Campaign Against Tuberculosis in New York City," in New York City Department of Health, *Annual Report of the Board of Health for the Year Ending December 31, 1908* (New York: 1909), I:557. See Emily K. Abel, "Taking the Cure to the Poor: Patients' Responses to New York City's Tuberculosis Program, 1894 to 1918," *American Journal of Public Health* 87 (1997): 1808–15.

48. Winslow, *The Life of Hermann M. Biggs*, 238–39.

49. New York City Department of Health, *Annual Report of the Board of Health . . . for the Years 1910 and 1911* (New York: 1912), 65, 69, 71; Duffy, *A History of Public Health in New York City: 1866–1966*, 540.

50. New York City Department of Health, *Annual Report 1923* (New York: n.d.), 43, 50.

51. Duffy, *A History of Public Health in New York City: 1866–1966*, 98–99; Teller, *The Tuberculosis Movement*, 21, 28, 61–62.

52. New York City Department of Health, *Annual Report for the Calendar Year 1919* (New York: 1920), 58–60.

53. Duffy, *A History of Public Health in New York City, 1866–1966*, 548; New York City Department of Health, *Advances in New York City's Health: Annual Report of the Department of Health of the City of New York for 1939* (New York: n.d.), 23, 170–74.

54. Laidlaw, *Population of the City of New York, 1890–1930*, 263; New York City Department of Health, *Annual Report of the Board of Health for the Year Ending December 31, 1905* (New York: 1906), I:328; New York City Department of Health, *An Account of Twelve Months of Health Defense: Containing the Activities of the Department of Health of the City of New York for 1940* (New York: 1941), 131, 55–56; Duffy, *A History of Public Health in New York City: 1866–1966*, 548–51.

55. Framingham Community Health and Tuberculosis Demonstration, *Framingham*

Monograph No. 10: Final Summary Report: 1917–1923 Inclusive, General Series IV (Framingham, MA: 1924), 16–17. See also Dublin, *A 40 Year Campaign Against Tuberculosis,* 80–95.

56. Jean M. Converse, *Survey Research in the United States: Roots and Emergence 1890—1960* (Berkeley: University of California Press, 1987), 11–16, 22–25; Maurine W. Greenwald and Margo Anderson, eds., *Pittsburgh Surveyed: Social Science and Social Reform in the Early Twentieth Century* (Pittsburgh, PA: University of Pittsburgh Press, 1996); Martin Bulmer, Kevin Bales, and Kathryn K. Sklar, eds., *The Social Survey in Historical Perspective, 1880–1940* (Cambridge: Cambridge University Press, 1991).

57. Richard K. Means, *A History of Health Education in the United States* (Philadelphia: Lea and Febiger, 1962), 135–36.

58. Framingham Community Health and Tuberculosis Demonstration, 19–22.

59. Also see Dublin, *A 40 Year Campaign Against Tuberculosis,* 88, 90.

60. Ibid., 92; Framingham Community Health and Tuberculosis Demonstration, 8.

61. Framingham Community Health and Tuberculosis Demonstration, 37–40; Dublin, *A 40 Year Campaign Against Tuberculosis,* 92.

62. Framingham Community Health and Tuberculosis Demonstration, 9, 40, 68–70.

Notes to Chapter 8

1. New York City Department of Health, *Annual Report of the Department of Health for the Calendar Year 1917* (New York: n.d.), 61.

2. Thomas Darlington, quoted in Ernest B. Hoag and Lewis M. Terman, *Health Work in the Schools* (Boston: Houghton Mifflin, 1914), 55.

3. New York City Department of Health, *Advances in New York City's Health: Annual Report of the Department of Health of the City of New York for 1939* (New York: n.d.), 77.

4. S. Josephine Baker, *Fighting for Life* (1939; New York: Arno Press, 1974), 58–59.

5. New York City Department of Health, *Annual Report 1923* (New York: n.d.), 67.

6. Baker, *Fighting for Life,* 91, 94–95; see also John Duffy, *A History of Public Health in New York City, 1866–1966* (New York: Russell Sage, 1974), 261.

7. Duffy, *A History of Public Health in New York City, 1866–1966* , 264, 642.

8. New York City Department of Health, *Annual Report of the Board of Health for the Year Ending December 31, 1912* (New York: 1913), 88; New York City Department of Health, *Annual Report 1927* (New York: n.d.), 16; New York City Department of Health, *Annual Report for the Calendar Year 1920* (New York: 1921), 164–65; New York City Department of Health, *Health for 7,500,000 People: Annual Report for 1937 and a Review of Developments from 1934 to 1938* (New York: n.d.), 197, 288.

9. For a description of the bacteriology of milk in New York City, see William H. Park and L. Emmett Holt, "Infant Feeding," in New York City Department of Health, *Annual Report of the Board of Health for the Year Ending Dec. 31, 1902* (New York: 1904), 275–92.

10. Milton J. Rosenau, *All About Milk* (New York: Metropolitan Life Insurance Company, 1922), 23–25.

11. Ibid., 3–4, 13.

12. Charles E. North, "Milk and its Relation to Public Health," in *A Half-Century of Public Health,* ed. Mazyck Ravenel (1921; New York: Arno Press, 1970), 270–77; Richard A. Meckel, *Save the Babies: American Public Health Reform and the Prevention of Infant Mortality, 1850–1929* (Baltimore: Johns Hopkins University Press, 1990), 89.

13. Duffy, *A History of Public Health in New York City, 1866–1966,* 135–36; New York City Department of Health, *Annual Report of the Board of Health for the Year Ending Dec. 31, 1905* (New York: 1906), I:75–82, 163–269; New York City Department of Health, *Annual Report of the Board of Health for the Year Ending December 31, 1912,* 12–13; New York City Department of Health, *Annual Report 1928* (New York: n.d.), 6.

14. North, "Milk and its Relation to Public Health," 279–78; Henry Koplik, "The History of the First Milk Depot or Gouttes de Lait with Consultations in America," *Journal of the American Medical Association* 63 (1914): 1574–75.

15. Straus served as president of the New York City Board of Health in 1898 but resigned within a year because the medical profession opposed his support for compulsory reporting of tuberculosis and other communicable diseases and the sale of vaccines and antitoxin by the city. Meckel, *Save the Babies,* 78–79; Park and Holt, "Infant Feeding," 282; S. Josephine Baker, *Child Hygiene* (New York: Harper, 1925), 214–15; Baker, *Fighting for Life,* 145; North, "Milk and Its Relation to Public Health," 279–80.

16. New York City Department of Health, *Annual Report of the Board of Health for the Year Ending December 31, 1905* (New York: 1906), I:331; New York City Department of Health, *Annual Report of the Board of Health for the Year Ending December 31, 1908* (New York: 1909), I:327; New York City Department of Health, *Annual Report of the Board of Health for the Years 1910 and 1911* (New York: 1912), 79; New York City Department of Health, *Annual Report of the Board of Health for the Year Ending December 31, 1912* (New York: 1913), 83–84, 90; New York City Department of Health, *Annual Report of the Department of Health for the Calendar Year 1920,* 147; New York City Department of Health, *Annual Report of the Department of Health for the Calendar Year 1922* (New York: 1923), 72.

17. Meckel, *Save the Babies,* 80.

18. Park and Holt, "Infant Feeding," 298; New York City Department of Health, *Annual Report 1923,* 70.

19. Robert M. Woodbury, *Causal Factors in Infant Mortality: A Statistical Study based on Investigations in Eight Cities* U.S. Children's Bureau Publication No. 142 (Washington: U.S. GPO: 1925), 88–90, 102, 156.

20. New York City Department of Health, *Annual Report of the Board of Health for the Year Ending Dec. 31, 1912,* 85; Park and Holt, "Infant Feeding," 296; New York City Department of Health, *Annual Report of the Board of Health for the Year Ending Dec. 31, 1907* (New York: 1908), 43–44.

21. Park and Holt, "Infant Feeding," 289.

22. Ibid., 296.

23. New York City Department of Health, *Annual Report for the Calendar Year 1918* (New York: 1919), 160–161; New York City Department of Health, *Annual Report for the Calendar Year 1919* (New York: 1920), 153–54.

24. Betsy Haughton, Joan Dye Gussow, and Janice M. Dodds, "An Historical Study of the Underlying Assumptions for United States Food Guides from 1917 through the Basic Four Food Group Guide," *Journal of Nutrition Education* 19 (1987): 170.

25. Michael M. Davis, Jr., *Immigrant Health and the Community* (1921; Montclair, NJ: Patterson Smith, 1971), 247–79.

26. New York City Department of Health, *Annual Report for the Calendar Year 1920,* 184.

27. Park and Holt, "Infant Feeding," 296.

28. Louis I. Dublin, *A Family of Thirty Million: The Story of the Metropolitan Life Insurance Company* (New York: 1943), 289–91; Marquis James, *The Metropolitan Life: A Study in Business Growth* (New York: Viking, 1947), 221–2, 431n.

29. New York City Department of Health, *Annual Report of the Board of Health for the Year Ending Dec. 31, 1905,* I:15–16; Duffy, *A History of Public Health in New York City: 1866–1966,* 263.

30. New York City Department of Health, *Annual Report for the Calendar Year 1920,* 139–41; New York City Department of Health, *Annual Report of the Board of Health for the Year Ending December 31, 1912,* 81; Baker, *Child Hygiene,* 113–14.

31. Duffy, *A History of Public Health in New York City: 1866–1966,* 259; Baker, *Fighting for Life,* 113; New York City Department of Health, *Annual Report for the Calendar Year 1914,* 77–78; New York City Department of Health, *Annual Report for the Calendar Year 1920,* 140; New York City Department of Health, *Guarding the Health of Seven Million People: Annual Report 1930–31* (New York: n.d.), 8; New York City Department of Health, *Health for 7,500,000 People,* 280.

32. New York City Department of Health, *Annual Report of the Board of Health for the Calendar Year 1915* (New York: 1916), 112.

33. Mary S. Gardner, *Public Health Nursing,* 3rd ed. (New York: Macmillan, 1936), 14–18, 27–29; Annie M. Brainard, *The Evolution of Public Health Nursing* (1922; New York: Garland, 1985), 207.

34. Brainard, *The Evolution of Public Health Nursing,* 273–81; New York City Department of Health, *Annual Report of the Board of Health for the Year Ending December 31, 1904* (New York: n.d.), 172–74; Hermann M. Biggs, "A Brief History of the Campaign Against Tuberculosis in New York City," in New York City Department of Health, *Annual Report of the Board of Health for the Year Ending December 31, 1908,* I:556–57; New York City Department of Health, *Annual Report of the Board of Health for the Years 1910 and 1911,* 65–66, 71. See Jessica M. Robbins, "Class Struggles in the Tubercular World: Nurses, Patients, and Physicians, 1903–1915," *Bulletin of the History of Medicine* 71 (1997): 412–34.

35. Lavinia L. Dock, "The History of Public Health Nursing," in *A Half Century of Public Health,* ed. Mazyck Ravenel (1921; New York: Arno Press, 1970), 441–42; Baker, *Child Hygiene,* 41–42; C.-E. A. Winslow, *The Life of Hermann M. Biggs: Physician and Statesman of the Public Health* (Philadelphia: Lea and Febiger, 1929), 186–87; Baker, *Fighting for Life,* 78–80; New York City Department of Health, *Annual Report of the Board of Health for the Year Ending Dec. 31, 1902* (New York: 1904), 15; New York City Department of Health, *Annual Report of the Board of Health for the Year Ending Dec. 31, 1903* (New York: 1905), 63–64; New York City Department of Health, *Annual Report of the Board of Health for the Year Ending Dec. 31, 1905,* I:419–22.

36. New York City Department of Health, *Annual Report of the Board of Health for the Year Ending Dec. 31, 1903,* 10–11; Baker, *Fighting for Life,* 85, 58.

37. Baker, *Fighting for Life,* 86. See New York City Department of Health, *Annual Report of the Board of Health for the Year Ending December 31, 1908,* I:328–35.

38. Baker, *Fighting for Health,* 84–87. See New York City Department of Health, *Annual Report of the Board of Health for the Year Ending December 31, 1908,* I:360–63, 326;

Walter Laidlaw, *Population of the City of New York, 1890–1930* (New York: 1932), 300.

39. New York City Department of Health, *Annual Report of the Board of Health for the Year Ending December 31, 1909* (New York: 1911), 170–71; New York City Department of Health, *Annual Report of the Board of Health for the Year Ending December 31, 1908,* I:360–61; New York City Department of Health, *Annual Report of the Board of Health for the Calendar Year 1918* (New York: 1919), 152–53; New York City Department of Health, *Annual Report for the Calendar Year 1920,* 180–81; New York City Department of Health, *Annual Report for the Calendar Year 1922,* 142.

40. New York City Department of Health, *Annual Report of the Board of Health for the Year Ending December 31, 1909,* 171; New York City Department of Health, *Annual Report of the Board of Health for the Year Ending December 31, 1912,* 87: New York City Department of Health, *Annual Report of the Board of Health for the Year Ending December 31, 1913* (New York: 1914), 61–62.

41. New York City Department of Health, *Annual Report for the Calendar Year 1915,* 63; New York City Department of Health, *Annual Report for the Calendar Year 1918,* 137–38, 152–53. See New York City Department of Health, *Annual Report for the Calendar Year 1920,* 147–50.

42. New York City Department of Health, *Annual Report for the Year Ending December 31, 1912,* 85: New York City Department of Health, *Annual Report for the Calendar Year 1918,* 154; New York City Department of Health, *Annual Report for the Calendar Year 1919,* 145–46.

43. Michael M. Davis and Mary C. Jarrett, *A Health Inventory of New York City* (New York: 1929), 17, 305.

44. New York City Department of Health, *Annual Report of the Board of Health for the Year Ending December 31, 1909,* 170–71. See Baker, *Child Hygiene,* 230–39.

45. New York City Department of Health, *Annual Report of the Board of Health for the Year Ending December 31, 1912,* 90; New York City Department of Health, *Annual Report for the Calendar Year 1920,* 179–80; Baker, *Fighting for Life,* 132–34.

46. Meckel, *Save the Babies,* 144–45; Baker, *Child Hygiene,* 233–39.

47. Baker, *Child Hygiene,* 276–78; New York City Department of Health, *Annual Report for the Calendar Year 1914,* 83–85; New York City Department of Health, *Annual Report 1923,* 78; New York City Department of Health, *Annual Report 1926* (NY: n.d.), 30–31.

48. New York City Department of Health, *Annual Report of the Board of Health for the Year Ending December 31, 1912,* 96; New York City Department of Health, *Annual Report for the Calendar Year 1914,* 85; New York City Department of Health, *Annual Report 1922* (New York: 1923), 80; Baker, *Fighting for Life,* 151; New York City Department of Health, *Annual Report 1923,* 77.

49. New York City Department of Health, *Annual Report for the Calendar Year 1920,* 186; Caroline F. Ware, *Greenwich Village, 1920–1930* (1935; New York: Octagon, 1977), 331.

50. New York City Department of Health, *Annual Report of the Board of Health for the Year Ending December 31, 1912,* 13, 83, 85–86.

51. New York City Department of Health, *Annual Report for the Calendar Year 1916* (New York: 1917), 49; New York City Department of Health, *Annual Report for the Calendar Year 1917,* 37; New York City Department of Health, *Annual Report for the Calendar Year 1919,* 130–32.

52. New York City Department of Health, *Annual Report of the Board of Health for the Year Ending December 31, 1918,* 150–51; New York City Department of Health, *Annual Report for the Calendar Year 1919,* 157–59; New York City Department of Health, *Annual Report for the Calendar Year 1920,* 166–68.

53. New York City Department of Health, *Annual Report for the Calendar Year 1918,* 147; New York City Department of Health, *Annual Report for the Calendar Year 1919,* 146–47; New York City Department of Health, *Annual Report for the Calendar Year 1920,* 173–74.

54. New York City Department of Health, *Annual Report for the Calendar Year 1919,* 144–46; New York City Department of Health, *Annual Report for the Calendar Year 1920,* 169–72.

55. New York City Department of Health, *Annual Report for the Calendar Year 1918,* 125, 153–54; New York City Department of Health, *Annual Report for the Calendar Year 1919,* 161–62; New York City Department of Health, *Annual Report for the Calendar Year 1920,* 182–84; Davis and Jarrett, *A Health Inventory of New York City,* 30.

56. New York City Department of Health, *Annual Report for the Calendar Year 1915,* 28, 30; New York City Department of Health, *Annual Report for the Calendar Year 1917,* 12–13; New York City Department of Health, *Health for 7,500,000 People,* 60; Duffy, *A History of Public Health in New York City, 1866–1966,* 268–69. Similar centers were also established in Los Angeles, Boston, and Baltimore: C.-E. A. Winslow and Savel Zimand, *Health under the "El,"* (New York: Harper, 1937), 35–36.

57. Pascal J. Imperato, *The Administration of a Public Health Agency: A Case Study of the New York City Department of Health* (New York: Human Sciences Press, 1983), 42–45; New York City Department of Health, *Annual Report for the Calendar Year 1922,* 139; New York City Department of Health, *Annual Report for the Calendar Year 1919,* 157.

58. New York City Department of Health, *Annual Report 1923,* 71; New York City Department of Health, *Annual Report 1924* (New York: n.d.), 77–78; New York City Department of Health, *Annual Report 1927,* 19.

59. Ware, *Greenwich Village, 1920–1930,* 175–77.

60. New York City Department of Health, *Annual Report 1926,* 35.

61. Imperato, *The Administration of a Public Health Agency: A Case Study of the New York City Department of Health,* 47; Evelynn M. Hammonds, *Childhood's Deadly Scourge: The Campaign to Control Diphtheria in New York City, 1880–1930* (Baltimore: Johns Hopkins University Press, 1999), 195–96; New York City Department of Health, *Advances in New York City's Health: Annual Report for 1939,* 21. For a history of the Bellevue-Yorkville center, see Winslow and Zimand, *Health under the "El,"* 116–17, 118–26.

62. New York City Department of Health, *Guarding the Health of Seven Million People: Annual Report 1929* (New York: n.d.), 16, 36–40, 43–49; New York City Department of Health, *Guarding the Health of Seven Million People: Annual Report 1930–31,* 81–82; New York City Department of Health, *Advances in New York City's Health: Annual Report for 1939,* 91–92, 167.

63. New York City Department of Health, *Health for 7,500,000 People,* 11, 59; New York City Department of Health, *Health for New York City's Millions: An Account of Activities for 1938* (New York: n.d.), 26, 30–32, 46–49, 76–79, 106; New York City Department of Health, *Advances in New York City's Health: Annual Report for 1939,* 18–23, 63–66; New York City Department of Health, *An Account of Twelve Months of Health Defense: Annual Report for 1940* (New York: n.d.), 201–2.

64. New York City Department of Health, *Advances in New York City's Health: Annual Report for 1939,* 21–22; New York City Department of Health, *Health for 7,500,000 People,* 65–71.

65. New York City Department of Health, *Health for 7,500,000 People,* 71–73; New York City Department of Health, *Health for New York City's Millions,* 79–81.

66. New York City Department of Health, *Health for 7,500,000 People,* 14.

67. New York City Department of Health, *Annual Report 1924,* 74–75; New York City Department of Health, *Annual Report 1925* (New York: n.d.), 15; New York City Department of Health, *Annual Report 1926,* 26; New York City Department of Health, *Guarding the Health of Seven Million People: Annual Report 1930–31,* 7.

68. New York City Department of Health, *Health for 7,500,000 People,* 193–94; New York City Department of Health, 99–100.

69. Duffy, *A History of Public Health in New York City, 1866–1966,* 264, 270.

70. New York City Department of Health, *Guarding the Health of Seven Million People: Annual Report 1929* (New York: n.d.), 74–84; New York City Department of Health, *Guarding the Health of Seven Million People: Annual Report 1930–31,* 74–89; New York City Department of Health, *Health for 7,500,000 People,* 214–25.

71. Imperato, *The Administration of a Public Health Agency: A Case Study of the New York City Department of Health,* 49–52, 63–99.

72. James, *The Metropolitan Life,* 222–26.

73. New York City Department of Health, *Health for New York City's Millions,* 107–8.

Notes to Chapter 9

1. Metropolitan Life Insurance Company, *An Epoch in Life Insurance: A Third of a Century of Achievement* (New York: 1924), xxxvii–iii.

2. Michael M. Davis and Mary C. Jarrett, *A Health Inventory of New York City* (New York: 1929), 276.

3. Richard K. Means, *Historical Perspectives on School Health* (Thorofare, NJ: Slack, 1975), 71–74, 51–52, 56–63.

4. Vincent Vinikas, *Soft Soap, Hard Sell: American Hygiene in an Age of Advertisement* (Ames: Iowa State University Press, 1992), xii, 10, 93–94.

5. Susan Strasser, *Satisfaction Guaranteed: The Making of the American Mass Market* (New York: Pantheon, 1989), 96; New York City Department of Health, *Annual Report of the Board of Health for the Year Ending December 31, 1909* (New York: 1911), 186; New York City Department of Health, *Annual Report 1923* (New York: n.d.), 82; New York City Department of Health, *Advances in New York City's Health: Annual Report of the Department of Health of the City of New York for 1939.* (New York: n.d.), 30.

6. Vinikas, *Soft Soap, Hard Sell,* 80–81, 85–90; Suellen Hoy, *Chasing Dirt: The American Pursuit of Cleanliness* (New York: Oxford University Press, 1995), 142–48.

7. James D. Norris, *Advertising and the Transformation of American Society, 1865—1920* (New York: Greenwood Press, 1990), 108–9.

8. Daniel Pope, *The Making of Modern Advertising* (New York: Basic Books, 1983), 41–46, 59, 229; Frank Presbrey, *The History and Development of Advertising* (1929; New York: Greenwood, 1968), 417–19, 428–30.

9. Richard S. Tedlow, *Keeping the Corporate Image: Public Relations and Business, 1900–1950* (Greenwich, CT: JAI Press, 1979), 5–7; Alan R. Raucher, *Public Relations and Business, 1900–1929* (Baltimore: Johns Hopkins Press, 1968), 113, 121.

10. Noobar R. Danielian, *A.T.&T.: The Story of Industrial Conquest* (1939; New York: Arno, 1974), 297–314; Horace Coon, *American Tel & Tel* (1939; Freeport, NY; Books for Libraries Press, 1971), 119–28; Raucher, *Public Relations and Business,* 49–57, 77–80; Tedlow, *Keeping the Corporate Image,* 45–48.

11. Roland Marchand, *Advertising the American Dream: Making Way for Modernity, 1920–1940* (Berkeley: University of California Press, 1985), 94–95.

12. H. Roger Grant, *Insurance Reform: Consumer Action in the Progressive Era* (Ames: Iowa State University Press, 1979), 28–54, 44, 59; Morton Keller, *The Life Insurance Enterprise, 1885–1910: A Study in the Limits of Corporate Power* (Cambridge, MA: Harvard University Press, 1963), 245–59, 290.

13. Keller, *The Life Insurance Enterprise, 1885–1910,* 14; Olivier Zunz, *Making America Corporate 1870–1920* (Chicago: University of Chicago Press, 1990), 92–100.

14. Marquis James, *The Metropolitan Life: A Study in Business Growth* (New York: Viking, 1947), 207–8; Metropolitan Life Insurance Company, *An Epoch in Life Insurance,* 71–72.

15. James, *The Metropolitan Life: A Study in Business Growth,* 168, 293; "Sixty Millions Hold Insurance Protection," *New York Times* July, 10, 1927, sec. 8, 12:1; Haley Fiske, "Metropolitan Accomplishment and Progress," *Addresses Delivered at the Triennial Conventions, Mangers' Annual Banquets and at Miscellaneous Gatherings of the Metropolitan Life Insurance Company,* Vol. III (New York: 1928), 445; "Metropolitan Life Insurance Company," *Fortune* 10 (Aug., 1934): 50.

16. Louis I. Dublin, *A Family of Thirty Million: The Story of the Metropolitan Life Insurance Company* (New York: 1943), 56–58; Haley Fiske, "The Light that Never Fails," *Addresses Delivered at the Triennial Conventions and Mangers' Annual Banquets of the Metropolitan Life Insurance Company,* Vol. I (New York: 1923), 7.

17. Shepard B. Clough, *A Century of American Life Insurance: A History of the Mutual Life Insurance Company of New York 1843–1943* (1946: reprint ed.: Westport CT: Greenwood Press, 1970), 11; Metropolitan Life Insurance Company, *An Epoch in Life Insurance,* 204.

18. Roland Marchand, *Creating the Corporate Soul: The Rise of Public Relations and Corporate Imagery in American Big Business* (Berkeley: University of California Press, 1998), 187.

19. Metropolitan Life Insurance Company, *An Epoch in Life Insurance,* 271–82; comment of George I. Cochran in *Addresses Delivered at the Triennial Conventions and Mangers' Annual Banquets of the Metropolitan Life Insurance Company,* Vol. II (New York: 1924), 389.

20. Dublin, *A Family of Thirty Million,* 51–58; "Metropolitan Life Insurance Company," 50; James, *The Metropolitan,* 213; Fiske, "The Light that Never Fails," 5; "Haley Fiske Dies at 77 in His Auto in Front of Home," *New York Times* March 4, 1929, 23:4. For a history of the infanticide issue, see Metropolitan Life Insurance Company, *Its History, Its Present Position in the Insurance World, Its Home Office Building and the Work Carried on Therein* (New York: Metropolitan Life Insurance Company, 1914), 156–61.

21. Dublin, *A Family of Thirty Million,* 58–62, 67–68; Metropolitan Life Insurance Company, *An Epoch in Life Insurance,* 21–22; Zunz, *Making America Corporate,* 96; Malvin E. Davis, *Industrial Life Insurance in the United States* (New York: McGraw-Hill, 1944), 11; Fiske, "The Light that Never Fails," 9; James, *The Metropolitan Life,* 226–31.

22. James, *The Metropolitan Life,* 173–74, 207; Haley Fiske, "Mother Metropolitan," *Addresses Delivered at the Triennial Conventions,* II: 107–8.

23. Haley Fiske, "Business Convention Address," 26, and Haley Fiske, "Metropolitan Opportunity and Responsibility," 12, both in *Addresses Delivered at the Triennial Conventions,* Vol. III; Haley Fiske, "Metropolitan Leads in Health Reform," *Delivered at the Triennial Conventions,* II: 88.

24. "Haley Fiske Dies at 77 in His Auto in Front of Home," 1:4 ff; "Haley Fiske," (editorial) *New York Times,* March 5, 1929, 30:4.

25. U.S. Bureau of the Census, *Historical Statistics of the United States, Colonial Times to 1970* (Washington, DC: U.S. GPO, 1975), II: 783.

26. Louis I. Dublin and Robert J. Vane, Jr., *Causes of Death by Occupation,* U.S. Bureau of Labor Statistics Bulletin No. 507 (Washington, DC; U.S. GPO, 1930), 7.

27. James, *The Metropolitan Life,* 183–85; "An Important Announcement to Our Policy-Holders" *Metropolitan* 25 (1909): n.p.

28. "Lee K. Frankel (1867–1931): A Leader in Public Health," *Statistical Bulletin of the Metropolitan Life Insurance Company* 12 (July 1931): 3–4.

29. Karen Buhler-Wilkerson, "Public Health Nursing: In Sickness or in Health?" *American Journal of Public Health* 75 (1985): 1158; comments of Mena Shipley in 1913 in *Addresses Delivered at the Triennial Conventions,* I: 193–94. See the comments of visiting nurses from Louisville, Kentucky and Buffalo, New York on 80 and 101.

30. James, *The Metropolitan Life,* 187; Donald B. Armstrong and Alma C. Haupt, "A Forty-Year Demonstration of Public Health Nursing by the Metropolitan Life Insurance Company," *Public Health Nursing* 43 (1951): 41–42; Metropolitan Life Insurance Company, *An Epoch in Life Insurance,* 26, 208–9; Mary S. Gardner, *Public Health Nursing,* 3rd ed. (New York: Macmillan, 1936), 35. See Diane Hamilton, "The Cost of Caring: The Metropolitan Life Insurance Company's Visiting Nurse Service, 1909–1953," *Bulletin of the History of Medicine* 63 (1989): 414–34.

31. "The Nursing Service of the Metropolitan," *The Metropolitan* 27 (1916?): 9. Emphasis in original.

32. Metropolitan Life Insurance Company, *An Epoch in Life Insurance,* 208.

33. Dublin, *A Family of Thirty Million,* 425–27; Lee K. Frankel and Louis I. Dublin, "Visiting Nursing and Life Insurance," *Publications of the American Statistical Association* 16 (June, 1918), 59–60.

34. Dublin, *A Family of Thirty Million,* 426–27; Metropolitan Life Insurance Company, *An Epoch in Life Insurance,* 216–18, 232.

35. Frankel and Dublin, "Visiting Nursing and Life Insurance," 59; Dublin, *A Family of Thirty Million,* 425–28; Armstrong and Haupt, "A Forty-Year Demonstration of Public Health Nursing by the Metropolitan Life Insurance Company," 42.

36. Frankel and Dublin, "Visiting Nursing and Life Insurance," 60, 62, 66–67, 82, 91, 93–94.

37. Ibid., 76, 78, 80, 86–87.

38. Metropolitan Life Insurance Company, *Nursing Manual,* rev. ed. (New York: Metropolitan Life Insurance Company, 1937), 5, 20–27; Metropolitan Life Insurance Company, *An Epoch in Life Insurance,* 208–9.

39. Metropolitan Life Insurance Company, *Greater New York Directory: Metropolitan Visiting Nurse Service* (New York: 1940s?), 1–2.

40. "Metropolitan Life Insurance Company," 51–2; Metropolitan Life Insurance

Company, *Educating for Longer Life* (New York: 1928), 11–12; "Plan Widens Survey of Funeral Costs," *New York Times* Jan. 30, 1926, I 7:4.

41. James, *The Metropolitan Life,* 187–88.

42. Haley Fiske, "An Epoch in Life Insurance," *Addresses Delivered at the Triennial Conventions,* II: 5; Metropolitan Life Insurance Company, *An Epoch in Life Insurance,* 56, 60–62.

43. *The Lady with the Lamp* (Metropolitan Life Insurance Company, n.d.), 3–8.

44. Dublin, *A Family of Thirty Million,* 427–28; "Metropolitan Life Insurance Company," 50; Comment of Mary Jones in *Addresses Delivered at the Triennial Conventions,* II: 503–4; Annie M. Brainard, *The Evolution of Public Health Nursing* (1922; New York: Garland, 1985), 306–7.

45. David Rothman, *Beginnings Count: The Technological Imperative in American Health Care* (New York: Oxford University Press, 1997), 37; "A Report of a Study of the Effect of the Termination of Metropolitan Nursing Contracts," *Public Health Nursing* 43 (1951): 285. The John Hancock Mutual Life Insurance Company discontinued its visiting nurse service at the same time as the Metropolitan. "Building Sources of Income for Voluntary Public Health Nursing Services," *Public Health Nursing* 44 (1952): 635.

46. Metropolitan Life Insurance Company, *An Epoch in Life Insurance,* 101–2; Louis I. Dublin, *A 40 Year Campaign Against Tuberculosis* (New York: 1952), 56.

47. Harry H. Moore, *Public Health in the United States* (New York: Harper, 1923), 338, 416; "Haley Fiske and the Public Health," *Statistical Bulletin* 10 (Mar. 1929): 3; Dublin, *A Family of Thirty Million,* 429; "Fifty Years of Health Conservation," *Statistical Bulletin* 40 (Jan., 1959): 3; Means, *Historical Perspectives on School Health* 128; Metropolitan Life Insurance Company, *An Epoch in Life Insurance,* 212.

48. Metropolitan Life Insurance Company, *An Epoch in Life Insurance,* 207; *The Metropolitan* 25:4 (1909): 1; 25:6 (1910): 5, 11.

49. A list of the principal pamphlets published through 1924 is in Metropolitan Life Insurance Company, *An Epoch in Life Insurance,* 209–11, 224.

50. Richard A. Meckel, *Save the Babies: American Public Health Reform and the Prevention of Infant Mortality, 1850–1929* (Baltimore: Johns Hopkins Press, 1990), 154; Stuart Galishoff, *Safeguarding the Public Health: Newark, 1895–1918* (Westport, CT: Greenwood Press, 1975), 115.

51. *Information for Expectant Mothers* (New York: Metropolitan Life Insurance Company, 1924), 1.

52. *Metropolitan Life Cook Book* (New York: Metropolitan Life Insurance Company, 1922), 3–4, passim; *The Child* (New York: Metropolitan Life Insurance Company, 1916), 10–11.

53. Metropolitan Life Insurance Company, *An Epoch in Life Insurance,* 240–42; Dublin, *A Family of Thirty Million,* 434; Dublin, *A 40 Year Campaign Against Tuberculosis,* 66; Marchand, *Creating the Corporate Soul,* 181–89, 187. This discussion also draws on materials in the Metropolitan Life Insurance Company archives.

54. George M. Wheatley, in U.S. Children's Bureau, *Proceedings of Conference on Rheumatic Fever* Publication No. 308 (Washington, D.C.: 1945), 107–8.

55. Dublin, *A 40 Year Campaign Against Tuberculosis,* 66–67; "More Calisthenics to go Upon the Air," *New York Times* Sept. 3, 1925, 23:2; "Radio Setting-Up Exercises Lauded by 39,000 Letters," *New York Times* May 17, 1925, sec. 9, 15:1; Marchand, *Creating the Corporate Soul,* 187.

56. Metropolitan Life Insurance Company, *An Epoch in Life Insurance,* 212, 221, 230.

57. Means, *Historical Perspectives on School Health,* 125–28; Metropolitan Life Insurance Company School Health Bureau—Welfare Division, *Health: the First Objective in Education* (New York: n.d.).

58. Dublin, *A 40 Year Campaign Against Tuberculosis,* 67–68; "12 American Health Heroes," *Health Bulletin for Teachers,* 1943–46, Vols. 15, 16, 17. The health heroes were Robert Koch, Louis Pasteur, Edward Jenner, Walter Reed, Florence Nightingale, William Osler, William H. Welch, Elizabeth Blackwell, Howard Ricketts, Hans Zinsser, Frederick Banting, William Sedgwick, Charles Chapin, Ellen Richards, William Gorgas, Lillian Wald, S. Josephine Baker, Theobald Smith, Walter Cannon, Florence Sabin, and Mabel Bragg. These were also published in individual pamphlets.

59. Dublin, *A Family of Thirty Million,* 175–77; Metropolitan Life Insurance Company, *An Epoch in Life Insurance,* 162–67; Haley Fiske, "The Metropolitan a Public Institution," *Addresses Delivered at the Triennial Conventions,* III: 202–3. See C.-E. A. Winslow, *The Health of the Worker: Dangers to Health in the Factory and Shop and How to Avoid Them* (New York: Metropolitan Life Insurance Company, 1913).

60. Metropolitan Life Insurance Company, *An Epoch in Life Insurance,* 243–66; James, *The Metropolitan Life,* 394.

61. Haley Fiske, "Manager's Annual Banquet," *Addresses Delivered at the Triennial Conventions,* III: 34–35; Dublin, *A Family of Thirty Million,* 432–33; Dublin, *A 40 Year Campaign Against Tuberculosis,* 73–77.

62. *Employment Survey Made by Agents of the Metropolitan Life Insurance Co.,* 71st Congress, 3rd session, Document No. 260. Jan. 24, 1931; Metropolitan Life Insurance Company, *An Epoch in Life Insurance,* 215–38; James, *The Metropolitan Life,* 206; Donald B. Armstrong, Louis I. Dublin and Elizabeth J. Steele, *The Cost of Medical Care: A Study of Costs in the Families of the Field Employees of the Metropolitan Life Insurance Company* (New York: Metropolitan Life Insurance Company, 1934); "Queen Anne or Mary Ann," *Adventure,* May 30, 1923, 7–8.

63. James, *The Metropolitan Life,* 215; Metropolitan Life Insurance Company, *An Epoch in Life Insurance,* 211–33. The monographs were published as the "Social Insurance Series."

64. Michael Kley, *How to Take Out Your First Papers: An Easy Book in Plain English for the Coming Citizen* (New York: Metropolitan Life Insurance Company, 1921); Michael Kley, *How to Take Out Your Second or Citizen Papers: An Easy Book in Plain English for the Coming Citizen* (New York: Metropolitan Life Insurance Company, 1921); Metropolitan Life Insurance Company, *An Epoch in Life Insurance,* 229–30.

65. "Metropolitan Life Makes Housing Pay," *Fortune,* April, 46, 133ff; "Profit in $9 a Room Flats," *New York Times,* July 26, 1925, sec. 8, p. 11:2; "Insurance Premiums and Infant Lives," (editorial) *New York Times,* Jan. 29, 1927, 14:6; Metropolitan Life Insurance Company, *An Epoch in Life Insurance,* 187–89; James, *The Metropolitan Life,* 252–55.

66. "Metropolitan Life Makes Housing Pay," 133ff; James, *The Metropolitan Life,* 306–7, 313–18, 384–87; "Well-Deserved Honor" (editorial) *New York Times,* Oct, 2, 1947, 26:3.

67. Richard Plunz, *A History of Housing in New York City: Dwelling Type and Social Change in the American Metropolis* (New York: Columbia University Press, 1990), 256; James, *The Metropolitan Life,* 338–39; Dublin, *A Family of Thirty Million,* 466. Evidence

concerning the Metropolitan's underwriting policies toward black applicants is conflicting. A 1924 company history stated that from 1881 to 1893 blacks with whole-life policies received two-thirds of the death benefits of whites, but beginning in 1893 blacks received the same death benefits as whites. Beginning in 1915, black whole-life policyholders insured before 1893 received the same death benefits as white policyholders insured at the same time. Metropolitan Life Insurance Company, *An Epoch in Life Insurance,* 12, 45.

68. Dublin, *A Family of Thirty Million,* 436–38; Waldemar Kaempffert, "This Week in Science: Germs on Phone Mouthpieces," *New York Times,* Oct. 3, 1937, sec. 12, p. 4:2.

69. "Cancer Increase is Small, Insurance Inquiry Finds," *New York Times,* Jan. 17, 1926, sec. 8, p. 13:1; John C. Burnham, "How the Discovery of Accidental Childhood Poisoning Contributed to the Development of Environmentalism in the United States," *Environmental History Review* 19 (Fall 1995): 62.

Notes to Chapter 10

1. U.S. Senate Subcommittee of the Committee on Labor and Public Welfare, *Hearings on National Heart Institute S.720 and S. 2215,* April 8–9, 1948, 80th Cong., 2nd sess. (Washington, DC: US GPO, 1948), 114.

2. Forrest E. Linder and Robert D. Grove, *Vital Statistics Rates in the United States: 1900–1940* (Washington, DC: U.S. Government Printing Office, 1943), 872, 998–99.

3. "Industrial Policy Written for 100,000,000th Person," *New York Times,* Oct. 27, 1928, 28:3; "Shows Death Rate Unchanged in 1929," *New York Times,* Jan. 25, 1930, 27:1; Louis I. Dublin and Alfred J. Lotka, *Twenty-five Years of Health Progress* (New York: Metropolitan Life Insurance Company, 1937), 7–8.

4. In 1920, 80% of the black population resided in southern states, mostly in rural areas. Thus the northern blacks who were Metropolitan policyholders or resided in the death registration area were highly unrepresentative of the black population and will not be examined here.

5. Dublin and Lotka, *Twenty-five Years of Health Progress,* 16, 47, 82, 122.

6. Ibid., 169, 236.

7. U.S. Bureau of the Census, *Historical Statistics of the United States, Colonial Times to 1970* (Washington, DC: U.S. GPO, 1975), I:10; Dublin and Lotka, *Twenty-Five Years of Health Progress,* 29.

8. Peter C. English, *Rheumatic Fever in America and Britain: A Biological, Epidemiological, and Medical History* (New Brunswick, NJ: Rutgers University Press, 1999), xvii; Michael M. Davis and Mary C. Jarrett, *A Health Inventory of New York City* (New York: 1929), 222.

9. Peter English, "Emergence of Rheumatic Fever in the Nineteenth Century," *Milbank Quarterly* 67 suppl. 1 (1999): 33–49; John R. Paul, *The Epidemiology of Rheumatic Fever,* 3rd ed. (New York: American Heart Association, 1957), 7–13.

10. Angelo Taranta and Milton Markowitz, *Rheumatic Fever,* 2nd ed. (Dordrecht: Kluwer, 1989), 66–69; Milton Markowitz and Leon Gordis, *Rheumatic Fever,* 2nd ed. (Philadelphia: Saunders, 1972), 62; Charles K. Friedberg, *Diseases of the Heart* (Philadelphia: Saunders, 1949), 752.

11. John R. Paul, *The Epidemiology of Rheumatic Fever* (New York: Metropolitan Life

Insurance Company, 1930), 13–14; Samuel A. Levine, *Clinical Heart Disease* (Philadelphia: Saunders, 1938), 25–33.

12. Paul, *The Epidemiology of Rheumatic Fever* (1930), 28, 41. See also "Encouraging Outlook in Rheumatic Fever," *Statistical Bulletin* 32 (Jan., 1951): 7–10.

13. Paul, *The Epidemiology of Rheumatic Fever* (1930), 21, 30; "New York Leads Defensive War Upon Heart Disease," *New York Times*, Mar. 15, 1925, IX, 19:3; Paul, *The Epidemiology of Rheumatic Fever* (1957), 99; "Heart Disease Rise in 12 Years Studied," *New York Times*, Mar. 13, 1932, II, 2:8.

14. Gene H. Stollerman, "Rheumatic Fever," *Lancet* 349 (1997): 941; English, *Rheumatic Fever in America and Britain*, 28; Ernst Boas, *The Unseen Plague: Chronic Disease* (New York: Augustin, 1940), 59–60.

15. Paul, *The Epidemiology of Rheumatic Fever* (1930), 52; Floyd W. Denny, Jr., "A 45-Year Perspective on the Streptococcus and Rheumatic Fever," *Clinical Infectious Diseases* 19 (1994): 1110–13.

16. May Sherman, *Rheumatic Fever and Rheumatic Heart Disease: A Review of Research Grants Supported by the National Heart Institute 1949 to 1966* (Bethesda, MD: National Institutes of Health, 1966), 95.

17. Taranta and Markowitz, *Rheumatic Fever*, 19. See English, *Rheumatic Fever in America and Britain*.

18. Markowitz and Gordis, *Rheumatic Fever*, 98; American Public Health Association Committee on Child Health, *Services for Children with Heart Disease and Rheumatic Fever* (New York: 1960), 28–31, 107.

19. Paul, *The Epidemiology of Rheumatic Fever* (1930), 64; Markowitz and Gordis, *Rheumatic Fever*, 198–99, 133–36.

20. "Work of City's 30 Heart Clinics," *New York Times*, Dec. 12, 1920, II, 10:1; "New York Leads Defensive War Upon Heart Disease," *New York Times*, Mar. 15, 1925, IX, 19:3; Joel D. Howell, "Hearts and Minds: The Invention and Transformation of American Cardiology," in *Grand Rounds: One Hundred Years of Internal Medicine*, Russell C. Maulitz and Diana C. Long, eds. (Philadelphia: University of Pennsylvania Press 1988), 245; New York City Department of Health, *Advances in New York City's Health: Annual Report of the Department of Health of the City of New York for 1939* (New York: n.d.), 113.

21. "Work of 30 City's Heart Clinics," 10:1; Paul, *The Epidemiology of Rheumatic Fever* (1930), 65; Friedberg, *Diseases of the Heart*, 764.

22. President's Commission on Heart Disease, Cancer and Stroke, *Report to the President: A National Program to Conquer Heart Disease, Cancer and Stroke*, Vol. 2 (Washington, DC: US GPO, 1965), 41, 61.

23. "Work of City's 30 Heart Clinics," 10:1; Paul, *The Epidemiology of Rheumatic Fever* (1957), 10; Robert Bolande, "Ritualistic Surgery—Circumcision and Tonsillectomy," *New England Journal of Medicine* 280 (1969): 591–96.

24. Howard A. Rusk, "Nation's Greatest Killer—Heart Disease—Challenged," *New York Times*, Feb. 9, 1947, I, 4:2; U.S. Senate Subcommittee of the Committee on Labor and Public Welfare, *Hearings on National Heart Institute S.720 and S. 2215*, 37, 75.

25. U.S. Senate Subcommittee of the Committee on Labor and Public Welfare, *Hearings on National Heart Institute S. 720 and S. 2215*, 115; Rusk, "Nation's Greatest Killer—Heart Disease—Challenged," 4:2; Howard A. Rusk, "Michigan Program is Hailed as Curb on Rheumatic Fever," *New York Times*, Oct. 26, 1947, I, 30:2; Robert K. Plumb, "New Drive is Due on Heart Disease," *New York Times*, Feb. 16, 1955, 33:6; W. Bruce Fye,

American Cardiology: The History of a Specialty and Its College (Baltimore: Johns Hopkins University Press, 1996), 100–1.

26. "Medical Enigma Seen," *New York Times,* Oct. 3, 1937, II, 10:5; Don W. Gudakunst, "Statement," U.S. Department of Labor, *Proceedings of Conference on Rheumatic Fever, 1943,* Children's Bureau Publication 308 (Washington, D.C.: 1944), 109, 121.

27. George M. Wheatley, "Statement," U.S. Department of Labor, *Proceedings of Conference on Rheumatic Fever, 1943,* 107–8, 125; Paul, *The Epidemiology of Rheumatic Fever* (1930), 1; "Rheumatic Fever a Major Health Problem Today," *Statistical Bulletin* 23 (Sept. 1942): 2–5.

28. Heart Disease Control Program, *Cardiovascular Disease: Data on Mortality, Prevalence and Control Activities* (Washington, DC: U.S. Public Health Service, 1955), 49–53.

29. American Public Health Association Committee on Child Health, *Services for Children with Heart Disease and Rheumatic Fever* (New York: 1960), 17–18; Rusk, "Michigan Program is Hailed as Curb on Rheumatic Fever," 30:2; President's Commission on Heart Disease, Cancer and Stroke, *Report to the President: A National Program to Conquer Heart Disease, Cancer and Stroke,* II:71.

30. Denny, Jr., "A 45–Year Perspective on the Streptococcus and Rheumatic Fever," 1114–17. See the comments by army and navy physicians in U.S. Department of Labor, *Proceedings of Conference on Rheumatic Fever,* 3–9.

31. Louis I. Dublin and Alfred J. Lotka, *Twenty-Five Years of Health Progress* (New York: Metropolitan Life Insurance Company, 1937), 376; Louis I. Dublin, *Health Progress, 1936 to 1945* (New York: Metropolitan Life Insurance Company, 1948), 54, 141; Leon Gordis, "The Virtual Disappearance of Rheumatic Fever in the United States: Lessons in the Rise and Fall of Disease," *Circulation* 72 (1985): 1155–62; Alan L. Bisno, "The Rise and Fall of Rheumatic Fever," *JAMA* 254 (1985): 538–41.

32. May G. Wilson, Wan N. Lim, and Ann M. Birch, "The Decline of Rheumatic Fever," *Journal of Chronic Diseases* 7 (1958): 183–94.

Notes to Chapter 11

1. Samuel A. Levine, *Clinical Heart Disease* (Philadelphia: Saunders, 1938), 18.

2. H. O. Lancaster, *Expectations of Life: A Study of the Demography, Statistics, and History of World Mortality* (New York: Springer-Verlag, 1990), 19–20.

3. Iwao M. Moriyama, Dean E. Krueger, and Jeremiah Stamler, *Cardiovascular Diseases in the United States* (Cambridge, MA: Harvard University Press, 1971), 31–32; Martha L. Slattery and D. Elizabeth Randall, "Trends in Coronary Heart Disease Mortality and Food Consumption in the United States Between 1909 and 1980," *American Journal of Clinical Nutrition* 47 (1988): 1061; Theodore D. Woolsley and I. M. Moriyama, "Statistical Studies of Heart Disease: II. Important Factors in Heart Disease Mortality Trends," *Public Health Reports* 63 (1948): 1254.

4. Kenneth G. Manton and Eric Stallard, *Recent Trends in Mortality Analysis* (Orlando, FL: Academic Press, 1984), 12–13; Iwao M. Moriyama, "Development of the Present Concept of Cause of Death," *American Journal of Public Health* 46 (1956): 436–37.

5. Moriyama, "Development of the Present Concept of Cause of Death," 437; Mary

Gover, "Statistical Studies of Heart Disease: VII. Mortality from Eight Specific Forms of Heart Disease Among White Persons," *Public Health Reports* 65 (1950): 821.

6. Edward A. Lew, "Some Implications of Mortality Statistics Relating to Coronary Artery Disease," *Journal of Chronic Diseases* 6 (1957): 192–94; Metropolitan Life Insurance Company, *The Mortality from the Principal Cardiovascular-Renal Diseases: A Study of the Experience Among the Industrial Policyholders of the Metropolitan Life Insurance Company 1911 to 1930*, Monograph 4 (New York: Metropolitan Life Insurance Company, 1938?), 16; Moriyama, "Development of the Present Concept of Cause of Death," 438.

7. Woolsley and Moriyama, "Statistical Studies of Heart Disease: II. Important Factors in Heart Disease Mortality Trends," 1253.

8. James Herrick, "Historical Note," 20, and Paul D. White, "The Clinical Significance of Cardiac Pain," 262, both in *Diseases of the Coronary Arteries and Cardiac Pain*, ed Robert L. Levy (New York: Macmillan, 1936).

9. A. D. Morgan, "Some Forms of Undiagnosed Coronary Disease in Nineteenth Century England," *Medical History* 12 (1968): 344–58; Robert A. Aronowitz, *Making Sense of Illness: Science, Society, and Disease* (Cambridge: Cambridge University Press, 1998), 84–105.

10. F. B. Smith, *The People's Health 1830–1910* (New York: Holmes and Meier, 1979), 325; L. Michaels, "Aetiology of Coronary Artery Disease: An Historical Approach," *British Heart Journal* 28 (1966): 258–60; Ernst Boas and Samuel Donner, "Coronary Artery Disease in the Working Classes," *Journal of the American Medical Association* 98 (1932): 2186; John A. Ryle and W. T. Russell, "The Natural History of Coronary Disease," *British Heart Journal* 11 (1949): 370.

11. Maurice Cassidy, "Coronary Disease," *Lancet* 2 (1946): 587–88; David E. Rogers, "A Postscript from the Physician as Patient: Some Observations on Having a Coronary," in *In Search of the Modern Hippocrates*, ed. Roger J. Bulger (Iowa City: University of Iowa Press, 1987), 235–36.

12. Samuel A. Levine, *Coronary Thrombosis: Its Various Clinical Features* (Baltimore: Williams and Wilkins, 1929), 17.

13. New York City Department of Health, *Annual Report for the Calendar Year 1915* (New York: 1916), 180–81, 186. A similar but less complete table was also published in the 1914 report: New York City Department of Health, *Annual Report for the Calendar Year 1914* (New York: 1915), 103–4.

14. New York City Department of Health, *Annual Report for the Calendar Year 1916* (New York: 1917), 122–23.

15. Woolsley and Moriyama, "Statistical Studies of Heart Disease: II. Important Factors in Heart Disease Mortality Trends," 1252–53.

16. Robert L. Levy, Howard G. Bruenn, and Dorothy Kurtz, "Facts on Disease of the Coronary Arteries, Based on a Survey of the Clinical and Pathologic Records of 762 Cases," *American Journal of the Medical Sciences* 187 (1934): 376; Alfred E. Cohn, "Heart Disease from the Point of View of the Public Health," *American Heart Journal* 2 (1927): 401.

17. H. O. Swartout and Robert G. Webster, "To What Degree are Mortality Statistics Dependable?" *American Journal of Public Health* 30 (1940): 811–15. See also Iwao M. Moriyama, "Factors in Diagnosis and Classification of Deaths from CVR Diseases," *Public Health Reports* 75 (1960): 189–95; George James, Robert E. Patton and A. Sandra Heslin, "Accuracy of Cause-of-Death Statements on Death Certificates," *Public Health Reports* 70 (1955): 39–51.

18. Levy, Bruenn, and Kurtz, "Facts on Disease of the Coronary Arteries," 376–90.

19. Henry M. Parrish, "Epidemiology of Ischemic Heart Disease Among White Males, II: Autopsy Incidence of Ischemic Heart Disease and Autopsy Prevalence of Coronary Atherosclerosis," *Journal of Chronic Diseases* 14 (1961): 326–38; Henry M. Parrish, "Epidemiology of Ischemic Heart Disease among White Males, III: Role of Coronary Atherosclerosis and Clot Formation in Patients with Ischemic Heart Disease," *Journal of Chronic Diseases* 14 (1961): 339–54; David M. Spain and Victoria A. Bradess, "The Relationship of Coronary Thrombosis to Coronary Atherosclerosis and Ischemic Heart Disease," *American Journal of the Medical Sciences* 240 (1960): 701–10.

20. Francis Denny, "The Increase in Coronary Disease and its Cause," *New England Journal of Medicine* 214 (1936): 769–73.

21. T. W. Anderson and W. H. LeRiche, "Ischaemic Heart Disease and Sudden Death, 1901–61," *British Journal of Preventive and Social Medicine* 24 (1970): 1–9.

22. David C. Miller, et al., "The Community Problem in Coronary Heart Disease: A Challenge for Epidemiologic Research," *American Journal of the Medical Sciences* 232 (1956): 336.

23. Paul Dudley White, *Heart Disease,* 3rd ed. (New York: Macmillan, 1944), 482; T. W. Anderson, "The Changing Pattern of Ischemic Heart Disease," *Canadian Medical Association Journal* 108 (1973): 1500–04.

24. Terence W. Anderson, "Mortality from Ischemic Heart Disease: Changes in Middle-Aged Men Since 1900," *JAMA* 224 (1973): 336–38; Terence W. Anderson and Mabel L. Halliday, "The Male Epidemic: 50 Years of Ischaemic Heart Disease," *Public Health, London* 93 (1979): 163–72.

25. Reuel A. Stallones, "Mortality Due to Ischemic Heart disease: Observations and Explanations," *Atherosclerosis Reviews* 9 (1982): 43–52.

26. William Osler, *The Principles and Practice of Medicine,* 8th ed. (New York: Appleton, 1914), 837; Paul D. White, "The Incidence of Heart Disease in Massachusetts," *Boston Medical and Surgical Journal* 196 (1927): 692.

27. "Decries Rising Toll of Heart Disease," *New York Times,* Oct. 29, 1931, 11:8; "Congress Warned Strain Brings 'Disease of the Intelligentsia,'" *New York Times,* July 25, 1937, II, 1:6.

28. William H. Gordon, Edward F. Bland, and Paul D. White, "Coronary Artery Disease Analyzed Post Mortem: With Special Reference to the Influence of Economic Status and Sex," *American Heart Journal* 17 (1939): 10–14; Levy, Bruenn, and Kurtz, "Facts on Disease of the Coronary Arteries," 383; Arthur M. Master, Simon Dack, and Harry L. Jaffe, "The Relation of Effort and Trauma," *Industrial Medicine* 9 (1940): 359–64; Boas and Donner, "Coronary Artery Disease in the Working Classes," 2187.

29. "Heart Disease and Socioeconomic Status" *Statistical Bulletin* 39 (March, 1958): 6–8.

30. Aaron Antonovsky, "Social Class and the Major Cardiovascular Diseases," *Journal of Chronic Diseases* 21 (1968): 65–106.

31. W. Melville Arnott, "The Changing Aetiology of Heart Disease," *British Medical Journal* 2 (1954): 890–1.

32. Levy, Bruenn, and Kurtz, "Facts on Disease of the Coronary Arteries," 390; New York City Department of Health, *Health for New York City's Millions: An Account of Activities for 1938* (New York: n.d.), 55.

33. W. Bruce Fye, "The Delayed Diagnosis of Myocardial Infarction: It Took Half a

Century!" *Circulation* 72 (1985): 262–71; Herrick, "Historical Note," 24; Paul Dudley White, *My Life and Medicine: An Autobiographical Memoir* (Boston: Gambit, 1971), 53, 81; "Survivorship in Heart Disease" *Statistical Bulletin* 31 (Sept, 1950): 8–10; "Survivorship after Recovery from Disability Due to Heart Disease," *Statistical Bulletin* 35 (Feb., 1954): 4–6; Richard S. Gubner, "The Changing Outlook in Heart Disease," in *Life Insurance and Medicine: The Prognosis and Underwriting of Disease,* ed. Harry E. Ungerleider and Richard S. Gubner (Springfield, IL: Thomas, 1958), 543–45.

34. W. Bruce Fye, "Acute Myocardial infarction: A Historical Summary," in *Acute Myocardial Infarction,* ed. Bernard J. Gersh and Shahbudin H. Rahimtoola (New York: Elsevier, 1991), 9–10; White, *Heart Disease* (1944), 501–2; Charles K. Friedberg, *Diseases of the Heart* (Philadelphia: Saunders, 1949), 483–85.

35. Friedberg, *Diseases of the Heart,* 483–84, 497–98; C. Warren Irwin, Jr. and Alexander M. Burgess, Jr., "The Abuse of Bed Rest in the Treatment of Myocardial Infarction," *New England Journal of Medicine* 243 (1950): 486–89; "Rest is Defended in Coronary Cases," *New York Times,* Oct. 2, 1946, 26:8; Samuel A. Levine, *Clinical Heart Disease* (Philadelphia: Saunders, 1938), 153; Samuel A. Levine, *Clinical Heart Disease,* 4th ed. (Philadelphia: Saunders, 1951), 129–30; Emanuel Goldberger, *Heart Disease: Its Diagnosis and Treatment* (Philadelphia: Lea and Febiger, 1951), 505.

36. Paul Dudley White, *Heart Disease* (New York: Macmillan, 1931), 612–13; Levine, *Clinical Heart Disease* (1938), 124.

37. Lawrence E. Davies, "New Head of AMA Hits Critics Within," *New York Times,* July 5, 1946, 21:8; White, *Heart Disease* (1931), 613.

38. New York City Department of Health, *Annual Report for the Calendar Year 1916,* 100; New York City Department of Health, *Annual Report for the Calendar Year 1915,* 115; Levine, *Clinical Heart Disease* (1938), 19.

39. Osler, *The Principles and Practice of Medicine,* 792; Albert S. Hyman and Aaron E. Parsonnet, *The Failing Heart of Middle Life: The Myocardosis Syndrome, Coronary Thrombosis, and Angina Pectoris* (Philadelphia: Davis, 1932), 3.

40. W. Bruce Fye, "A History of the Origin, Evolution, and Impact of Electrocardiography," *American Journal of Cardiology* 73 (1994): 937–49; "Historical Highlights of ALIMD, 1889–1964," *Transactions of the Association of Life Insurance Medical Directors of America,* 73th annual meeting (New York: 1965), 283; W. Bruce Fye, *American Cardiology: The History of a Specialty and Its College* (Baltimore: Johns Hopkins University Press, 1996), 62.

41. Fye, *American Cardiology,* 60, 68; White, *Heart Disease* (1931), 223; Lawrence E. Davies, "New Head of AMA Hits Critics Within," *New York Times,* July 5, 1946, 21:8; George E. Burch and Nicholas DePasquale, *A History of Electrocardiography* (1964; San Francisco: Norman, 1990), 15–18; I. T. T. Higgins, A. L. Cochrane, and A. J. Thomas, "Epidemiological Studies of Coronary Disease," *British Journal of Preventive and Social Medicine* 17 (1963): 156–57.

42. Cohn, "Heart Disease from the Point of View of the Public Health," 403; Friedberg, *Diseases of the Heart,* 339; Robert L. Levy, "Arteriosclerosis, Including Thrombosis of the Coronary Arteries," in *Diseases of the Coronary Arteries and Cardiac Pain,* ed. Robert L. Levy (New York: Macmillan, 1936), 201.

43. Louis I Dublin, Alfred J. Lotka, and Mortimer Spiegelman, *Length of Life: A Study of the Life Table,* rev. ed. (New York: Ronald, 1949), 195.

44. Marquis James, *The Metropolitan Life: A Study in Business Growth* (New York: Viking, 1947), 393–94; Metropolitan Life Insurance Company archives.

45. Peter N. Stearns, *Fat History: Bodies and Beauty in the Modern West* (New York: New York University Press, 1997), 12, 25–47.

46. White, *Heart Disease* (1944), 433; Arthur M. Fishberg, *Hypertension and Nephritis* (Philadelphia: Lea and Febiger, 1930), 463.

47. White, *Heart Disease* (1931), 400; Theodore C. Janeway, *The Clinical Study of Blood-Pressure: A Guide to the Use of the Sphygmomanometer* (New York: Appleton, 1904), 143.

48. Fishberg, *Hypertension and Nephritis,* 461; Arthur M. Master, Charles I. Garfield, and Max B. Walters, *Normal Blood Pressure and Hypertension: New Definitions* (Philadelphia: Lea and Febiger, 1952), 81–82.

49. Master, Garfield, and Walters, *Normal Blood Pressure and Hypertension,* 45–46, 71–72; George W. Norris, Henry C. Bazett, Thomas M. McMillan, *Blood-Pressure: Its Clinical Applications,* 4th ed. (Philadelphia: Lea and Febiger, 1927), 125–43.

50. Fishberg, *Hypertension and Nephritis,* 518.

51. Ibid., 519–20; White, *Heart Disease* (1931), 401.

Notes to Chapter 12

1. D. W. Forrest, *Francis Galton: The Life and Work of a Victorian Genius* (London: Elek, 1974), 199.

2. This discussion is based on the references below and on Alfred S. Evans, *Causation and Disease: A Chronological Journey* (New York: Plenum, 1993), and Elliot G. Mishler, et al., *Social Contexts of Health, Illness, and Patient Care* (Cambridge: Cambridge University Press, 1981).

3. Henrik R. Wulff, *Rational Diagnosis and Treatment: An Introduction to Clinical Decision-Making,* 2nd ed. (Oxford: Blackwell, 1981), 46–51. See Alvan R. Feinstein, *Clinical Judgment* (Baltimore: Williams and Wilkens, 1967).

4. Robert A. Aronowitz, *Making Sense of Illness: Science, Society, and Disease* (Cambridge: Cambridge University Press, 1998), 8.

5. Henrik R. Wulff, "The Causal Basis of the Current Disease Classification," in *Health, Disease, and Causal Explanations in Medicine,* ed. Lennart Nordenfelt and Ingemar B. Lindahl (Dordrecht: Reidel, 1984), 174; Christoph Gradmann, "Robert Koch and the Pressures of Scientific Research: Tuberculosis and Tuberculin," *Medical History* 45 (2000): 1–32; Robert Koch, *Essays of Robert Koch* (Westport, CT: Greenwood Press, 1987), 149; Karl Pearson, *The Fight Against Tuberculosis and the Death-rate from Phthisis* (London: Cambridge University Press, 1911), 19–23.

6. Rene Dubos, *The World of Rene Dubos: A Collection from His Writings* (New York: Holt, 1990), 126.

7. Rene J. Dubos, "Infection Into Disease," in *Life and Disease: New Perspectives in Biology and Medicine,* ed. Dwight J. Ingle (New York Basic Books: 1963), 108.

8. Wulff, "The Causal Basis of the Current Disease Classification," 169, 172.

9. Dubos, *The World of Rene Dubos,* 238–40.

10. Margaret L. Grimshaw, "Scientific Specialization and the Poliovirus Controversy in the Years Before World War II," *Bulletin of the History of Medicine* 69 (1995): 44–65. See also John R. Paul, *A History of Poliomyelitis* (New Haven: Yale University Press, 1971).

11. Galton also invented two other widely used tools in social science research: percentiles and mathematical regression. See Nicholas W. Gillham, *A Life of Sir Francis Galton: From African Exploration to the Birth of Eugenics* (New York: Oxford University Press, 2001).

12. Gio Batta Gori, "The Regulation of Carcinogenic Hazards," *Science* 208 (1980): 256—61.

13. See Mervyn Susser, *Causal Thinking in the Health Sciences* (New York: Oxford University Press, 1973), 140–62 and passim.

14. A. Bradford Hill, *Principles of Medical Statistics* (London: Lancet, 1937), 3. The definition is that of George U. Yule.

15. Intersalt Cooperative Research Group, "Intersalt: An International Study of Electrolyte Excretion and Blood Pressure: Results for 24 Hour Urinary Sodium and Potassium Excretion," *British Medical Journal* 297 (1988): 319–28; Paul Elliott, et al., "Intersalt Revisited: Further Analyses of 24 Hour Sodium Excretion and Blood Pressure Within and Across Populations," *British Medical Journal* 312 (1996): 1249–53; American Heart Association Nutrition Committee, "Rationale of the Diet-Heart Statement of the American Heart Association," *Circulation* 88 (1993): 3019.

16. Martin Muntzel and Tilman Drueke, "A Comprehensive Review of the Salt and Blood Pressure Relationship," *American Journal of Hypertension* 5 (April 1992) suppl., 7S.

17. Aronowitz, *Making Sense of Illness,* 125, 112.

18. Theodore M. Porter, *The Rise of Statistical Thinking: 1820–1900* (Princeton, NJ: Princeton University Press, 1986), 236.

19. Stephen J. Haines, "Randomized Clinical Trials in the Evaluation of Surgical Innovations," *Journal of Neurosurgery* 51 (1979): 6–7.

20. L. J. Witts, "Introduction," in *Medical Surveys and Clinical Trials,* ed. L. J. Witts, 2nd ed. (London: Oxford University Press, 1964), 5; Harry F. Dowling, "The Emergence of the Cooperative Clinical Trial," *Transactions and Studies of the College of Physicians of Philadelphia* 43 (1975): 20–29; J. Rosser Matthews, *Quantification and the Quest for Medical Certainty* (Princeton: Princeton University Press, 1995), 139 and passim; Harry M. Marks, *The Progress of Experiment: Science and Therapeutic Reform in the United States, 1900–1990* (Cambridge: Cambridge University Press, 1997).

21. James D. Neaton, et al., "Total and Cardiovascular Mortality in Relation to Cigarette Smoking, Serum Cholesterol Concentration, and Diastolic Blood Pressure among Black and White Males Followed up for Five Years," *American Heart Journal* 108 (1984): 760–62.

22. David Freedman, et al., *Statistics,* 2nd. ed. (New York: Norton, 1991), 12–14; Coronary Drug Project Research Group, "Influence of Adherence to Treatment and Response of Cholesterol on Mortality in the Coronary Drug Project," *New England Journal of Medicine* 303 (1980): 1038–41.

23. Richard Doll, "Smoking and Death Rates," *JAMA* 251 (1984): 2856; Edward A. Lew, "Biostatistical Pitfalls in Studies of Atherosclerotic Heart Disease," *Federation Proceedings* 21 (4) pt. 2 (July-Aug. 1962): 63.

24. Forrest, *Francis Galton: The Life and Work of a Victorian Genius,* 188–89; Freedman et al., *Statistics,* 159–64.

25. Prospective Studies Collaboration, "Cholesterol, Diastolic Blood Pressure, and Stroke," *Lancet* 346 (1995): 1649.

26. P. O. Korner, et al., "Untreated Mild Hypertension," *Lancet* 1 (1982): 185–91.

Notes to Chapter 13

1. Peter Taylor, *The Smoke Ring: Tobacco, Money, and Multinational Politics* (New York: Pantheon, 1984), 33.

2. Richard Kluger, *Ashes to Ashes: America's Hundred-Year Cigarette War, the Public Health, and the Unabashed Triumph of Philip Morris* (New York: Knopf, 1996), 617. This chapter relies heavily on Kluger's book.

3. W. Gilman Thompson, *The Occupational Diseases: Their Causation, Symptoms, Treatment, and Prevention* (New York: Appleton, 1914), 609; Kluger, *Ashes to Ashes,* 132.

4. "Urban Life Cited in Heart Ailments," *New York Times,* June 10, 1937, 16:1; Charles K. Friedberg, *Diseases of the Heart* (Philadelphia: Saunders, 1949), 407, 486; "Death Comes to the Average Man," *Fortune* 16 (Nov. 1937): 154.

5. "Cancer of the Lung a Growing Health Problem," *Statistical Bulletin* 20 (Nov. 1939): 7–9.

6. Lauren V. Ackerman and Juan A. del Regato, *Cancer: Diagnosis, Treatment, and Prognosis* (St. Louis: Mosby, 1947), 437–38; R. A. Willis, *Pathology of Tumours* (St. Louis, MO: Mosby, 1948), 362–64.

7. Robert D. Grove and Alice M. Hetzel, *Vital Statistics Rates in the United States, 1940–1960* (Washington, DC: U.S. Department of Health, Education, and Welfare, 1968), 368.

8. Kluger, *Ashes to Ashes,* 160–62, 349–58.

9. Ibid., 191–95, 225–26.

10. Jerome Cornfield, et al., "Smoking and Lung Cancer: Recent Evidence and a Discussion of Some Questions," *Journal of the National Cancer Institute* 22 (1959): 177–80.

11. Sarah C. Darby and Jonathan M. Samet, "Radon," in *Epidemiology of Lung Cancer,* ed. Jonathan M. Samet (New York: Dekker, 1994), 220–21, and other articles in this book; W. Keith Morgan and Anthony Seaton, *Occupational Lung Diseases,* 3rd ed. (Philadelphia: Saunders, 1995), 629–35; Cornfield, et al., "Smoking and Lung Cancer: Recent Evidence and a Discussion of Some Questions," 179.

12. U.S. Surgeon General's Advisory Committee on Smoking and Health, *Smoking and Health* (Washington, D.C.: U.S. Department of Health, Education, and Welfare, 1964), 45. U.S. Bureau of the Census, *Statistical Abstract of the United States: 1960* (Washington, DC), p. 803.

13. See Jean M. Converse, *Survey Research in the United States: Roots and Emergence 1890–1960* (Berkeley: University of California Press, 1987) and Herbert H. Hyman, *Taking Society's Measure: A Personal History of Survey Research* (New York: Russell Sage Foundation, 1991).

14. U.S. Surgeon General's Advisory Committee on Smoking and Health, *Smoking and Health,* 361–65; Grove and Hetzel, *Vital Statistics Rates in the United States, 1940–1960,* 307.

15. Ernst L. Wynder and Evarts A. Graham, "Tobacco Smoking as a Possible Etiologic Factor in Bronchiogenic Carcinoma," *JAMA* 143 (1950): 329–36; Ernst L. Wynder, "Tobacco as a Cause of Lung Cancer," *Pennsylvania Medical Journal* 57 (1954): 1082–83.

16. E. Cuyler Hammond, "Smoking in Relation to Lung Cancer," *Connecticut State Medical Journal* 18 (1954): 6; Wynder, "Tobacco as a Cause of Lung Cancer," 1081.

17. E. Cuyler Hammond and Daniel Horn, "The Relationship between Human Smoking Habits and Death Rates," *JAMA* 155 (1954): 1316–28; Hammond, "Smoking in

Relation to Lung Cancer," 6–9; "Text of the American Cancer Society's Report on the Effects of Tobacco Smoking," *New York Times,* June 5, 1957, 24:1; Richard Doll, "Smoking and Death Rates," *JAMA* 251 (1984): 2854–57.

18. James T. Patterson, *The Dread Disease: Cancer and Modern American Culture* (Cambridge, MA: Harvard University Press, 1987), 211; Kluger, *Ashes to Ashes,* 222; Morris Kaplan, "Pipe Users Make Report on Cancer," *New York Times,* June 5, 1957, 25:1.

19. Harold F. Dorn, "Tobacco Consumption and Mortality from Cancer and Other Diseases," *Public Health Reports* 74 (1959): 581–93.

20. Richard Doll and A. Bradford Hill, "Lung Cancer and Other Causes of Death in Relation to Smoking," *British Medical Journal* 2 (1956): 1071–81; Richard Doll and Austin B. Hill, "Mortality in Relation to Smoking: Ten Years' Observations of British Doctors," *British Medical Journal* 1 (1964): 1399–1410, 1460–67.

21. Dorn, "Tobacco Consumption and Mortality from Cancer and Other Diseases," 585; Hammond and Horn, "The Relationship between Human Smoking Habits and Death Rates," 1320.

22. U.S. Surgeon General's Advisory Committee on Smoking and Health, *Smoking and Health,* 89–93; R. B. McConnell, K. C. T. Gordon, and Thelwall Jones, "Occupational and Personal Factors in the Aetiology of Carcinoma of the Lung," *Lancet* 2 (1952): 654.

23. Dorn, "Tobacco Consumption and Mortality from Cancer and Other Diseases," 591; Cornfield, et al., "Smoking and Lung Cancer," 177–79.

24. E. Cuyler Hammond, "Smoking in Relation to Heart Disease," *American Journal of Public Health* 50 suppl. (Mar. 1960): 25; Robert N. Proctor, *Cancer Wars: How Politics Shapes What We Know and Don't Know About Cancer* (New York: Basic Books, 1995), 153–73.

25. Cornfield, et al., "Smoking and Lung Cancer: Recent Evidence and a Discussion of Some Questions," 186–87; John Higginson, Calum S. Muir, and Nubia Munoz, *Human Cancer: Epidemiology and Environmental Causes* (Cambridge: Cambridge University Press, 1992), xxi.

26. Morris Kaplan, "Full Cancer Data on Tobacco Urged," *New York Times,* June 23, 1954, I, 17:3; Howard A. Rusk, "Cigarette-Cancer Question is Left Open in Report," *New York Times,* June 27, 1954, I, 53:3; W.K. [Waldemar Kaempffert], "Cigarette Habit: Cause and Effect," *New York Times,* June 27, 1954, IV, 7:6.

27. Harold M. Schmeck, Jr., "7 Experts Find Cigarettes A Factor in Lung Cancer," *New York Times,* Mar. 23, 1957, 1:5; 12:6; "Text of the American Cancer Society's Report on the Effects of Tobacco Smoking," *New York Times,* June 5, 1957, 24:6.

28. Elizabeth M. Whelan, *A Smoking Gun: How the Tobacco Industry Gets Away with Murder* (Philadelphia: Stickley, 1984), 99–100; Patterson, *The Dread Disease: Cancer and Modern American Culture,* 216.

29. U.S. Surgeon General's Advisory Committee on Smoking and Health, *Smoking and Health,* 20–21.

30. Ibid., 21.

31. Ibid., 26–31.

32. Ibid., 37–39.

33. U.S. National Clearing House for Smoking and Health, *The Health Consequences of Smoking: A Public Health Service Review: 1967* (Washington, DC: U.S. Public Health Service, 1968), 4, 26.

34. U.S. National Clearing House for Smoking and Health, *The Health Consequences*

of Smoking: A Public Health Service Review: 1968 supplement to the 1967 Public Health Service Review (Washington, DC: U.S. Public Health Service, 1968), 24, 28; U.S. National Clearing House for Smoking and Health, *The Health Consequences of Smoking: A Report of the Surgeon General: 1971* (Washington, DC: U.S. Public Health Service, 1971), 8–14.

35. U.S. Public Health Service, *The Health Consequences of Involuntary Smoking: A Report of the Surgeon General* (Rockville, MD: U.S. Public Health Service, 1986), 7 and passim.

36. Ernst L. Wynder, "Tobacco and Health: a Review of the History and Suggestions for Public Health Policy," *Public Health Reports* 103 (1988), 11.

37. Thomas Whiteside, *Selling Death: Cigarette Advertising and Public Health* (New York: Liveright, 1971), 46–47, 74.

38. Robert H. Miles, *Coffin Nails and Corporate Strategies* (Englewood Cliffs, NJ: Prentice-Hall, 1982), 32–34.

39. Morris Kaplan, "Full Cancer Data on Tobacco Urged," *New York Times,* June 23, 1954, 17:3; "Smokers Assured in Industry Study," *New York Times,* Aug 17, 1964, 27:5; Alix M. Freedman and Laurie Cohen, "Smoke and Mirrors: How Cigarette Makers Keep Health Question 'Open' Year After Year," *Wall Street Journal,* Feb. 11, 1993, A1; Kenneth E. Warner, "Tobacco Industry Scientific Advisors: Serving Society or Selling Cigarettes?" *American Journal of Public Health* 81 (1991): 839–42.

40. Kluger, *Ashes to Ashes,* 375, 434, 438, 708–9, 735–37; Howard M. Leichter, *Free to be Foolish: Politics and Health Promotion in the United States and Great Britain* (Princeton: Princeton University Press, 1991), 137–38; Peter S. Arno, et al., "Tobacco Industry Strategies to Oppose Federal Regulation," *JAMA* 275 (1996): 1258–62.

41. A. Lee Fritschler, *Smoking and Politics,* 3rd ed. (Englewood Cliffs, NJ: Prentice-Hall, 1983), 38.

42. Ibid., 32–33; Kluger, *Ashes to Ashes,* 301, 369, 439–41.

43. Maurine B. Neuberger, *Smoke Screen: Tobacco and the Public Welfare* (Englewood Cliffs, NJ: Prentice-Hall, 1963), 51–53; Kluger, *Ashes to Ashes,* 436.

44. Neuberger, *Smoke Screen,* 50–51; Food and Drug Administration et al. v. Brown & Williamson Tobacco Corp. et al., 529 U.S. 23 (2000), 23.

45. Patterson, *The Dread Disease,* 242, 252–53; Proctor, *Cancer Wars,* 109; Kluger, *Ashes to Ashes,* 425–27, 465; Donald R. Shopland and Marianne Haenlein, "Reducing Lung Cancer Through Smoking Prevention and Control," in *Epidemiology of Lung Cancer,* ed. Jonathan M. Samet, (New York: Dekker, 1994), 451–52; personal communication from Donald R. Shopland, Feb. 22, 1999.

46. Whiteside, *Selling Death,* 46–47; Fritschler, *Smoking and Politics,* 31, 83–84, 135–38; Miles, *Coffin Nails and Corporate Strategies,* 43–44.

47. Miles, *Coffin Nails and Corporate Strategies,* 44, 75; Fritschler, *Smoking and Politics,* 112–16.

48. Miles, *Coffin Nails and Corporate Strategies,* 45–46; Kevin Sack, "For the Nation's Politicians, Big Tobacco No Longer Bites," *New York Times,* April 22, 1997, A1.

49. Walter S. Ross, *Crusade: The Official History of the American Cancer Society* (New York: Arbor House, 1987), 56–57; W. Bruce Fye, *American Cardiology: The History of a Specialty and Its College* (Baltimore: Johns Hopkins University Press, 1996), 55–56, 70, 100–1; Philip Benjamin, "Rival Health Camps Fight for Charity Dollar in U.S." *New York Times,* June 15, 1959, 20:5.

50. Robert K. Plumb, "Cancer Unit Asks a Smoking Parley," *New York Times,* Oct. 23, 1954, 17:1; Ross, *Crusade: The Official History of the American Cancer Society,* 49–56, 61; Kluger, *Ashes to Ashes,* 169, 204, 222, 308, 506–10.

51. William W. Moore, *Fighting for Life: The Story of the American Heart Association 1911–1975* (n.p.: American Heart Association, 1983), 78, 133, 220; "Heart Study Pressed," *New York Times,* Mar. 15, 1956, 33:4; Lawrence E. Davies, "Heart Unit Plans $50,000,000 Drive," *New York Times,* Oct. 24, 1958, 20:5; Alfred E. Clark, "Heart Society Maps Drive on Cigarettes," *New York Times,* June 9, 1963, 1:6, 76:1; Pat McGrady, *The Savage Cell: A Report on Cancer and Cancer Research* (New York: Basic Books, 1964), 71.

52. Howard Wolinsky and Tom Brune, *The Serpent on the Staff: The Unhealthy Politics of the American Medical Association* (New York: Putnam, 1994), 148–49.

53. Ibid., 150–55; Susan Wagner, *Cigarette Country: Tobacco in American History and Politics* (New York: Praeger, 1971), 141–42; Kluger, *Ashes to Ashes,* 286, 360–61, 448.

54. Wolinsky and Brune, *The Serpent on the Staff,* 151–52, 161; Kenneth E. Warner, *Selling Smoke: Cigarette Advertising and Public Health* (Washington, DC: American Public Health Association, 1986), 32–33.

55. Wolinsky and Brune, *The Serpent on the Staff,* 152–54, 162; Warner, *Selling Smoke,* 32.

56. Gallup News Services, "Nine of Ten Americans View Smoking as Harmful," Oct. 7, 1999, *www.gallup.com.*

57. Kenneth E. Warner, "Reactions to Perceived Risk: Changes in the Behavior of Cigarette Smokers," in *The Analysis of Actual Versus Perceived Risks,* ed. Vincent T. Covello, et al., (New York: Plenum, 1983), 185; National Center for Health Statistics, *Health United States, 1999* (Hyattsville, MD: 1999), 212–13.

58. Beth Schucker, et al., "Change in Physician Perspective on Cholesterol and Heart Disease," *JAMA* 258 (1987): 3522; *Tobacco and the Clinician: Interventions for Medical and Dental Practice,* monograph no. 5 (n.p.: National Institutes of Health, 1994), 15.

59. Anne N. Thorndike, et al., "National Patterns in the Treatment of Smokers by Physicians," *JAMA* 279 (1998): 604–8; Robert M. Saywell, Jr., et al., "Indiana Family Physician Attitudes and Practices Concerning Smoking Cessation," *Indiana Medicine* 89 (1996): 149–56; Jack L. Franklin, et al., "Smoking Cessation Interventions by Family Physicians in Texas," *Texas Medicine* 88 (1992): 60–64; Robert F. Anda, et al., "Are Physicians Advising Smokers to Quit? The Patient's Perspective," *JAMA* 257 (1987): 1916–19; Patrick E. McBride, et al., "Smoking Screening and Management in Primary Care Practices," *Archives of Family Medicine* 6 (1997): 165–72.

60. Thorndike, et al., "National Patterns in the Treatment of Smokers by Physicians," 607; Henry Wechsler, et al., "The Physician's Role in Health Promotion: A Survey of Primary-Care Practitioners," *New England Journal of Medicine* 308 (1983): 99; McBride, et al., "Smoking Screening and Management in Primary Care Practices," 169–70; Steven R. Cummings, et al., "Smoking Counseling and Preventive Medicine," *Archives of Internal Medicine* 149 (1989): 346.

61. Miles, *Coffin Nails and Corporate Strategies,* 120–53; Kluger, *Ashes to Ashes,* 617.

62. Gallup News Services, "Nine of Ten Americans View Smoking as Harmful," Nov. 1, 1999, *www.gallup.com*; Kluger, *Ashes to Ashes,* 632.

63. Sack, "For the Nation's Politicians, Big Tobacco No Longer Bites"; Arno, et al., "Tobacco Industry Strategies to Oppose Federal Regulation," 1259–60.

Notes to Chapter 14

1. R. D. C. Brackenridge, *Medical Selection of Life Risks: A Comprehensive Guide to Life Expectancy for Underwriters and Clinicians,* 2nd ed. (New York: Nature Press, 1985), 160.

2. Lawrence E. Ramsey, et al., "Interpretation of Prospective Trials in Hypertension: Do Treatment Guidelines Accurately Reflect Current Evidence?" *Journal of Hypertension* 14 suppl. 5 (1996): S189–90.

3. Robert D. Grove and Alice M. Hetzel, *Vital Statistics Rates in the United States, 1940–1960* (Washington, DC: U.S. Department of Health, Education, and Welfare, 1968), 374, 393, 408, 455.

4. W. R. Houston, "Psychic Factors in Essential Hypertension," in *The Diagnosis and Treatment of Cardiovascular Disease,* ed. William D. Stroud, 4th ed. (Philadelphia: Davis, 1950), I:928.

5. George Pickering, "Hypertension: Definitions, Natural Histories and Consequences," in *Hypertension Manual,* ed. John H. Laragh (New York: Yorke, 1974), 20.

6. George Pickering, *The Nature of Essential Hypertension* (New York: Grune and Stratton, 1961), 10–21; George Pickering, *High Blood Pressure* (New York: Grune and Stratton, 1955), 154–56, 171, 244; Pickering, "Hypertension: Definitions, Natural Histories and Consequences," 25. See also J. D. Swales, ed., *Platt Versus Pickering: An Episode in Recent Medical History,* (n.p.: Keynes Press, 1985).

7. Pickering, *The Nature of Essential Hypertension,* 136; George Pickering, "Normo and Hypertension," *American Journal of Medicine* 65 (1983): 562.

8. Pickering, *High Blood Pressure,* 181; John A. Morsell, "The Problem of Hypertension: A Critical Review of the Literature Dealing with its Extent," in *A Symposium on Essential Hypertension: An Epidemiologic Approach to the Elucidation of its Natural History in Man* (Boston, 1951), 28.

9. Arthur M. Master, Charles I. Garfield, and Max B. Walters, *Normal Blood Pressure and Hypertension: New Definitions* (Philadelphia: Lea and Febiger, 1952), 124.

10. Irvine H. Page, "Arterial Hypertension," in *Diagnosis and Treatment of Cardiovascular Disease,* ed. William D. Stroud, 4th ed., II:1033.

11. Martin Muntzel and Tilman Drueke, "A Comprehensive Review of the Salt and Blood Pressure Relationship," *American Journal of Hypertension* 5 (suppl. April 1992): 11S; Jay. S. Skyler, "Walter Kempner: A Biographical Note," *Archives of Internal Medicine* 133 (1974): 752–755: Eugene A. Stead, "Walter Kempner: A Perspective," *Archives of Internal Medicine* 133 (1974): 756–57.

12. Karl H. Beyer, "Chlorothiazide: How the Thiazides Evolved as Antihypertensive Therapy," *Hypertension* 22 (1993): 388–91; William I. Gefter, Bernard H. Pastor, and Ralph M. Myerson, *Synopsis of Cardiology* (St. Louis, MO: Mosby, 1965), 503–4.

13. Edward D. Freis, "The Role of Hypertension," *American Journal of Public Health* 50 suppl. (Mar. 1960): 11.

14. Veterans Administration Cooperative Study Group on Antihypertensive Agents, "Effects of Treatment on Morbidity in Hypertension," *JAMA* 202 (1967): 116–22; Veterans Administration Cooperative Study Group on Antihypertensive Agents, "Effects of Treatment on Morbidity in Hypertension II," *JAMA* 213 (1970): 1143–52.

15. Veterans Administration Study Group, "Effects of Treatment on Morbidity in Hypertension II," 1143–51.

16. Julian T. Hart, *Hypertension; Community Control of High Blood Pressure,* 2nd ed. (Edinburgh: Churchill Livingstone, 1987), 53; Veterans Administration Study Group, "Effects of Treatment on Morbidity in Hypertension II," 1151.

17. Roger A. Rosenblatt, et al., "The Content of Ambulatory Care in the United States," *New England Journal of Medicine* 309 (1983): 892–97.

18. Mitchell H. Charap, "The Periodic Health Examination: Genesis of a Myth," *Annals of Internal Medicine* 95 (1981): 733–35.

19. G. A. Rose, "Hypertension in the Community," in *Epidemiology of Hypertension,* ed. C. J. Bulpitt (Amsterdam: Elsevier, 1985), 9.

20. Norman M. Kaplan, *Clinical Hypertension,* 6th ed. (Baltimore: Williams and Wilkens, 1994), 27–36.

21. S. W. Rabkin, F. A. Mathewson, and R. B. Tate, "Relationship of Blood Pressure in 20–39–Year-Old Men to Subsequent Blood Pressure and Incidence of Hypertension over a 30–year Period," *Circulation* 65 (1982): 291–300.

22. Ibid., 294–95.

23. Ibid., 293.

24. See Hypertension Detection and Follow-up Program Cooperative Group, "Five-Year Findings of the Hypertension Detection and Follow-up Program," *JAMA* 242 (1979): 2572–77; Treatment of Mild Hypertension Research Group, "The Treatment of Mild Hypertension," *Archives of Internal Medicine* 151 (1991): 1413–23; James D. Neaton, et al., "The Treatment of Mild Hypertension Study: Final Results," *JAMA* 270 (1993): 713–24.

25. "The Australian Therapeutic Trial in Mild Hypertension," *Lancet* 1 (1980): 1261–67; "Untreated Mild Hypertension," *Lancet* 1 (1982): 185–91.

26. Medical Research Council Working Party, "MRC Trial of Treatment of Mild Hypertension: Principal Results," *British Medical Journal* 291 (1985): 97–104; W. E. Miall and Gillian Greenberg, *Mild Hypertension: Is There Pressure to Treat?* (Cambridge: Cambridge University Press, 1987), 4, 43, 46, 105, 111, 116–17.

27. Miall and Greenberg, *Mild Hypertension,* 41.

28. "Untreated Mild Hypertension," 187.

29. Edward D. Freis, "Should Mild Hypertension be Treated?" *New England Journal of Medicine* 307 (1982): 308–9.

30. Miall and Greenberg, *Mild Hypertension,* 71; Neaton, et al., "The Treatment of Mild Hypertension Study: Final Results," 1417.

31. Robin M. Henig, "Defining Hypertension" *New York Times Magazine,* Jan. 24, 1988, VI, 32. "The 1988 Report of the Joint National Committee on Detection, Evaluation, and Treatment of High Blood Pressure," *Archives of Internal Medicine* 148 (1988): 1024; "Fifth Report of the Joint National Committee on Detection, Evaluation, and Treatment of High Blood Pressure," *Archives of Internal Medicine* 153 (1993): 161; "The Sixth Report of the Joint National Committee on Detection, Evaluation, and Treatment of High Blood Pressure," *Archives of Internal Medicine* 157 (1997): 2417.

32. "The 1988 Report of the Joint National Committee," 1026–27; "Fifth Report of the Joint National Committee," 167; "Sixth Report of the Joint National Committee," 2420.

33. Medical Research Council Working Party, "Stroke and Coronary Heart Disease in Mild Hypertension: Risk Factors and the Value of Treatment," *British Medical Journal* 296 (1988): 1568; William B. Kannel, "Contribution of the Framingham Study to Preventive Cardiology," *Journal of the American College of Cardiology* 15 (1990): 210; "The 1988

Report of the Joint National Committee," 1026; "Fifth Report of the Joint National Committee," 162; "Sixth Report of the Joint National Committee," 2423.

34. "The 1988 Report of the Joint National Committee," 1032; "Fifth Report of the Joint National Committee," 161; "Sixth Report of the Joint National Committee," 2427.

35. British Hypertension Society Working Party, "Treating Mild Hypertension" *British Medical Journal* 298 (1989): 694–98; British Hypertension Society Second Working Party, "Management Guidelines in Essential Hypertension," *British Medical Journal* 306 (1993): 983–87; Martin G. Myers, et al., "Recommendations from the Canadian Hypertension Society Consensus Conference on the Pharmacologic Treatment of Hypertension," *Canadian Medical Association Journal* 140 (1989): 1141–46. See also Lawrence E. Ramsay, et al., "Interpretation of Prospective Trials in Hypertension: Do Treatment Guidelines Accurately Reflect Current Evidence?" *Journal of Hypertension* 14 suppl. 5 (1996): S191.

36. "Summary of 1993 World Health Organization-International Society of Hypertension Guidelines for the Management of Mild Hypertension," *BMJ* 307 (1993): 1541–46.

37. Stephen Fortmann, et al., "Attitudes and Practices of Physicians Regarding Hypertension and Smoking: the Stanford Five City Project" *Preventive Medicine* 14 (1985): 70–80.

38. W. T. Friedewald, "Implementation in the USA," in *Screening for Risk of Coronary heart Disease,* ed. Michael Oliver, Michael Ashley-Miller, and David Wood (Chichester: Wiley, 1987), 82.

39. Hart, *Hypertension: Community Control of High Blood Pressure,* 2; "Sixth Report of the Joint National Committee" 2414.

40. Glen R. Elliott and Carl Eisdorfer, eds., *Stress and Human Health: Analysis and Implications of Research* (New York: Springer, 1982), 11, 17, 149; "The 1988 Report of the Joint National Committee," 1026; "Sixth Report of the Joint National Committee," 2423.

41. Arthur C. Guyton, "Personal Views on Mechanisms of Hypertension," in *Hypertension: Physiopathology and Treatment,* ed. Jacques Genest, Erich Koiw, and Otto Kuchel (New York: McGraw-Hill, 1977), 566–68, 574.

42. H. C. Trowell and D. Burkitt, eds., *Western Diseases: Their Emergence and Prevention* (Cambridge, MA: Harvard University Press, 1981), 3–12; Muntzel and Drueke, "A Comprehensive Review of the Salt and Blood Pressure Relationship," 7S.

43. Reay Tannahill, *Food in History,* 2nd ed. (New York: Crown, 1988), 175–81. See also Robert Multhauf, *Neptune's Gift: A History of Common Salt* (Baltimore: Johns Hopkins University Press, 1978) and John Burnett, *Plenty and Want: A Social History of Diet in England from 1815 to the Present Day,* rev. ed. (London: Scolar Press, 1979), 135–37.

44. Paul Elliott, et al., "Intersalt Revisited: Further Analyses of 24 Hour Sodium Excretion and Blood Pressure within and across Populations," *British Medical Journal* 312 (1996): 1252; Matthew A. Boegehold and Theodore A. Kotchen, "Importance of Dietary Chloride for Salt Sensitivity of Blood Pressure," *Hypertension* 17 Supp. 1 (1991): I-158–I-161.

45. Jay M. Sullivan, "Salt Sensitivity: Definition, Conception, Methodology, and Long-Term Issues," *Hypertension* 17 Supp. 1 (1991): I:61–68; Muntzel and Drueke, "A Comprehensive Review of the Salt and Blood Pressure Relationship," 22S–28S.

46. Muntzel and Drueke, "A Comprehensive Review of the Salt and Blood Pressure Relationship," 17S–18S; Michael H. Alderman and Bernard Lamport, "Moderate Sodium Restriction: Do the Benefits Justify the Hazards?" *American Journal of Hypertension* 3 (1990): 501.

47. Alderman and Lamport, "Moderate Sodium Restriction," 500.

48. Muntzel and Drueke, "A Comprehensive Review of the Salt and Blood Pressure Relationship," 10S–11S; Thomas R. Dawber, et al., "Environmental Factors in Hypertension, in *The Epidemiology of Hypertension,* ed. Jeremiah Stamler, Rose Stamler, and Theodore N. Pullman (New York Grune and Stratton, 1967), 270–71.

49. George Pickering, "Salt Intake and Essential Hypertension," *Cardiovascular Reviews and Reports* 1 (April, 1980): 16; Muntzel and Drueke, "A Comprehensive Review of the Salt and Blood Pressure Relationship," 20S–22S.

50. U.S. Senate Select Committee on Nutrition and Human Needs, *Dietary Goals for the United States—Supplemental Views,* 95th Congress, 1st sess. (Washington, DC: U.S. GPO, 1977), 674–75, 679, 682; American Medical Association Council on Scientific Affairs, "American Medical Association Concepts of Nutrition and Health," *JAMA* 242 (1979): 2337; American Heart Association Nutrition Committee, "Rationale of the Diet-Heart Statement of the American Heart Association," *Circulation* 88 (1993): 3019; American Heart Association Nutrition Committee, "Dietary Guidelines for Healthy American Adults," *Circulation* 94 (1996): 1797.

51. U.S. Surgeon General, *The Surgeon General's Report on Nutrition and Health, 1988* (Washington, DC: Public Health Service, 1988), 141; U.S. Senate Select Committee on Nutrition and Human Needs, *Hearings* (90th Congress, 2nd sess., and 91st Congress, 1st sess., 1969), 4088; Wayne Callaway, "Reexamining Cholesterol and Sodium Recommendations," *Nutrition Today* 29 (Sept.–Oct., 1994): 35–36; Food and Nutrition Board, National Academy of Sciences, *Toward Healthful Diets* (Washington, DC: National Academy of Sciences, 1980), 13.

52. National Research Council Committee on Diet and Health, *Diet and Health: Implications for Reducing Chronic Disease Risk* (Washington, DC: National Academy Press, 1989), 415, 660, 673–74; Institute of Medicine, *Improving America's Diet and Health: From Recommendations to Action* (Washington, DC: National Academy Press, 1991), 104.

53. Virginia L. Wilkening, "FDA's Regulations to Implement the NLEA," *Nutrition Today* 31 (Sept.–Oct., 1993): 17–19.

Notes to Chapter 15

1. William Kannel, et al., "Epidemiology of Coronary Heart Disease," *Geriatrics* 17 (1962): 675–76.

2. Robert J. Goldberg, "Coronary Heart Disease: Epidemiology and Risk Factors," in *Prevention of Coronary Heart Disease,* ed. Ira S. Ockene and Judith K. Ockene (Boston: Little, Brown, 1992), 5.

3. Thomas Dawber, Gilcin F. Meadors, and Felix E. Moore, Jr., "Epidemiological Approaches to Disease: The Framingham Study," *American Journal of Public Health* 41 (1951): 280; Thomas R. Dawber, *The Framingham Study: The Epidemiology of Atherosclerotic Disease* (Cambridge, MA: Harvard University Press, 1980), 15–17. This book contains a bibliography of all study publications to that time.

4. Dawber, Meadors, and Moore, Jr., "Epidemiological Approaches to Heart Disease," 279–86.

5. Ibid., 281–83; Tavia Gordon and William B. Kannel, "The Framingham, Massa-

chusetts, Study Twenty Years Later," in *The Community as an Epidemiological Laboratory*, ed. Irving I. Kessler and Morton L. Levin (Baltimore: Johns Hopkins Press, 1970), 123–44.

6. William B. Kannel, et al., "Risk Factors in Coronary Heart Disease," *Annals of Internal Medicine* 61 (1964): 888–89; Gordon and Kannel, "The Framingham, Massachusetts Study Twenty Years Later," 135. Different Framingham study reports provide slightly different numbers for these groups.

7. Tavia Gordon, et al., "Some Methodological Problems in the Long-Term Study of Cardiovascular Disease: Observations on the Framingham Study," *Journal of Chronic Diseases* 10 (1959): 189–91, 195; Gordon and Kannel, "The Framingham, Massachusetts Study Twenty Years Later," 129–35.

8. Donald Lloyd-Jones, et al., "Accuracy of Death Certificates for Coding Coronary Heart Disease as the Cause of Death," *Annals of Internal Medicine* 129 (1998): 1020–26.

9. Tavia Gordon and William B. Kannel, "Premature Mortality from Coronary Heart Disease," *JAMA* 215 (1971): 1617–25.

10. William B. Kannel and Robert D. Abbott, "Incidence and Prognosis of Unrecognized Myocardial Infarction," *New England Journal of Medicine* 311 (1984): 1144–47; William B. Kannel, "Hypertension: Relationship with Other Risk Factors," *Drugs* 31 suppl. 1 (1986): 3–4. Very similar findings occurred in a study in Reykjavik, Iceland: Emil Sigurdsson, et al., "Unrecognized Myocardial infarction: Epidemiology, Clinical Characteristics, and the Prognostic Role of Angina Pectoris," *Annals of Internal Medicine* 122 (1995): 96–102.

11. Kannel, et al., "Epidemiology of Coronary Heart Disease," 676–77.

12. John A. Morsell, "The Problem of Hypertension: A Critical Review of the Literature Dealing with its Extent," in *Symposium on Essential Hypertension: An Epidemiologic Approach to the Elucidation of its Natural History in Man* (Boston, 1951), 27.

13. Mark E. Rushefsky, *Making Cancer Policy* (Albany: State University of New York Press, 1986), 211; Jack Siemiatycki, ed. *Risk Factors for Cancer in the Workplace* (Boca Raton, FL: CRC Press, 1991), 3–4.

14. George V. Mann, "The Clinical Trials," in *Coronary Heart Disease: the Dietary Sense and Nonsense,* ed. George V. Mann (London: Janus, 1993), 74; Dawber, Meadors, and Moore, "Epidemiological Approaches to Heart Disease," 280; Thomas R. Dawber, et al., "Some Factors Associated with the Development of Coronary Heart Disease," *American Journal of Public Health* 49 (1959): 1350; William B. Kannel, et al., "Factors of Risk in the Development of Coronary Heart Disease—Six-Year Follow-up Experience: The Framingham Study," *Annals of Internal Medicine* 55 (1961): 33, 47.

15. Kannel, et al., "Epidemiology of Coronary Heart Disease," 675–90.

16. See Dawber, *The Framingham Study: The Epidemiology of Atherosclerotic Disease.*

17. Thomas R. Dawber, et al., "Dietary Assessment in the Epidemiologic Study of Coronary Heart Disease: The Framingham Study," *America Journal of Clinical Nutrition* 11 (1962): 226–34; Tavia Gordon, "The Framingham Diet Study: Diet and the Regulation of Serum Cholesterol," Section 24, The Framingham Study: an Epidemiological Investigation of Cardiovascular Disease (Washington, DC: National Institutes of Health, 1970?); Thomas R. Dawber, et al., "Environmental Factors in Hypertension," in *The Epidemiology of Hypertension,* ed. Jeremiah Stamler, Rose Stamler, and Theodore N. Pullman (New York Grune and Stratton, 1967), 270–71.

18. William B. Kannel and Paul R. Sorlie, "Some Health Benefits of Physical Activity," *Archives of Internal Medicine* 139 (1979): 857–61.

19. Dawber, et al., "Some Factors Associated with the Development of Coronary Heart Disease," 1351–52; Dawber, et al., "Environmental Factors in Hypertension," 259–61.

20. Kannel, et al., "Epidemiology of Coronary Heart Disease," 685.

21. W. B. Kannel, "The Framingham Experience" in *Coronary Heart Disease Epidemiology: From Aetiology to Public Health,* ed. Michael Marmot and Paul Elliott (Oxford: Oxford University Press, 1992), 67.

22. Kannel, "Epidemiology of Coronary Heart Disease," 676–77.

Notes to Chapter 16

1. Klim McPherson, "Why Do Variations Occur?" in *The Challenges of Medical Practice Variations,* ed. Tavs F. Andersen and Gavin Mooney (London: Macmillan, 1990), 17.

2. W. Bruce Fye, "The Delayed Diagnosis of Myocardial Infarction: It Took Half a Century!" *Circulation* 72 (1985): 262–71.

3. A. Bleakley Chandler, et al., "Coronary Thrombosis in Myocardial Infarction," *American Journal of Cardiology* 34 (1974): 823–33.

4. William F. Enos, Robert H. Holmes, and James Beyer, "Coronary Disease among United States Soldiers Killed in Action in Korea," *JAMA* 152 (1953): 1090–93; Jack Strong, "Coronary Atherosclerosis in Soldiers: A Clue to the Natural History of Atherosclerosis in the Young," *JAMA* 256 (1986): 2863.

5. Esmond R. Long, "The Development of Our Knowledge of Arteriosclerosis," in *Arteriosclerosis: A Survey of the Problem,* ed. Edmund V. Cowdry (New York: Macmillan, 1933), 19–52; Strong, "Coronary Atherosclerosis in Soldiers: A Clue to the Natural History of Atherosclerosis in the Young," 2864; Franz M. Groedel, "Observations on the Circulatory System of Combatants During World War I," *Experimental Medicine and Surgery* 1 (1943): 97–99.

6. William H. Gordon, Edward F. Bland, and Paul D. White, "Coronary Artery Disease Analyzed Post Mortem: With Special Reference to the Influence of Economic Status and Sex," *American Heart Journal* 17 (1939): 10–11; Henry M. Parrish, "Epidemiology of Ischemic Heart Disease among White Males, II: Autopsy Incidence of Ischemic Heart Disease and Autopsy Prevalence of Coronary Atherosclerosis" *Journal of Chronic Diseases* 14 (1961): 329; J. Judson McNamara, et al., "Coronary Artery Disease in Combat Casualties in Vietnam," *JAMA* 216 (1971): 1185–87.

7. Michael J. Gibney, *Nutrition, Diet and Health* (Cambridge: Cambridge University Press, 1986), 103–6.

8. W. Ophuls, "The Pathogenesis of Arteriosclerosis," in *Arteriosclerosis: A Survey of the Problem,* 251–53; Strong, "Coronary Atherosclerosis in Soldiers: A Clue to the Natural History of Atherosclerosis in the Young," 2864–65; Albert S. Hyman and Aaron E. Parsonnet, *The Failing Heart of Middle Life: The Myocardosis Syndrome, Coronary Thrombosis, and Angina Pectoris* (Philadelphia: Davis, 1932), 24–30.

9. J. B. Duguid, "Thrombosis as a Factor in the Pathogenesis of Coronary Atherosclerosis," *Journal of Bacteriology and Pathology* 58 (1946): 207–12.

10. Meyer Texon, "The Hemodynamic Basis of Atherosclerosis," in *Coronary Heart Disease: The Dietary Sense and Nonsense,* ed. George V. Mann (London: Janus, 1993), 109–

18; William E. Stehbens, "The Lipid Hypothesis and the Role of Hemodynamics in Athero-genesis," *Progress in Cardiovascular Diseases* 33 (1990): 119–36; W. Linda Cashin, et al., "Accelerated Progression of Atherosclerosis in Coronary Vessels with Minimal Lesions that are Bypassed," *New England Journal of Medicine* 311 (1984): 824–28.

11. A. D. Morgan, "Some Forms of Undiagnosed Coronary Disease in Nineteenth Century England," *Medical History* 12 (1968): 355; Duguid, "Thrombosis as a Factor in the Pathogenesis of Coronary Atherosclerosis," 210–11.

12. J. R. A. Mitchell, "Anticoagulants in Coronary Heart Disease: Retrospect and Prospect," *Lancet* 1 (1981): 257–62.

13. Sol Sherry, "The Origin of Thrombolytic Therapy," *Journal of the American College of Cardiology* 14 (1989): 1085–92; Louis J. Acierno, *The History of Cardiology* (London: Parthenon, 1994), 670; S. Yusuf, et al., "Intravenous and Intracoronary Fibrinolytic Therapy in Acute Myocardial Infarction," *European Heart Journal* 6 (1985): 556–85: Sol Sherry, "Revisiting the Development of Thrombolytic Therapy: An Historical Perspective," *Transactions and Studies of the College of Physicians of Philadelphia,* ser. 5, vol. 11 (1989): 337–54; Glenn L. Laffel and Eugene Braunwald, "Thrombolytic Therapy: A New Strategy for the Treatment of Acute Myocardial infarction," *New England Journal of Medicine* 311 (1984): 710–17, 770–76; Baruch A. Brody, *Ethical Issues in Drug Testing, Approval, and Pricing: The Clot-Dissolving Drugs* (New York: Oxford University Press, 1995), 9–29.

14. Sherry, "The Origin of Thrombolytic Therapy," 1090–91.

15. Thomas Killip, "Twenty Years of Coronary Bypass Surgery," *New England Journal of Medicine* 319 (1988): 367; National Center for Health Statistics, *Health United States 1995* (Hyattsville, MD: Public Health Service, 1996), 205; U.S. Census Bureau, *Statistical Abstract of the United States: 1999* (Washington, DC: 1999), 139.

16. Debra L. Sherman and Thomas J. Ryan, "Coronary Angioplasty Versus Bypass Grafting," *Medical Clinics of North America* 79 (1995): 1085; "Heart Bypasses are Often Unnecessary, Study Says," *New York Times,* Mar. 10, 1977, 18:2; Jane E. Brody, "Personal Health," *New York Times,* Feb. 8, 1978, C8:1; Jane E. Brody, "Findings are in Conflict on Value of Coronary Bypass Operations," *New York Times,* Nov. 18, 1990, C2; "Study Warns Surgeons to Wait on Bypasses," *New York Times,* Oct. 3, 1984, A19:4.

17. Kenneth M. Kent, "Percutaneous Transluminal Coronary Angioplasty in Chronic Coronary Heart Disease," in *Trends in Coronary Heart Disease Mortality: The Influence of Medical Care,* ed. Millicent W. Higgins and Russell V. Luepker (New York: Oxford University Press, 1988), 245–46; W. Bruce Fye, *American Cardiology: The History of a Specialty and Its College* (Baltimore: Johns Hopkins University Press, 1996), 302–4; Sherman and Ryan, "Coronary Angioplasty Versus Bypass Grafting," 1085–86.

18. Sherman and Ryan, "Coronary Angioplasty Versus Bypass Grafting," 1087–88.

19. "Report Assails Emergency Heart Procedures," *New York Times,* Nov. 16, 1988, A22:2; Jane E. Brody, "Findings are in Conflict on Value of Coronary Bypass Operations," *New York Times,* Nov. 18, 1980, C2; "Many Men with Angina Don't Need Bypass Surgery," *New York Times,* Nov. 20, 1990, C2:3; "Study Finds Angioplasty as Good as Heart Bypass," *New York Times,* Nov. 11, 1993, A19:1; "No Difference Seen in Death Rates for 2 Heart Attack Treatments," *New York Times,* Oct. 24, 1996, A21:1.

20. David S. Jones, "Visions of a Cure: Visualization, Clinical Trials, and Controversy in Cardiac Therapeutics, 1968–98," *Isis* 91 (2000): 504–41; "A Debate on Coronary Bypass," *New England Journal of Medicine* 297 (1977): 1464–70.

21. "U.S. Study Backs Bypass Surgery," *New York Times,* Dec. 6, 1980, 9:4; Lawrence

K. Altman, "Experts Advise Caution on Using Balloons to Clear Arteries," *New York Times,* Aug. 2, 1988, C3:1; Working Party of the British Cardiac Society, "Coronary Angioplasty in the United Kingdom," *British Heart Journal* 66 (1991): 325; "Many Men with Angina Don't Need Bypass Surgery," *New York Times,* Nov. 20, 1990, C2:3.

22. "Experts Split on Two Ways to Treat Heart Attack," *New York Times* Mar. 22, 1995, C11:1; Fye, *American Cardiology: The History of a Specialty and Its College,* 318–20; Lawrence K. Altman, "New Recommendations on Clot-Busting Drugs for Heart Victims," *New York Times,* Feb. 9, 1994, C8:1.

23. "Use of Balloons to Unclog Arteries Soars Among the Very Old," *New York Times,* Mar. 21, 1995, C7:1; Warren E. Leary, "Study Urges Less Heart Surgery for Elderly," *New York Times,* Sept. 26, 1994, B9:1.

Notes to Chapter 17

1. Irvine H. Page, et al., "Atherosclerosis and the Fat Content of the Diet," *Circulation* 16 (1957): 164.

2. Martha D. Wilson and Lawrence L. Rudel, "Review of Cholesterol Absorption with Emphasis on Dietary and Biliary Cholesterol," *Journal of Lipid Research* 35 (1994): 943–55.

3. John W. Gofman, *What We Do Know about Heart Attacks* (New York: Putnam's Sons, 1958), 23–28; Corinne H. Robinson, et al., *Normal and Therapeutic Nutrition,* 17th ed. (New York: Macmillan, 1986), 91; "Report of the National Cholesterol Education Program Expert Panel on Detection, Evaluation, and Treatment of High Blood Cholesterol in Adults," *Archives of Internal Medicine* 148 (1988): 39.

4. Lars A. Solberg and Jack Strong, "Risk Factors and Atherosclerotic Lesions: A Review of Autopsy Studies," *Arteriosclerosis* 3 (1983): 187–98.

5. Keaven M. Anderson, William Castelli, and Daniel Levy, "Cholesterol and Mortality: 30 Years of Follow-up from the Framingham Study," *JAMA* 257 (1987): 2176–80.

6. Uri Goldbourt and Shomit Yaari, "Cholesterol and Coronary Heart Disease Mortality: A 23–year Follow-up Study of 9902 Men in Israel," *Arteriosclerosis* 10 (1990): 512–19; Michael J. Klag, et al., "Serum Cholesterol in Young Men and Subsequent Cardiovascular Disease," *New England Journal of Medicine* 328 (1993): 313–18; George D. Smith, et al., "Plasma Cholesterol Concentration and Mortality: The Whitehall Study," *JAMA* 267 (1992): 70–76.

7. "U.S. to Use Drug on Cholesterol," *New York Times,* Feb. 28, 1967, 23:3; "Lowering Blood Cholesterol to Prevent Heart Disease," *JAMA* 253 (1985): 2082; Gina Kolata, "Major Study Aims to Learn Who Should Lower Cholesterol," *New York Times,* Sept. 26, 1989, C1:1; Diane K. Wysowski, Dianne L. Kennedy, and Thomas Gross, "Prescribed Use of Cholesterol-Lowering Drugs in the United States 1978 through 1988," *JAMA* 263 (1990): 2185–88.

8. James Shepherd, et al., "Prevention of Coronary Heart Disease with Pravastatin in Men with Hypercholesterolemia," *New England Journal of Medicine* 333 (1995): 1301–7.

9. John R. Downs, et al., "Primary Prevention of Acute Coronary Events with Lovastatin in Men and Women with Average Cholesterol Levels," *JAMA* 279 (1996): 1615–1622.

10. Allan S. Brett, "Treating Hypercholesterolemia: How Should Practicing Physicians Interpret the Published Data for Patients?" *New England Journal of Medicine* 321 (1989): 679; Gina Kolata, "Report Calls Cholesterol Tests in Young Unjustified," *New York Times,* Mar. 17, 1993, B8:3.

11. American Medical Association Council on Foods and Nutrition, "Diet and Coronary Heart Disease," *JAMA* 222 (1972): 1647; "Rationale of the Diet-Heart Statement of the American Heart Association," *Arteriosclerosis* 4 (1982): 180; American Heart Association Nutrition Committee, "Rationale of the Diet-Heart Statement of the American Heart Association," *Circulation* 88 (1993): 3010–11; "Report of the National Cholesterol Education Program," 36.

12. American Heart Association, *1997 Heart and Stroke Statistical Update* (Dallas, TX: American Heart Association, 1996), 22; "Report of the National Cholesterol Education Program," 36.

13. Stephen Fortmann, et al., "Attitudes and Practices of Physicians Regarding Hypertension and Smoking: The Stanford Five Cities Project" *Preventive Medicine* 14 (1985): 70–80; Colleen E. O'Keefe, Donna F. Hahn, Nancy M. Betts, "Physicians' Perspectives on Cholesterol and Heart Disease," *Journal of the American Dietetic Association* 91 (Feb., 1991): 189–92; Beth Schucker, et al., "Change in Cholesterol Awareness and Action," *Archives of Internal Medicine* 151 (1991): 666–73.

14. Schucker, et al., "Change in Cholesterol Awareness and Action," 670–71.

15. James C. Roberts, Jr. and Reuben Straus, eds., *Comparative Atherosclerosis* (New York: Hoeber, 1965), 274–76 and passim.

16. Ancel Keys, "Atherosclerosis: A Problem in Newer Public Health," *Journal of the Mount Sinai Hospital New York* 20 (1953): 125–26; Ancel Keys, et al., "Diet and Serum Cholesterol in Man," *Journal of Nutrition* 59 (1956): 39–56.

17. Tavia Gordon, "The Framingham Diet Study: Diet and the Regulation of Serum Cholesterol," Sec. 24, The Framingham Study: An Epidemiological Investigation of Cardiovascular Disease (Washington, DC: National Institutes of Health, 1970?), 24–28; Paul N. Hopkins, "Effects of Dietary Cholesterol on Serum Cholesterol: A Meta-analysis and Review," *American Journal of Clinical Nutrition* 55 (1992): 1060–70; Ancel Keys, [letter], *New England Journal of Medicine* 325 (1991): 584.

18. American Heart Association, *Epidemiology of Atherosclerosis and Hypertension* (New York: 1956), 21; John A. Osmundsen, "Heart Cases Wary of Egg Diet, But Medical Opinion is Divided," *New York Times,* June 1, 1959, 33:6; Jane E. Brody, "Heart Association Strengthens Its Advice: Cut Down on Fats," *New York Times,* June 28, 1973, 54:1; American Heart Association Nutrition Committee, "Dietary Guidelines for Healthy American Adults," *Circulation* 94 (1996): 1797; Frederick J. Stare, Robert E. Olson, and Elizabeth M. Whelan, *Balanced Nutrition: Beyond the Cholesterol Scare* (Holbrook, MA: Bob Adams, 1989), 118. See Raymond Reiser, "A Commentary on the Rationale of the Diet-Heart Statement of the American Heart Association," *American Journal of Clinical Nutrition* 40 (1984): 654–58.

19. Robinson, et al., *Normal and Therapeutic Nutrition,* 86–88.

20. Germain J. Brisson, *Lipids in Human Nutrition: An Appraisal of Some Dietary Concepts* (Englewood Cliffs, NJ: Burgess, 1981), 5, 32–40.

21. British Nutrition Foundation, *Unsaturated Fatty Acids: Nutritional and Physiological Significance* (London: Chapman and Hall, 1992), 6–11.

22. Edward H. Ahrens, Jr., "Nutritional Factors and Serum Lipid Levels," *American*

Journal of Medicine 23 (1957): 935; Penny M. Kris-Etherton and Shaomei Yu, "Individual Fatty Acid Effects on Plasma Lipids and Lipoproteins: Human Studies," *American Journal of Clinical Nutrition* 65 (suppl.) (1997): 1628S–44S.

23. S. Boyd Eaton and Melvin Konner, "Paleolithic Nutrition," *New England Journal of Medicine* 312 (1985): 283–89; Mark N. Cohen, "The Significance of Long-Term Changes in Human Diet and Food Economy," in *Food and Evolution: Toward a Theory of Human Food Habits,* ed. Marvin Harris and Eric B. Ross (Philadelphia: Temple University Press, 1987), 269–70, 273–75; Broda O. Barnes and Charlotte W. Barnes, *Heart Attack Rareness in Thyroid-Treated Patients* (Springfield, IL: Thomas, 1972), 3–4.

24. Richard O. Cummings, *The American and His Food: A History of Food Habits in the United States,* rev. ed. (Chicago: University of Chicago Press, 1941), 53–78, 89–90, 114; James D. Norris, *Advertising and the Transformation of American Society, 1865–1920* (New York: Greenwood Press, 1990), 111–12.

25. Letitia Brewster and Michael F. Jacobson, *The Changing American Diet* (Washington, DC: Center for Science in the Public Interest, 1983), passim; Berta Friend, Louise Page, and Ruth Marston, "Food Consumption Patterns in the United States: 1909–13 to 1976," in *Nutrition, Lipids, and Coronary Heart Disease: A Global View,* ed. Robert I. Levy, et al. (New York: Raven, 1979), 489–98.

26. National Research Council Committee on Diet and Health, *Diet and Health: Implications for Reducing Chronic Disease Risk* (Washington, DC: National Academy Press, 1989), 53; Brewster and Jacobson, *The Changing American Diet,* passim; U.S. Bureau of the Census, *Statistical Abstract of the United States: 1999* (Washington, DC: 1997), 157.

27. Brewster and Jacobson, *The Changing American Diet,* 8–9.

28. Page, et al., "Atherosclerosis and the Fat Content of the Diet," 173; Alison M. Stephen and Nicholas J. Wald, "Trends in Individual Consumption of Dietary Fat in the United States, 1920–1984," *American Journal of Clinical Nutrition* 52 (1990): 460.

29. Page, et al., "Atherosclerosis and the Fat Content of the Diet," 174.

30. M. G. Marmot, "Affluence, Urbanization and Coronary Heart Disease," in *Disease and Urbanization,* ed. E. J. Clegg and J. Garlick (London: Taylor and Francis, 1980), 140.

31. J. Yerushalmy and Herman E. Hilleboe, "Fat in the Diet and Mortality from Heart Disease," *New York State Journal of Medicine* 57 (1957): 2343–54.

32. Ancel Keys, et al., *Seven Countries: A Multivariate Analysis of Death and Coronary Heart Disease* (Cambridge, MA: Harvard University Press, 1980), 3–10; Mary G. Enig, "Diet, Serum Cholesterol, and Coronary Heart Disease," in *Coronary Heart Disease: The Dietary Sense and Nonsense,* ed. George V. Mann (London: Janus, 1993), 55. See also Ancel Keys, ed., "Coronary Heart Disease in Seven Countries," *Circulation* 41 suppl. (April, 1970).

33. Keys, *Seven Countries,* 107, 135, 137–38, 153, 164, 193.

34. Gordon, "The Framingham Diet Study: Diet and the Regulation of Serum Cholesterol."

35. Richard B. Shekelle, et al., "Diet, Serum Cholesterol, and Death from Coronary Heart Disease: The Western Electric Study," *New England Journal of Medicine* 304 (1981): 65–70.

36. [Robert K. Plumb], "Diet Related to Heart Disease," *New York Times,* June 19, 1954, IV, 11:6; Robert K. Plumb, "Animal Fats Tied to Fatal Disease," *New York Times,* April 17, 1956, 33:8; William L. Laurence, "Science in Review," *New York Times,* Jan. 12, 1958, IV, 11:6; William K. Laurence, "Science in Review," *New York Times,* Mar. 17, 1957, IV, 11:6; William L. Laurence, "Diet and Arteries," *New York Times,* Dec. 18, 1960, IV, 7:7.

37. Jane E. Brody, "6–Year Study of Heart Ailments Seeks 12,000 Middle-Age Men," *New York Times,* Jan. 25, 1974, 30:1; Joan Cook, "Thousands Take Heart Tests," *New York Times,* Nov. 10, 1973, 94:3; William J. Zukel, Oglesby Paul, and Harold W. Schnaper, "The Multiple Risk Factor Intervention Trial: 1. Historical Perspectives," *Preventive Medicine* 10 (1981): 387–401; Multiple Risk Factor Intervention Trial Research Group, "Mortality Rates after 10.5 Years for Participants in the Multiple Risk Factor Intervention Trial," *JAMA* 263 (1990): 1795; Jerry Bishop, "Heart Attacks: A Test Collapses," *Wall Street Journal,* Oct. 6, 1982, 32.

38. Multiple Risk Factor Intervention Trial Research Group, "Multiple Risk Factor Intervention Trial," *JAMA* 248 (1982): 1465–77; Multiple Risk Factor Intervention Trial Research Group. "Mortality Rates after 10.5 Years," 1795–1801.

39. Donald B. Hunninghake, et al., "The Efficacy of Intensive Dietary Therapy Alone or in Combination with Lovastatin in Outpatients with Hypercholesterolemia," *New England Journal of Medicine* 328 (1993): 1213–19.

40. Ancel Keys, Joseph T. Anderson, and Francisco Grande, "Prediction of Serum-Cholesterol Responses of Man to Changes in Fats in the Diet," *Lancet* 2 (1957): 959.

41. L. E. Ramsay, W. W. Yeo, R. Jackson, "Dietary Reduction of Serum Cholesterol Concentration: Time to Think Again," *British Medical Journal* 303 (1991): 953–57.

42. Ibid., 956.

43. "Lowering Blood Cholesterol to Prevent Heart Disease," *JAMA* 253 (1985): 2082–83; Beverly Merz, "Low-Fat Diet May be Imprudent for Some, Say Opponents of Population-Based Cholesterol Control," *JAMA* 256 (1986): 2779; Lipid Research Clinics Program, "The Lipid Research Clinics Coronary Primary Prevention Trial Results 1. Reduction in Incidence of Coronary Heart Disease," *JAMA* 251 (1984): 351–64.

44. Thomas C. Chalmers, "Mortality Rate versus Funeral Rate in Clinical Medicine," *Gastroenterology* 46 (1964): 788–91.

45. Arnold M. Weissler, Brian I. Miller, and Harisios Boudoulas, "The Need for Clarification of Percent Risk Reduction Data in Clinical Cardiovascular Trial Reports," *Journal of the American College of Cardiology* 13 (1989): 764–66; Richard A. Kronmal, "Commentary on the Published Results of the Lipid Research Clinics Coronary Primary Prevention Trial," *JAMA* 253 (1985): 2091–93; U. Ravnskov, "Cholesterol Lowering Trials in Coronary Heart Disease: Frequency of Citation and Outcome," *British Medical Journal* 305 (1992): 15–19.

Notes to Chapter 18

1. John Carey, et al., "Snap, Crackle, Stop: States Crack down on Misleading Food Claims," *Business Week,* Sept. 25, 1989, 42.

2. Sanford A. Miller and Marilyn G. Stephenson, "Scientific and Public Health Rationale for the Dietary Guidelines for Americans," *American Journal of Clinical Nutrition* 42 (1985): 742.

3. Peter N. Stearns, *Fat History: Bodies and Beauty in the Modern West* (New York: New York University Press, 1997), 8, 12–17, 71–85, 98–101; Harvey Levenstein, *Paradox of Plenty: A Social History of Eating in Modern America* (New York: Oxford University Press, 1993), 136.

4. Betsy Haughton, Joan D. Gussow, and Janice M. Dodds, "An Historical Study of the Underlying Assumptions for United States Food Guides from 1917 through the Basic Four Food Group Guide," *Journal of Nutrition Education* 19 (1987): 169–75.

5. American Heart Association, *Epidemiology of Atherosclerosis and Hypertension* (New York: 1956), 21; Central Committee for Medical and Community Programs of the American Heart Association, "Dietary Fat and Its Relation to Heart Attacks and Stroke," *Circulation* 23 (1961): 134–35; "Heart Unit Backs Reduction in Fat," *New York Times,* Dec. 11, 1960, I, 57:1.

6. Donald Janson, "A.M.A. Suggests Cholesterol Cut: Report Calls for Reduction in the Saturated Fats for Artery Patients' Diets," *New York Times,* Aug. 3, 1962, 25:8; Austin C. Wehrwein, "Antifat 'Food Fad' Assailed by A.M.A.," *New York Times,* Oct. 12, 1962, 1: 7; "AMA Blows Whistle on Fat-Free Diets," *Business Week,* Oct. 20, 1962, 46.

7. Harrison Wellford, *Sowing the Wind* (New York: Bantam, 1973), 24.

8. Senator Warren G. Magnuson, "Consumerism and the Emerging Goals of a New Society," in *Consumerism: Viewpoints from Business, Government, and the Public Interest,* ed. Ralph M. Gaedeke and Warren W. Etcheson (San Francisco: Canfield, 1972), 4.

9. Detlof von Winterfeldt, "Expert Knowledge and Public Values in Risk Management: The Role of Decision Analysis," in *Social Theories of Risk,* ed. Sheldon Krimsky and Dominic Golding (Westport, CT: Praeger, 1992), 322–23; Jacqueline Verrett and Jean Carper, *Eating May be Hazardous to your Health* (Garden City, NY: Anchor, 1975), 10–12, 174–82; Frank Graham, Jr., *Since Silent Spring* (Boston: Houghton Mifflin, 1970), 104, 222.

10. Seymour M. Lipset and William Schneider, *The Confidence Gap: Business, Labor, and Government in the Public Mind* (New York: Free Press, 1983), 17, 48–49.

11. John D. Graham and Jonathan B. Wiener, "Confronting Risk Tradeoffs," in *Risk Versus Risk: Tradeoffs in Protecting Health and the Environment,* ed. John D. Graham and Jonathan B. Wiener (Cambridge, MA: Harvard University Press, 1995), 6–7.

12. William W. Moore, *Fighting for Life: The Story of the American Heart Association 1911–1975* (n.p.: American Heart Association, 1983), 219–220; Jane E. Brody, "Heart Experts Disagree on Desirability of a Diet That is Low in Saturated Fats," *New York Times,* Nov. 13, 1970, 14:1; Jane E. Brody, "Heart Association Strengthens Its Advice: Cut Down on Fats," *New York Times,* June 28, 1973, 54:1.

13. "Fat and Oil Ads Disputed by U.S." *New York Times,* Dec. 11, 1959, 26:2; James J. Nagle, "Vegetable Oils are Enjoying a Boom," *New York Times,* Mar. 4, 1962 III:1:1; "F.D.A. Acts to Drop Ban on Disclosures of Content of Fats," *New York Times,* June 14, 1971, 22:1.

14. Martha C. Howard, "The Margarine Industry in the United States: Its Development Under Legislative Control" (Ph.D. diss., Columbia University, 1951), 7–8, 20. See also J. H. van Stuyvenberg, ed., *Margarine: An Economic, Social and Scientific History 1869–1969* (Toronto: University of Toronto Press, 1969).

15. Howard, "The Margarine Industry in the United States," 49–50, 317; van Stuyvenberg, *Margarine: An Economic, Social and Scientific History 1869–1969,* passim.

16. Howard, "The Margarine Industry in the United States," 22–23, 199–200; van Stuyvenberg, *Margarine: An Economic, Social and Scientific History 1869–1969,* 227–327; Vincent Vinikas, *Soft Soap, Hard Sell: American Hygiene in an Age of Advertisement* (Ames: Iowa State University Press, 1992), 93–94; Susan Strasser, *Satisfaction Guaranteed: The Making of the American Mass Market* (New York: Pantheon, 1989), 7–14.

17. Howard, "The Margarine Industry in the United States," 284, 286, 318–19, 327a, 337.

18. "Heart Motif Puts Margarine One Up," *Business Week,* Jan. 28, 1961, 98.

19. Letitia Brewster and Michael F. Jacobson, *The Changing American Diet* (Washington, DC: Center for Science in the Public Interest, 1983), 22–23, 78; Frances Cerra, "Complaints on Ads Get Slow Response," *New York Times,* Sept. 3, 1975, 46:7; "Two Products Must Halt Claims of Endorsement," *New York Times,* Jan. 8, 1981, C15:3.

20. National Research Council, National Academy of Sciences, *The Role of Dietary Fat in Human Health* (Washington, DC: 1958), 17; National Research Council Food and Nutrition Board, *Dietary Fat and Human Health* (Washington, DC: National Academy of Sciences, 1966), 43.

21. Jane E. Brody, "Federal Heart Panel Asks Public to Eat Fewer Fats," *New York Times,* Dec. 16, 1970, 1:6; "Typical Fat-Rich American Diet has Long Been Suspect in Heart Disease Studies" *New York Times,* Dec. 16, 1970, 37:1.

22. National Heart and Lung Institute Task Force on Arteriosclerosis, *Arteriosclerosis* (Washington, DC: U.S. GPO, 1971), I:14.

23. American Medical Association Council on Foods and Nutrition, "Diet and Coronary Heart Disease," *JAMA* 222 (1972): 1647; "Diet and Coronary Heart Disease," *Preventive Medicine* 1 (1972): 559–61.

24. A. Stewart Truswell, "Dietary Goals and Guidelines: National and International Perspectives," in *Modern Nutrition in Health and Disease,* 8th ed., ed. Maurice E. Shils, James A. Olson, and Moshe Shike (Philadelphia: Lea and Febiger, 1994), II:1615; A. Stewart Truswell, "Evolution of Dietary Recommendations, Goals, and Guidelines," *American Journal of Clinical Nutrition* 45 (1987): 1064–65.

25. U.S. Senate Select Committee on Nutrition and Human Needs, *Dietary Goals for the United States: Supplemental Views,* 95th Congress, 1st sess. (Washington, DC: U.S. GPO, 1977), 680–84, 688, 692, 700–6.

26. Ibid., 676–77; "Dietary Goals for the United States," *Rhode Island Medical Journal* 60 (1977): 576–81; American Medical Association Council on Scientific Affairs, "American Medical Association Concepts of Nutrition and Health," *JAMA* 242 (1979): 2335–38.

27. U.S. Senate Select Committee, *Dietary Goals for the United States:Supplemental Views,* 17, 34, 48, 175–76.

28. U.S. Senate Select Committee on Nutrition and Human Needs, *Dietary Goals for the United States,* 2d ed. (Washington, DC: U.S. GPO, 1977), xv, 4; Kristen McNutt, "Dietary Advice to the Public: 1957 to 1980," *Nutrition Reviews* 38 (1980): 354.

29. Jane E. Brody, "Panel Reports Healthy Americans Need Not Cut Intake of Cholesterol," *New York Times,* May 28, 1980, A1:1; Food and Nutrition Board, Nation Research Council, *Toward Healthful Diets* (Washington, DC: National Academy Press, 1980), 9–10, 17, 6, 19–20.

30. Brody, "Panel Reports Healthy Americans Need Not Cut Intake of Cholesterol," A1:1; Lawrence K. Altman, "Report about Cholesterol Draws Agreement and Dissent," *New York Times,* May 28, 1980, A16:1; Jane E. Brody, "Experts Assail Report Declaring Curb on Cholesterol Isn't Needed," *New York Times,* June 1, 1980, 1; Jane E. Brody, "When Scientists Disagree, Cholesterol is in Fat City," *New York Times,* June 1, 1980, IV, 7:3; "A Confusing Diet of Fact," *New York Times,* June 3, 1980, 18:1; Karen De Witt, "Scientists Clash on Academy's Cholesterol Advice," *New York Times,* June 20, 1980, 15:2; Suzanne Garment, "Science Academy's Cholesterol Report Spatters in Capital," *Wall Street Journal,* June 27, 1980, 24:3.

31. Jane E. Brody, "Experts Assail Report Declaring Curb on Cholesterol Isn't Needed," *New York Times,* June 1, 1980, 1:1; Nicholas Wade, "Food Board's Fat Report Hits Fire," *Science* 209 (1980): 248–50; Phillip M. Boffey, *The Brain Bank of America: An Inquiry into the Politics of Science* (New York: McGraw-Hill, 1975), 166–69.

32. Marian Burros, "U.S. Diet Guideline Will Be Assayed," *New York Times,* Oct. 14, 1981, III, C10; Michele M. Bradley, "The States' Role in Regulating Food Labeling and Advertising: The Effect of the Nutrition Labeling and Education Act of 1990," *Food and Drug Law Journal* 49 (1994): 651–52.

33. "Lowering Blood Cholesterol to Prevent Heart disease: NIH Consensus Development Conference Statement," *Arteriosclerosis* 5 (1985): 404–12; Consensus Conference, "Lowering Blood Cholesterol to Prevent Heart Disease," *JAMA* 253 (1985): 2080–86; Albert R. Karr, "Cholesterol Risks Cited by National Institutes of Health," *Wall Street Journal,* Dec. 13, 1984, 24; Jane E. Brody, "Panel Says Cholesterol Level in Many is Dangerously High," *New York Times,* Dec. 13, 1984, 1:3.

34. Gina Kolata, "Heart Panel's Conclusions Questioned," *Science* 227 (1985): 40–41; E.H. Ahrens, Jr., "The Diet-Heart Question in 1985: Has It Really Been Settled?" *Lancet* (May 11, 1985): 1085–87; Beverly Merz, "Low-Fat Diet May be Imprudent for Some, Say Opponents of Population-Based Cholesterol Control," *JAMA* 256 (1986): 2779–80.

35. Claude Lenfant, "A New Challenge for America: The National Cholesterol Education Program," *Circulation* 73 (1986): 855–56; Philip M. Boffey, "Cholesterol: Debate Flares Over Wisdom in Widespread Reductions," *New York Times,* July 14, 1987, C1:6. See Thomas J. Moore, "The Cholesterol Myth," *Atlantic Monthly* 264 (Sept. 1989): 37ff.

36. U.S. Surgeon General, *The Surgeon General's Report on Nutrition and Health, 1988* (Washington, DC: US GPO, 1988), 102–4, 120, 86, 94; "Report of the National Cholesterol Education Program Expert Panel on Detection, Evaluation, and Treatment of High Blood Cholesterol in Adults," *Archives of Internal Medicine* 148 (1988): 36–37.

37. National Research Council Committee on Diet and Health, *Diet and Health: Implications for Reducing Chronic Disease Risk* (Washington, DC: National Academy Press, 1989), 31, 13–14.

38. Ibid, 31.

39. "Heart Groups Reaffirm The Health Benefits of Lower Cholesterol," *New York Times,* Nov. 16, 1989, B19:1.

40. "Report of the Expert Panel on Detection, Evaluation and Treatment of High Blood Cholesterol in Adults."

41. U.S. House of Representatives Committee on Energy and Commerce, Subcommittee on Health and the Environment, *Hearing on Cholesterol Education Program,* 101st Congress, 1st sess. Dec. 7, 1989, Serial No. 101–107 (Washington, DC: US GPO, 1990), 127, 17, 118.

42. Warren J. McIsaac, David Naylor, and Antoni Basinski, "Mismatch of Coronary Risk and Treatment Intensity under the National Cholesterol Education Program Guidelines," *Journal of General Internal Medicine* 6 (1991): 518–23; Ron Winslow, "Critics Assail New Cholesterol-Test Guidelines," *Wall Street Journal,* Mar. 1, 1996, B1.

43. American Heart Association Nutrition Committee, "Rationale of the Diet-Heart Statement of the American Heart Association," *Circulation* 88 (1993): 3010, 3012, 3108, 3021, 3023,

44. American Heart Association Nutrition Committee, "Dietary Guidelines for Health American Adults," *Circulation* 94 (1996): 1796, 1798.

45. Jane Kirby, "Nutrition Education: A Food Editor's Perspective," *Nutrition Today* 29 (May–June, 1994): 7; Bruce R. Stillings, "Trends in Foods," *Nutrition Today* 29 (Sept.–Oct., 1994): 11.

46. Patricia Hausman, *Jack Spratt's Legacy: The Science and Politics of Fat and Cholesterol* (New York: Marek, 1981), 204; Peter Bart: Advertising: Dairy Men Open Counterattack," *New York Times*, Aug. 7, 1962, 36:3; Jonathan Probber, "Is Nothing Sacred? Milk's American Appeal Fades," *New York Times*, Feb. 18, 1987, C1:2; Zachary Schiller, et al., "The Great American Health Pitch," *Business Week*, Oct. 9, 1989, 119; U.S. Bureau of the Census, *Statistical Abstract of the United States 1994* (Washington, DC: 1994), 147; U.S. Bureau of the Census, *Statistical Abstract of the United States 1997* (Washington, DC: 1997), 149.

47. U.S. Bureau of the Census, *Statistical Abstract of the United States 1994,* 147; U.S. Bureau of the Census, *Statistical Abstract of the United States 1997,* 149; "Ads Push Merits of Red Meat," *New York Times*, Jan. 21, 1987, C14:4; Keith Schneider, "Panel Suggests a Leaner Look for U.S. Meat," *New York Times*, April 6, 1988, A1:5.

48. Anthony Ramirez, "Getting Burned by the Frying Pan," *New York Times*, Mar. 20, 1990, IV, D1:3; Marian Burros, "Fast-Food Chains Try to Slim Down," *New York Times*, April, 11, 1990, C1; Anthony Ramirez, "Low-Fat McDonald's Burger Is Planned to Answer Critics," *New York Times*, Mar. 13, 1991, A1; Anthony Ramirez, "Fast Food Lightens Up But Sales are Often Thin," *New York Times*, Mar. 19, 1991, D1; Glenn Collins, "Low-Fat Food: Feeding Frenzy for Marketers," *New York Times*, Sept. 27, 1995, D1.

49. James J. Nagle, "Vegetable Oils are Enjoying a Boom," *New York Times*, Mar. 4, 1962 III, 1:1; Alix M. Freedman and Michael Waldholz, "A Different Oil War Breaks Out, and Now the Fat is in the Fire," *Wall Street Journal*, Nov. 17, 1987 1:4; Shoba Purushothaman, "Soy Industry's Negative Ads Damp Tropical-Oil Imports," *Wall Street Journal*, Jan. 17, 1989, B1; Douglas C. McGill, "Tropical-Oil Exporters Seek Reprieve in U.S.," *New York Times*, Feb. 3, 1989, D1:4; Dena Kleiman, "For Amber Waves of . . . Canola?" *New York Times*, Sept. 5, 1990, C1.

50. Marion Nestle, *Food Politics: How the Food Industry Influences Nutrition and Health* (Berkeley: University of California Press. 2002), 123–25; Marian Burros, "Heart Group Begins Food Labeling Amid Outcry," *New York Times*, Feb. 1, 1990, A1:2; Natalie Angier, "Heart Association Cancels Its Program to Rate Foods," *New York Times*, April 3, 1990, A1:1; Marian Burros, "Is a 'Good Food' Logo a Good Idea?" *New York Times*, Aug. 11, 1993, C4:1; Marian Burros, "Endorsements Raise Money and Questions," *New York Times*, Oct. 22, 1997, F3:3; Milt Freudenheim, "Marriage of Necessity: Nonprofit Groups and Drug Makers," *New York Times*, Aug. 20, 1996, D2.

51. Philip J. Hilts, "In Reversal, White House Backs Curbs on Health Claims for Food," *New York Times*, Feb. 9, 1990, I, A1:1; Kurt Eichenwald, "Biotechnology Food: From the Lab to a Debacle," *New York Times*, Jan. 25, 2001, A1:2ff.

52. Hilts, "In Reversal, White House Backs Curbs on Health Claims for Food"; Schiller, "The Great American Health Pitch," 116; Alix M. Freedman, "FTC Alleges Campbell Ad is Deceptive," *Wall Street Journal*, Jan. 27, 1989, B1; N. R. Kleinfield, "Catching the Anti-Cholesterol Fever," *New York Times*, April 16, 1989, III, 1:2.

53. John E. Calfee, "FDA Underestimates Food Shoppers" *Wall Street Journal*, May 29, 1991, A10; Anthony Ramirez, "3 Companies Cited on Cholesterol Claims," *New York Times*, May 15, 1991, D1.

54. Kleinfield, "Catching the Anti-Cholesterol Fever," 1:2.

55. Schiller, "The Great American Health Pitch," 118; Richard Gibson, "Kellogg Tries to Blunt the Attacks on Cereal Makers' Health Claims," *Wall Street Journal,* Aug. 31, 1989, B4; "Kellogg May Use Disputed Ingredient," *New York Times,* Aug. 30, 1989, C4:1; "F.D.A. Questions Use of Grain in 3 Cereals," *New York Times,* Oct. 1, 1989, A28:2.

56. Bradley, "The States' Role in Regulating Food Labeling and Advertising: The Effect of the Nutrition Labeling and Education Act of 1990," 652–53; Jeff Bailey, "Quaker Oats Co. is Sued by Texas Over Health Claims in Cereal Ads," *Wall Street Journal,* Sept. 8, 1989, B4; Richard Gibson, "Kellogg Tries to Blunt the Attacks on Cereal Makers' Health Claims," *Wall Street Journal,* Aug. 31, 1989, B4; "Texas Embargoes A Cereal," *New York Times,* Sept. 5, 1990, C11:1; "5 More States Accuse Kellogg of Deceptive Claims," *New York Times,* Dec. 30, 1990, A19:1.

57. Carey, et al., "Snap, Crackle, Stop: States Crack down on Misleading Food Claims," 443.

58. Hilts, "In Reversal, White House Backs Curbs on Health Claims for Food," I:1.

59. Haughton, Gussow, and Dodds, "An Historical Study of the Underlying Assumptions for United States Food Guides from 1917 through the Basic Four Food Group Guide," 169–75. See also Marion Nestle, *Food Politics: How the Food Industry Influences Nutrition and Health* (Berkeley: University of California Press, 2002), 34–50.

60. Truswell, "Dietary Goals and Guidelines," II:1612–13; Karil Bialostosky and Sachiko T. St. Jeor, "The 1995 Dietary Guidelines for Americans," *Nutrition Today* 31 (Jan.–Feb. 1996): 6–7.

61. Truswell, "Dietary Goals and Guidelines," II:1621–22.

62. Anthony Ramirez, "F.D.A. to Examine Food Label Claims Over Cholesterol," *New York Times,* May 12, 1991, I, 1:3; Virginia L. Wilkening, "FDA's Regulations to Implement the NLEA," *Nutrition Today* 31 (Sept.–Oct., 1993): 13–20; Donna V. Porter, "Health Claims on Food Products: NLEA," *Nutrition Today* 31 (Jan.–Feb. 1996): 35–38.

63. Wilkening, "FDA's Regulations to Implement the NLEA," 19.

64. Michael Fumento, *The Fat of the Land: The Obesity Epidemic and How Overweight Americans Can Help Themselves* (New York: Viking, 1997), 58–59, 77.

65. Jane Kirby, "Nutrition Education: A Food Editor's Perspective," 7.

66. Nestle, *Food Politics: How the Food Industry Influences Nutrition and Health,* 111, 127, 111–36; Marian Burros, "Additives in Advice on Food?" *New York Times,* Nov. 15, 1995, C1.

67. Institute of Medicine, *Improving America's Diet and Health* (Washington, DC: National Academy Press, 1991), 48–49: Kenneth E. Warner, "Tobacco Industry Scientific Advisors: Serving Society or Selling Cigarettes?" *American Journal of Public Health* 81 (1991): 841.

68. Michael S. Goldstein, *The Health Movement: Promoting Fitness in America* (New York: Twayne, 1992), 76–77; Stearns, *Fat History: Bodies and Beauty in the Modern West,* 52–53.

69. Jesse A. Berlin and Graham A. Colditz, "A Meta-Analysis of Physical Activity in the Prevention of Coronary Heart Disease," *American Journal of Epidemiology* 132 (1990): 612–28; Henry A. Solomon, *The Exercise Myth* (San Diego: Harcourt Brace Jovanovich, 1984), 52–53.

70. National Center for Health Statistics, *Health United States 1996–97* (Hyattsville, MD: 1997), 192–93.

71. "Overweight Shortens Life," *Statistical Bulletin,* 32 (Oct., 1951), 1–4; Caren G.

Solomon and JoAnne E. Manson, "Obesity and Mortality: A Review of the Epidemiologic Data," *American Journal of Clinical Nutrition* 66 suppl. (1997): 1044S–50S.

72. "Mortality Among Overweight Men," *Statistical Bulletin* 41 (Feb. 1960): 6–10; "Mortality Among Overweight Women," *Statistical Bulletin* 41 (Mar. 1960): 1–4.

73. "Mortality of Overweights with Impairments," *Statistical Bulletin* 41 (May 1960): 3—6.

74. "Handicaps of Overweight" *Statistical Bulletin* 33 (Aug. 1952): 3–5.

75. "Overweights Benefit from Weight Reduction," *Statistical Bulletin,* 41 (Apr. 1960): 1–3.

76. Expert Panel on Detection, Evaluation, and Treatment of High Blood Cholesterol in Adults, "Executive Summary of the Third Report of the National Cholesterol Education Program (NCEP) Expert Panel on Detection, Evaluation, and Treatment of High Blood Cholesterol in Adults (Adult Treatment Panel III)," *JAMA* 285 (2001): 2486–88.

77. Nestle, *Food Politics: How the Food Industry Influences Nutrition and Health,* 21–22, 315–17.

Notes to Chapter 19

1. Harry M. Rosenberg and A. Joan Klebba, "Trends in Cardiovascular Mortality with a Focus on Ischemic Heart Disease: United States, 1950–1976," in *Proceedings of the Conference on the Decline in Coronary Heart Disease Mortality,* ed. Richard J. Havlik and Manning Feinleib (Bethesda, MD: National Institutes of Health, 1978), 15.

2. William B. Kannel and Thomas J. Thom, "Declining Cardiovascular Mortality," *Circulation* 70 (1984): 335.

3. Robert R. Kohn, "Cause of Death in Very Old People," *JAMA* 247 (1982): 2793, 2797.

4. Rosenberg and Klebba, "Trends in Cardiovascular Mortality," 17–22.

5. Kathleen E. Ragland, Steve Selvin, and Deane W. Merrill, "The Onset of Decline in Ischemic Heart Disease Mortality in the United States," *American Journal of Epidemiology* 127 (1988): 516–31.

6. Eugene Rogot and Zdenek Hrubec, "Trends in Mortality from Coronary Heart Disease and Stroke among U.S. Veterans, 1954–79," *Journal of Clinical Epidemiology* 42 (1989): 245–56.

7. Sidney Pell and William Fayerweather, "Trends in the Incidence of Myocardial Infarction and in Associated Mortality and Morbidity in a Large Employed Population, 1957–1983," *New England Journal of Medicine* 312 (1985): 1005–11: Lila R. Elveback, Daniel C. Connolly, and L. Joseph Melton, "Coronary Heart Disease in Residents of Rochester, Minnesota. VII: Incidence, 1950 through 1982," *Mayo Clinic Proceedings* 61 (1986): 896–900.

8. Lewis H. Kuller, et al., "Sudden Death and the Decline in Coronary Heart Disease Mortality," *Journal of Chronic Diseases* 39 (1986): 1001–9.

9. Robert J. Goldberg, et al., "A Communitywide Perspective of Sex Differences and Temporal Trends in the Incidence and Survival Rates After Acute Myocardial Infarction and Out-of-Hospital Deaths Caused by Coronary Heart Disease," *Circulation* 87 (1993): 1947–53; Gary D. Friedman, "Decline in Hospitalizations for Coronary Heart Disease and

Stroke: the Kaiser-Permanente Experience in Northern California, 1971–1977," in *Proceedings of the Conference on the Decline in Coronary heart disease Mortality*, ed. Havlik and Feinleib, 109–14; Eve Weinblatt, et al., "Mortality after First Myocardial infarction," *JAMA* 247 (1982): 1576–81.

10. Kazuo Uemura and Zbynek Pisa, "Trends in Cardiovascular Disease Mortality in Industrialized Countries Since 1950," *World Health Statistics Quarterly* 41 (1988): 155–78; Thomas J. Thom, "International Mortality from Heart Disease: Rates and Trends," *International Journal of Epidemiology* 18, suppl. 1 (1989): S20–S28; M. G. Marmot and J. F. Mustard, "Coronary Heart Disease from a Population Perspective," in *Why Are Some People Healthy and Others Not?* ed. Robert G. Evans, Morris L. Barer, and Theodore R. Marmor (New York: Aldine de Gruyer, 1994), 196–97.

11. Lawrence E. Meltzer and J. Roderick Kitchell, "The Development and Current Status of Coronary Care," in *Textbook of Coronary Care*, ed. Lawrence E. Meltzer and Arend J. Dunning (Philadelphia: Charles Press, 1972), 7–10, 18–20; American College of Cardiology, *The Current State of Intensive Coronary Care* (New York: Charles Press, 1966); Robert J. Goldberg, "Temporal Trends and Declining Mortality Rates from Coronary Heart Disease in the United States," in *Prevention of Coronary Heart Disease*, ed. Ira S. Ockene and Judith K. Ockene (Boston: Little, Brown, 1992), 58–59.

12. National Center for Health Statistics, *Health United States 1996–97* (Washington, DC: U.S. GPO, 1997), 140, 111.

13. Ibid., 190–92.

14. J. Stamler, "Established Major Coronary Risk Factors," in *Coronary Heart Disease Epidemiology: From Aetiology to Public Health*, ed. Michael Marmot and Paul Elliott (Oxford: Oxford University Press, 1992), 35.

15. National Center for Health Statistics, *Health United States 1996–97* (Washington, DC: U.S. GPO, 1997), 191.

16. Sidney Pell and C. Anthony D'Alonzo, "Acute Myocardial Infarction in a Large Industrial Population," *JAMA* 185 (1963): 831–38.

17. M. G. Marmot, et al., "Employment Grade and Coronary Heart Disease in British Civil Servants," *Journal of Epidemiology and Community Health* 32 (1978): 244–49.

18. Carl C. Seltzer and Seymour Jablon, "Army Rank and Subsequent Mortality by Cause: 23-Year Follow-up," *American Journal of Epidemiology* 108 (1977): 559–66.

19. George A. Kaplan and Julian E. Keil, "Socioeconomic Factors and Cardiovascular Disease: A Review of the Literature," *Circulation* 88, no. 4 pt. 1 (Oct., 1993): 1973, 1990.

20. David R. Williams and Chiquita Collins, "U.S. Socioeconomic and Racial Differences in Health: Patterns and Explanations," *Annual Review of Sociology* 21 (1995): 349–86; Nancy E. Adler, et al., "Socioeconomic Status and Health: The Challenge of the Gradient," *American Psychologist* 49 (1994): 15–24; Barry M. Popkin, Anna M. Siega-Riz, and Pamela S. Haines, "A Comparison of Dietary Trends among Racial and Socioeconomic Groups in the United States," *New England Journal of Medicine* 335 (1996): 716–20.

21. Thomas R. Dawber, et al., "Some Factors Associated with the Development of Coronary Heart Disease," *American Journal of Public Health* 49 (1959): 1351–52; Jing Fang, Shantha Madhavan, and Michael H. Alderman, "The Association Between Birthplace and Mortality from Cardiovascular Causes among Black and White Residents of New York City," *New England Journal of Medicine* 335 (1996): 1545–51.

Notes to Chapter 20

1. John-Arne Skolbekken, "The Risk Epidemic in Medical Journals," *Social Science and Medicine* 40 (1995): 298.

2. J. Rosser Matthews, *Quantification and the Quest for Medical Certainty* (Princeton: Princeton University Press, 1995), 138–39; Harry M. Marks, *The Progress of Experiment: Science and Therapeutic Reform in the United States, 1900–1990* (Cambridge: Cambridge University Press, 1997), 129.

3. David H. Spodick, "Revascularization of the Heart—Numerators in Search of Denominators," *American Heart Journal* 81 (1971): 150; Stephen J. Haines, "Randomized Clinical Trials in the Evaluation of Surgical Innovation," *Journal of Neurosurgery* 51 (1979): 5–11; Lawrence I. Bonchek, "Are Randomized Trials Appropriate for Evaluating New Operations?" *New England Journal of Medicine* 301 (1979): 44–45.

4. Alvan R. Feinstein, "Scientific Standards in Epidemiologic Studies of the Menace of Daily Life," *Science* 242 (1988): 1257; Robert A. Aronowitz, *Making Sense of Illness: Science, Society, and Disease* (Cambridge: Cambridge University Press, 1998), 111–12, 117.

5. Aronowitz, *Making Sense of Illness,* 112. See John D. Graham, Laura C. Green, and Marc J. Roberts, *In Search of Safety: Chemicals and Cancer Risk* (Cambridge, MA: Harvard University Press, 1988); National Research Council, *Science and Judgment in Risk Assessment* (Washington, DC: National Academy Press, 1994); Charles Walker, Leroy C. Gould, and Edward J. Woodhouse, eds., *Too Hot to Handle? Social and Policy Issues in the Management of Radioactive Wastes* (New Haven, CT: Yale University Press, 1983).

6. Vincent T. Covello and Miley W. Merkhofer, *Risk Assessment Methods: Approaches for Assessing Health and Environmental Risks* (New York: Plenum, 1993), 1–3; Skolbekken, "The Risk Epidemic in Medical Journals," 292–93.

7. Michael S. Goldstein, *Alternative Health Care: Medicine, Miracle, or Mirage?* (Philadelphia, PA: Temple University Press, 1999), 28–29; Charles C. Mann, "Press Coverage: Leaving Out the Big Picture," *Science* 269 (1995): 166.

8. *Preventive Medicine USA* (New York: Prodist, 1976), 7–20.

9. *Report of the President's Committee on Health Education* (New York, 1973), 2.

10. Michael S. Goldstein, *The Health Movement: Promoting Fitness in America* (New York: Twayne, 1992), xi–xii, 13, 18.

11. *Report of the President's Committee on Health Education,* p, 11; Howard M. Leichter, *Free to Be Foolish: Politics and Health Promotion in the United States and Great Britain* (Princeton: Princeton University Press, 1991), 92–93; T. Abelin, Z.J. Brzezinski, Vera D.L. Carstairs, eds., *Measurement in Health Promotion and Protection,* WHO Regional Publications, European Series No. 22 (Copenhagen: World Health Organization Regional Office for Europe, 1987), 653.

12. *Healthy People: The Surgeon General's Report on Health Promotion and Disease Prevention, 1979* (Washington, DC: U.S. Department of Health, Education, and Welfare, 1979), 6, 7, 13.

13. *Report of the President's Committee on Health Education,* 17.

14. Aronowitz, *Making Sense of Illness,* 142–43; William R. Harlan and Jeoffrey K. Stross, "An Educational View of a National Initiative to Lower Plasma Lipid Levels" *JAMA* 253 (1985): 2087–90.

15. Lester B. Lave, "Health and Safety Risk Analyses: Information for Better Decisions," *Science* 236 (1987): 291–95.

16. *Preventive Medicine USA,* 85–86.

17. Cary Gross, et al., "The Relation between Funding by the National Institutes of Health and the Burden of Disease," *New England Journal of Medicine* 340 (1999): 1881–87.

18. Thomas R. Dawber, *The Framingham Study: The Epidemiology of Atherosclerotic Disease* (Cambridge, MA: Harvard University Press, 1980), 8. See also Martin J. Gardner and Douglas G. Altman, "Confidence Intervals Rather than P Values: Estimation Rather than Hypothesis Testing," *British Medical Journal* 292 (1986): 746–50: Kenneth J. Rothman, "A Show of Confidence," *New England Journal of Medicine* 299 (1978): 1362–63.

19. Paul C. Stern and Harvey V. Fineberg, eds., *Understanding Risk: Informing Decisions in a Democratic Society* (Washington, DC: National Academy Press, 1996), 26.

20. Marion Nestle, *Food Politics: How the Food Industry Influences Nutrition and Health* (Berkeley: University of California Press, 2002), 219–93.

—

BIBLIOGRAPHY

Abel, Emily K., "Taking the Cure to the Poor: Patients' Responses to New York City's Tuberculosis Program, 1894 to 1918," *American Journal of Public Health* 87 (1997): 1808–15.

Abelin, T., Z. J. Brzezinski, Vera D. L. Carstairs, eds., *Measurement in Health Promotion and Protection,* WHO Regional Publications, European Series No. 22 (Copenhagen: World Health Organization Regional Office for Europe, 1987).

Abrams, Philip, *The Origins of British Sociology: 1834–1914* (Chicago: University of Chicago Press, 1968).

Abstracts of the Proceedings of the Meetings of the Association of Life Insurance Medical Directors of America, also *Proceedings of the Association of Life Insurance Medical Directors of America* (New York: n.p.).

Acierno, Louis J., *The History of Cardiology* (London: Parthenon, 1994).

Ackerman, Lauren V., and Juan A. del Regato, *Cancer: Diagnosis, Treatment, and Prognosis* (St. Louis: Mosby, 1947).

Ackerman, S. B., *Industrial Life Insurance: Its History, Statistics and Plans,* 2nd ed. (Chicago: Spectator Co., 1926).

Addresses Delivered at the Triennial Conventions and Mangers' Annual Banquets of the Metropolitan Life Insurance Company. 3 Vols. (New York: 1923, 1924, 1928).

Adler, Nancy E., et al., "Socioeconomic Status and Health: The Challenge of the Gradient," *American Psychologist* 49 (1994): 15–24.

Ahrens, E. H. Jr., "The Diet-Heart Question in 1985: Has It Really Been Settled?" *Lancet* (11 May 1985): 1085–87.

Ahrens, Edward H. Jr., "Nutritional Factors and Serum Lipid Levels," *American Journal of Medicine* 23 (1957): 928–52.

Albert, Michael R., Kristen G. Ostheimer, and Joel G. Breman, "The Last Smallpox Epidemic in Boston and the Vaccination Controversy, 1901–1903," *New England Journal of Medicine* 344 (2001): 375–79.

Alderman, Michael H., and Bernard Lamport, "Moderate Sodium Restriction: Do the Benefits Justify the Hazards?" *American Journal of Hypertension* 3 (1990): 499–504.

Alter, George C., and Ann G. Carmichael, "Classifying the Dead: Toward a History of the Registration of Causes of Death," *Journal of the History of Medicine and Allied Sciences* 54 (1999): 114–32.

American College of Cardiology, *The Current State of Intensive Coronary Care* (New York: Charles Press, 1966).

American Heart Association, *Epidemiology of Atherosclerosis and Hypertension* (New York: 1956).

———, *1997 Heart and Stroke Statistical Update* (Dallas, TX: American Heart Association, 1996).

American Heart Association Nutrition Committee, "Dietary Guidelines for Healthy American Adults," *Circulation* 94 (1996): 1795–800.

———, "Rationale of the Diet-Heart Statement of the American Heart Association," *Circulation* 88 (1993): 3008–29.

American Medical Association Council on Foods and Nutrition, "Diet and Coronary Heart Disease: A Council Statement," *JAMA* 222 (1972): 1647.

American Medical Association Council on Scientific Affairs, "American Medical Association Concepts of Nutrition and Health," *JAMA* 242 (1979): 2335–38.

American Public Health Association Committee on Child Health, *Services for Children with Heart Disease and Rheumatic Fever* (New York: 1960).

Anda, Robert F. et al., "Are Physicians Advising Smokers to Quit? The Patient's Perspective," *JAMA* 257 (1987): 1916–19.

Andersen, Tavs F., and Gavin Mooney, eds., *The Challenges of Medical Practice Variations* (London: Macmillan, 1990).

Anderson, Keaven M., William P. Castelli, and Daniel Levy, "Cholesterol and Mortality: 30 Years of Follow-up from the Framingham Study," *JAMA* 257 (1987): 2176–80.

Anderson, T. W., "The Changing Pattern of Ischemic Heart Disease," *Canadian Medical Association Journal* 108 (1973): 1500–04.

Anderson, T. W., and W. H. LeRiche, "Ischaemic Heart Disease and Sudden Death, 1901–61," *British Journal of Preventive and Social Medicine* 24 (1970): 1–9.

Anderson, Terence W., "Mortality from Ischemic Heart Disease: Changes in Middle-Aged Men Since 1900," *JAMA* 224 (1973): 336–38.

Anderson, Terence W., and Mabel L. Halliday, "The Male Epidemic: 50 Years of Ischaemic Heart Disease," *Public Health, London* 93 (1979): 163–72.

Annual Report of the Board of Health of the City of New York.

Antonovsky, Aaron, "Social Class and the Major Cardiovascular Diseases," *Journal of Chronic Diseases* 21 (1968): 65–106.

Armstrong, Donald B., Louis I. Dublin, and Elizabeth J. Steele, *The Cost of Medical Care: A Study of Costs in the Families of the Field Employees of the Metropolitan Life Insurance Company* (New York: Metropolitan Life Insurance Company, 1934).

Armstrong, Donald B., and Alma C. Haupt, "A Forty-Year Demonstration of Public Health Nursing by the Metropolitan Life Insurance Company," *Public Health Nursing* 43 (1951): 41–42.

Arno, Peter S. et al., "Tobacco Industry Strategies to Oppose Federal Regulation," *JAMA* 275 (1996): 1258–62.

Arnott, W. Melville, "The Changing Aetiology of Heart Disease," *British Medical Journal* 2 (1954): 887–91.

Aronowitz, Robert A., *Making Sense of Illness: Science, Society, and Disease* (Cambridge: Cambridge University Press, 1998).

Association of Life Insurance Presidents, *Birth and Death Bookkeeping: Need for Better Vital Statistics* (New York: 1912).

"The Australian Therapeutic Trial in Mild Hypertension: Report by the Management Committee," *Lancet* 1 (1980): 1261–67.

Baker, Josephine, *Child Hygiene* (New York: Harper, 1925).

Baker, S. Josephine, *Fighting for Life* (1939: New York: Arno Press, 1974).

Bates, Barbara, *Bargaining for Life: A Social History of Tuberculosis, 1876–1938* (Philadelphia: University of Pennsylvania Press, 1992).

Barnes, Broda O., and Charlotte W. Barnes, *Heart Attack Rareness in Thyroid-Treated Patients* (Springfield, IL: Thomas, 1972).

Beito, David T., *From Mutual Aid to the Welfare State: Fraternal Societies and Social Services, 1890–1967* (Chapel Hill: University of North Carolina Press, 2000).

Berenson, Abram S., ed. *Control of Communicable Diseases in Man,* 15th ed. (Washington, DC: American Public Health Association, 1990).

Berlin, Jesse A., and Graham A. Colditz, "A Meta-Analysis of Physical Activity in the Prevention of Coronary Heart Disease," *American Journal of Epidemiology* 132 (1990): 612–28.

Bernard, Claude, *An Introduction to the Study of Experimental Medicine* (1865; New York: Schuman, 1949).

Beyer, Karl H., "Chlorothiazide: How the Thiazides Evolved as Antihypertensive Therapy," *Hypertension* 22 (1993): 388–91.

Bialostosky, Karil, and Sachiko T. St. Jeor, "The 1995 Dietary Guidelines for Americans," *Nutrition Today* 31 (Jan.–Feb. 1996): 6–11.

Bideau, Alain, Bertrand Desjardins, and Hector P. Brignoli, eds., *Infant and Child Mortality in the Past,* (Oxford: Clarendon Press, 1997).

Bisno, Alan L., "The Rise and Fall of Rheumatic Fever," *JAMA* 254 (1985): 538–41.

Boas, Ernst P., *The Unseen Plague: Chronic Disease* (New York: Augustin, 1940).

Boas, Ernst P., and Samuel Donner, "Coronary Artery Disease in the Working Classes," *Journal of the American Medical Association* 98 (1932): 2186–89.

Boegehold, Matthew A., and Theodore A. Kotchen, "Importance of Dietary Chloride for Salt Sensitivity of Blood Pressure," *Hypertension* 17 Supp. 1 (1991): I-158–I-161.

Boffey, Phillip M., *The Brain Bank of America: An Inquiry into the Politics of Science* (New York: McGraw-Hill, 1975).

Bolande, Robert P., "Ritualistic Surgery—Circumcision and Tonsillectomy," *New England Journal of Medicine* 280 (1969): 591–96.

Bonchek, Lawrence I., "Are Randomized Trials Appropriate for Evaluating New Operations?" *New England Journal of Medicine* 301 (1979): 44–45.

Brace, Charles Loring, *The Dangerous Classes of New York, and Twenty Years' Work Among Them* (1872; Washington, DC: NASW Classics, 1973).

Brackenridge, R. D. C., *Medical Selection of Life Risks: A Comprehensive Guide to Life Expectancy for Underwriters and Clinicians,* 2nd ed. (New York: Nature Press, 1985).

Bradley, Michele M., "The States' Role in Regulating Food Labeling and Advertising: The Effect of the Nutrition Labeling and Education Act of 1990," *Food and Drug Law Journal* 49 (1994): 649–74.

Brainard, Annie M., *The Evolution of Public Health Nursing* (1922; New York: Garland, 1985).

Brett, Allan S., "Treating Hypercholesterolemia: How Should Practicing Physicians Interpret the Published Data for Patients?" *New England Journal of Medicine* 321 (1989): 676–80.

Brewster, Letitia, and Michael F. Jacobson, *The Changing American Diet* (Washington, DC: Center for Science in the Public Interest, 1983).

Brisson, Germain J., *Lipids in Human Nutrition: An Appraisal of Some Dietary Concepts* (Englewood Cliffs, NJ: Burgess, 1981).

British Hypertension Society Second Working Party, "Management Guidelines in Essential Hypertension," *British Medical Journal* 306 (1993): 983–87.

British Hypertension Society Working Party, "Treating Mild Hypertension," *British Medical Journal* 298 (1989): 694–98.

British Nutrition Foundation, *Unsaturated Fatty Acids: Nutritional and Physiological Significance* (London: Chapman and Hall, 1992).

Brody, Baruch A., *Ethical Issues in Drug Testing, Approval, and Pricing: The Clot-Dissolving Drugs* (New York: Oxford University Press, 1995).

Buhler-Wilkerson, Karen, "Public Health Nursing: In Sickness or in Health?" *American Journal of Public Health* 75 (1985): 000–000.

"Building Sources of Income for Voluntary Public Health Nursing Services," *Public Health Nursing* 44 (1952): 635–36.

Bulger, Roger J., ed., *In Search of the Modern Hippocrates* (Iowa City: University of Iowa Press, 1987).

Bulmer, Martin, Kevin Bales, and Kathryn K. Sklar, eds., *The Social Survey in Historical Perspective: 1880–1940* (Cambridge: Cambridge University Press, 1991).

Bulpitt, C. J. ed., *Epidemiology of Hypertension* (Amsterdam: Elsevier, 1985).

Burnett, John *Plenty and Want: A Social History of Diet in England from 1815 to the Present Day,* rev. ed. (London: Scolar Press, 1979).

Burch, George E., and Nicholas P. DePasquale, *A History of Electrocardiography* (1964; San Francisco: Norman, 1990).

Burnham, John C., "How the Discovery of Accidental Childhood Poisoning Contributed to the Development of Environmentalism in the United States," *Environmental History Review* 19 (Fall 1995): 57–81.

Callaway, Wayne, "Reexamining Cholesterol and Sodium Recommendations," *Nutrition Today* 29 (Sept.–Oct., 1994): 32–36.

Cancer of the Lung a Growing Health Problem," *Statistical Bulletin* 20 (Nov. 1939): 7–9.

Carpenter, Niles, *Immigrants and their Children* (1927; New York: Arno Press, 1969).

Cashin, W. Linda, et al., "Accelerated Progression of Atherosclerosis in Coronary Vessels with Minimal Lesions that are Bypassed," *New England Journal of Medicine* 311 (1984): 824–28.

Cassedy, James H., *American Medicine and Statistical Thinking, 1800–1860* (Cambridge, MA: Harvard University Press, 1984).

———, *Demography in Early America: Beginnings of the Statistical Mind, 1600–1800* (Cambridge, MA: Harvard University Press, 1969).

———, "The Registration Area and American Vital Statistics," *Bulletin of the History of Medicine* 39 (1965): 221–31.

Cassidy, Maurice, "Coronary Disease," *Lancet* 2 (1946): 587–88.

"Causes of the Recent Decline in Tuberculosis and Outlook for the Future," *Statistical Bulletin* 4 (June, 1923): 1–4.

Central Committee for Medical and Community Programs of the American Heart Association, "Dietary Fat and Its Relation to Heart Attacks and Stroke," *Circulation* 23 (1961): 389–91.

Chadwick, Henry D., and David Zacks, "The Incidence of Tuberculous Infection in School Children," *New England Journal of Medicine* 200 (1929): 332–37.

Chalmers, Thomas C., "Mortality Rate versus Funeral Rate in Clinical Medicine," *Gastroenterology* 46 (1964): 788–91.

Chandler, A. Bleakley, "Coronary Thrombosis in Myocardial Infarction," *American Journal of Cardiology* 34 (1974): 823–33.

Chapin, Robert C., *The Standard of Living Among Workingmen's Families in New York City* (New York: Russell Sage Foundation, 1909).

Charap, Mitchell H., "The Periodic Health Examination: Genesis of a Myth," *Annals of Internal Medicine* 95 (1981): 733–35.

Cinel, Dino, *From Italy to San Francisco: The Immigrant Experience* (Stanford, CA: Stanford University Press, 1982).

Cinel, Dino, *The National Integration of Italian Return Migration, 1870–1929* (Cambridge: Cambridge University Press, 1991).

Clegg, E. J., and J. P. Garlick, eds., *Disease and Urbanization* (London: Taylor and Francis, 1980).

Clough, Shepard B., *A Century of American Life Insurance: A History of the Mutual Life Insurance Company of New York 1843–1943* (1946: reprint, Westport CT: Greenwood Press, 1970).

Cohen, Patricia Cline, *A Calculating People: The Spread of Numeracy in Early America* (Chicago: University of Chicago Press, 1982). .

Cohn, Alfred E., "Heart Disease from the Point of View of the Public Health," *American Heart Journal* 2 (1927): 386–407.

Coleman, William, *Death is a Social Disease: Public Health and Political Economy in Early Industrial France* (Madison: University of Wisconsin Press, 1982). .

Condran, Gretchen A., and Ellen A. Kramarow, "Child Mortality Among Jewish Immigrants to the United States," *Journal of Interdisciplinary History* 22 (1991): 223–54.

Consensus Conference, "Lowering Blood Cholesterol to Prevent Heart Disease," *JAMA* 253 (1985): 2080–86.

Converse, Jean M., *Survey Research in the United States: Roots and Emergence 1890–1960* (Berkeley: University of California Press, 1987).

Coon, Horace, *American Tel & Tel* (1939; Freeport, NY; Books for Libraries Press, 1971).

Covello, Vincent T., et al., eds., *The Analysis of Actual Versus Perceived Risks* (New York: Plenum, 1983).

Covello, Vincent T., and Miley W. Merkhofer, *Risk Assessment Methods: Approaches for Assessing Health and Environmental Risks* (New York: Plenum, 1993).

Cowing, W. H., *Blood Pressure: Technique Simplified,* 3rd. ed. (Rochester, NY: Taylor Instrument Companies, 1912).

Coronary Drug Project Research Group, "Influence of Adherence to Treatment and Response of Cholesterol on Mortality in the Coronary Drug Project," *New England Journal of Medicine* 303 (1980): 1038–41.

Cornfield, Jerome, et al., "Smoking and Lung Cancer: Recent Evidence and a Discussion of Some Questions," *Journal of the National Cancer Institute* 22 (1959): 173–202. .

Cowdry, Edmund V. ed., *Arteriosclerosis: A Survey of the Problem* (New York: Macmillan, 1933).

Cullen, M.J., *The Statistical Movement in Early Victorian Britain: The Foundations of Empirical Social Research* (New York: Barnes and Noble, 1975). .

Cummings, Richard O., *The American and His Food: A History of Food Habits in the United States,* rev. ed. (Chicago: University of Chicago Press, 1941).

Cummings, Steven R., et al., "Smoking Counseling and Preventive Medicine: A Survey of Internists in Private Practice and a Health Maintenance Organization," *Archives of Internal Medicine* 149 (1989): 345–49.

Cushing, Harvey, "On Routine Determinations of Arterial Tension in Operating Room and Clinic," *Boston Medical and Surgical Journal* 148 (1903): 254, 250–56.

Daley, Robert M., Harry E. Ungerleider, and Richard S. Gubner, "Prognosis in Hypertension," *Journal of the American Medical Association* 121 (1943): 383–89.

Daniel, Thomas M., *Captain of Death: The Story of Tuberculosis* (Rochester, NY: University of Rochester Press, 1997).

Danielian, Noobar R., *A.T.&T.: The Story of Industrial Conquest* (1939; New York: Arno, 1974).

Daston, Lorraine, *Classical Probability in the Enlightenment* (Princeton, NJ: Princeton University Press, 1988).

Dawber, Thomas R., *The Framingham Study: The Epidemiology of Atherosclerotic Disease* (Cambridge, MA: Harvard University Press, 1980).

Dawber, Thomas R., et al., "Dietary Assessment in the Epidemiologic Study of Coronary Heart Disease: The Framingham Study," *American Journal of Clinical Nutrition* 11 (1962): 226–34.

——, "Some Factors Associated with the Development of Coronary Heart Disease," *American Journal of Public Health* 49 (1959): 1349–56.

Dawber, Thomas, Gilcin F. Meadors, and Felix E. Moore, Jr., "Epidemiological Approaches to Disease: The Framingham Study," *American Journal of Public Health* 41 (1951): 279–86.

Davis, Audrey B. "Life Insurance and the Physical Examination: A Chapter in the Rise of American Medical Technology," *Bulletin of the History of Medicine* 55 (1981): 392–406.

Davis, Malvin E., *Industrial Life Insurance in the United States* (New York: McGraw-Hill, 1944).

Davis, Michael M. Jr., *Immigrant Health and the Community* (1921; Montclair, NJ: Patterson Smith, 1971).

Davis, Michael M., and Mary C. Jarrett, *A Health Inventory of New York City* (New York, 1929).

"Death Comes to the Average Man," *Fortune* 16 (Nov. 1937), 140ff.

"A Debate on Coronary Bypass," *New England Journal of Medicine* 297 (1977): 1464–70.

DeForest, Robert W., and Lawrence Veiller, eds., *The Tenement House Problem* (1903; New York: Arno Press, 1970).

Denny, Floyd W. Jr., "A 45–Year Perspective on the Streptococcus and Rheumatic Fever," *Clinical Infectious Diseases* 19 (1994): 1110–22.

Denny, Francis P., "The Increase in Coronary Disease and its Cause," *New England Journal of Medicine* 214 (1936): 769–73.

"Diet and Coronary Heart Disease," *Preventive Medicine* 1 (1972): 559–61.

"Dietary Goals for the United States," *Rhode Island Medical Journal* 60 (1977): 576–81.

Doll, Richard, "Smoking and Death Rates," *JAMA* 251 (1984): 2854–57.

Doll, Richard, and A. Bradford Hill, "Lung Cancer and Other Causes of Death in Relation to Smoking," *British Medical Journal* 2 (1956): 1071–81 .

Doll, Richard, and Austin B. Hill, "Mortality in Relation to Smoking: Ten Years' Observations of British Doctors," *British Medical Journal* 1 (1964): 1399–1410, 1460–67.

Dorn, Harold F., "Tobacco Consumption and Mortality from Cancer and Other Diseases," *Public Health Reports* 74 (1959): 581–93.

Dowling, Harry F., "The Emergence of the Cooperative Clinical Trial," *Transactions and Studies of the College of Physicians of Philadelphia* 43 (1975): 20–29.

Downs, John R., et al., "Primary Prevention of Acute Coronary Events with Lovastatin in Men and Women with Average Cholesterol Levels," *JAMA* 279 (1996): 1615–1622.

Dublin, Louis, *After Eighty Years: The Impact of Life Insurance on the Public Health* (Gainesville, FL: University of Florida Press, 1966).

Dublin, Louis I., *A Family of Thirty Million: The Story of the Metropolitan Life Insurance Company* (New York: 1943).

———, *A 40 Year Campaign Against Tuberculosis* (New York: Metropolitan Life Insurance Company, 1952).

———, *Health and Wealth: A Survey of the Economics of World Health* (New York: Harper, 1928).

———, *Health Progress, 1936 to 1945* (New York: Metropolitan Life Insurance Company, 1948).

———, *Mortality Statistics of Insured Wage-Earners and Their Families* (New York: Metropolitan Life Insurance Company, 1919).

Dublin, Louis I., and Gladys W. Baker, "The Mortality of Race Stocks in Pennsylvania and New York, 1910," *Quarterly Publications of the American Statistical Association* 17 (1920): 13–44.

Dublin, Louis I., and Alfred J. Lotka, *Twenty-five Years of Health Progress* (New York: Metropolitan Life Insurance Company, 1937).

Dublin, Louis I., Alfred J. Lotka, and Mortimer Spiegelman, *Length of Life: A Study of the Life Table,* revised ed. (New York: Ronald, 1949).

Dublin, Louis I., and Robert J. Vane, Jr., *Causes of Death by Occupation,* U.S. Bureau of Labor Statistics Bulletin No. 507 (Washington, DC; U.S. GPO, 1930).

———, "Occupational Mortality Experience of Insured Wage Earners," *Monthly Labor Review* 64 (1947): 1003–18.

Dubos, Rene, *The World of Rene Dubos: A Collection from His Writings* (New York: Holt, 1990).

Dubos, Rene, and Jean Dubos, *The White Plague: Tuberculosis, Man and Society* (Boston: Little, Brown, 1952).

Duffy, John, *Epidemics in Colonial America* (Baton Rouge: Louisiana State University Press, 1953) .

———, *A History of Public Health in New York City: 1866–1966* (New York: Russell Sage, 1974).

Duguid, J. B., "Thrombosis as a Factor in the Pathogenesis of Coronary Atherosclerosis," *Journal of Bacteriology and Pathology* 58 (1946): 207–12.

Eaton, S. Boyd, and Melvin Konner, "Paleolithic Nutrition," *New England Journal of Medicine* 312 (1985): 283–89.

Edwards, Lydia B., and Carroll E. Palmer, *Tuberculosis* (Cambridge, MA: Harvard University Press, 1969).

Elliott, Glen R., and Carl Eisdorfer, eds., *Stress and Human Health: Analysis and Implications of Research* (New York: Springer, 1982).

Elliott, Paul, et al., "Intersalt Revisited: Further Analyses of 24 Hour Sodium Excretion and Blood Pressure Within and Across Populations," *British Medical Journal* 312 (1996): 1249–53.

Ellison, David L., *Healing Tuberculosis in the Woods: Medicine and Science at the End of the Nineteenth Century* (Westport, CT: Greenwood, 1994).

Elveback, Lila R., Daniel C. Connolly, and L. Joseph Melton, "Coronary Heart Disease in Residents of Rochester, Minnesota. VII: Incidence, 1950 through 1982," *Mayo Clinic Proceedings* 61 (1986): 896–900.

Employment Survey Made by Agents of the Metropolitan Life Insurance Co., 71st Congress, 3rd session, Document No. 260. Jan. 24, 1931.

English, Peter, "Emergence of Rheumatic Fever in the Nineteenth Century," *Milbank Quarterly* 67 suppl. 1 (1999): 33–49.

English, Peter C., *Rheumatic Fever in America and Britain: A Biological, Epidemiological, and Medical History* (New Brunswick, NJ: Rutgers University Press, 1999).

———, *Shock, Physiological Surgery, and George Washington Crile: Medical Innovation in the Progressive Era* (Westport, CT: Greenwood Press, 1980), 96–113.

"Encouraging Outlook in Rheumatic Fever," *Statistical Bulletin* 32 (Jan., 1951): 7–10.

Enos, William F., Robert H. Holmes, and James Beyer, "Coronary Disease Among United States Soldiers Killed in Action in Korea," *JAMA* 152 (1953): 1090–93.

Evans, Alfred S., *Causation and Disease: A Chronological Journey* (New York: Plenum, 1993).

Evans, Hughes, "Losing Touch: The Controversy over the Introduction of Blood Pressure Instruments into Medicine," *Technology and Culture* 34 (1993): 784–807.

Evans, Robert G., Morris L. Barer, and Theodore R. Marmor, eds., *Why Are Some People Healthy and Others Not?* (New York: Aldine de Gruyer, 1994).

Expert Panel on Detection, Evaluation, and Treatment of High Blood Cholesterol in Adults, "Executive Summary of the Third Report of the National Cholesterol Education Program (NCEP) Expert Panel on Detection, Evaluation, and Treatment of High Blood Cholesterol in Adults (Adult Treatment Panel III)," *JAMA* 285 (2001): 2486–88.

Eyler, John M., *Sir Arthur Newsholme and State Medicine, 1885–1935* (Cambridge: Cambridge University Press, 1997).

Eyler, John M., *Victorian Social Medicine: The Ideas and Methods of William Farr* (Baltimore: Johns Hopkins University Press, 1979).

Fairchild, Henry P., *Immigration: A World Movement and Its American Significance,* rev. ed. (New York: Macmillan, 1925).

Fang, Jing, Shantha Madhavan, and Michael H. Alderman, "The Association Between Birthplace and Mortality from Cardiovascular Causes Among Black and White Residents of New York City," *New England Journal of Medicine* 335 (1996): 1545–51.

Faught, Francis A., *Blood-Pressure: From the Clinical Standpoint* (Philadelphia: Saunders, 1913).

———, "The Status of the Blood Pressure Observation in Life Insurance Examinations" *New York Medical Journal* 92 (1910): 168–71.

Feinstein, Alvan R., *Clinical Judgment* (Baltimore: Williams and Wilkens, 1967).

———, "Meta-Analysis: Statistical Alchemy for the 21st Century," *Journal of Clinical Epidemiology* 48 (1995): 71–79.

———, "Scientific Standards in Epidemiologic Studies of the Menace of Daily Life," *Science* 242 (1988): 1257–63.

"Fifth Report of the Joint National Committee on Detection, Evaluation, and Treatment of High Blood Pressure," *Archives of Internal Medicine* 153 (1993): 154–83.

"Fifty Years of Health Conservation," *Statistical Bulletin* 40 (Jan., 1959): 1–4.

"Fifty Years of Life Conservation," *Statistical Bulletin* 40 (Jan., 1959): 1–4.

Fishberg, Arthur M., *Hypertension and Nephritis* (Philadelphia: Lea and Febiger, 1930).

Fisher, J. W., "The Diagnostic Value of the Sphygmomanometer in Examinations for Life Insurance," *Journal of the American Medical Association* 63 (1914): 1752–54.

Floud, Roderick, Kenneth Wachter, and Annabel Gregory, *Height, Health and History: Nutritional Status in the United Kingdom, 1750–1980* (Cambridge: Cambridge University Press, 1990).

Food and Drug Administration et al. v. Brown & Williamson Tobacco Corp. et al., 529 U.S. 23 (2000).

Food and Nutrition Board, National Academy of Sciences, *Toward Healthful Diets* (Washington, DC: National Academy of Sciences, 1980).

Forrest, D. W., *Francis Galton: The Life and Work of a Victorian Genius* (London: Elek, 1974).

Fortmann, Stephen P., et al., "Attitudes and Practices of Physicians Regarding Hypertension and Smoking: The Stanford Five City Project" *Preventive Medicine* 14 (1985): 70–80.

Fox, Daniel M., "Social Policy and City Politics: Tuberculosis Reporting in New York, 1889–1900," *Bulletin of the History of Medicine* 49 (1975): 169–75.

Framingham Community Health and Tuberculosis Demonstration, *Framingham Monograph No. 10: Final Summary Report: 1917–1923 Inclusive* General Series IV (Framingham, MA: 1924).

Frankel, Lee K., and Louis I. Dublin, *Heights and Weights of New York City Children: A Study of Measurements of Boys and Girls Granted Employment Certificates* (New York: Metropolitan Life Insurance Company, 1916) .

———, "Visiting Nursing and Life Insurance," *Publications of the American Statistical Association* 16 (June, 1918).

Franklin, Jack L., et al., "Smoking Cessation Interventions by Family Physicians in Texas," *Texas Medicine* 88 (1992): 60–64.

Freedman, David, et al., *Statistics,* 2nd. ed. (New York: Norton, 1991).

Freis, Edward D., "The Role of Hypertension," *American Journal of Public Health* 50, suppl. (Mar. 1960): 11–13.

———, "Should Mild Hypertension be Treated?" *New England Journal of Medicine* 307 (1982): 306–9.

Friedberg, Charles K., *Diseases of the Heart* (Philadelphia: Saunders, 1949).

Fritschler, A. Lee, *Smoking and Politics,* 3rd ed.(Englewood Cliffs, NJ: Prentice-Hall, 1983).

Fumento, Michael, *The Fat of the Land: The Obesity Epidemic and How Overweight Americans Can Help Themselves* (New York: Viking, 1997).

Fye, W. Bruce, *American Cardiology: The History of a Specialty and Its College* (Baltimore: Johns Hopkins University Press, 1996).

———, "The Delayed Diagnosis of Myocardial Infarction: It Took Half a Century!" *Circulation* 72 (1985): 262–71.

———, "A History of the Origin, Evolution, and Impact of Electrocardiography," *American Journal of Cardiology* 73 (1994): 937–49 .

Gaedeke, Ralph M., and Warren W. Etcheson, eds., *Consumerism: Viewpoints from Business, Government, and the Public Interest* (San Francisco: Canfield, 1972).

Galdston, Iago, ed., *The Epidemiology of Health,* (New York: Health Education Council, 1953).

Galishoff, Stuart, *Safeguarding the Public Health: Newark, 1895–1918* (Westport, CT: Greenwood Press, 1975).

Gardner, Martin J., and Douglas G. Altman, "Confidence Intervals Rather than P Values: Estimation Rather than Hypothesis Testing," *British Medical Journal* 292 (1986): 746–50.

Gardner, Mary S., *Public Health Nursing,* 3rd ed. (New York: Macmillan, 1936).

Gefter, William I., Bernard H. Pastor, and Ralph M. Myerson, *Synopsis of Cardiology* (St. Louis, MO: Mosby, 1965).

Genest, Jacques, Erich Koiw, and Otto Kuchel, eds., *Hypertension: Physiopathology and Treatment* (New York: McGraw-Hill, 1977).

Gersh, Bernard J., and Shahbudin H. Rahimtoola, eds., *Acute Myocardial Infarction* (New York: Elsevier, 1991).

Gibney, Michael J., *Nutrition, Diet and Health* (Cambridge: Cambridge University Press, 1986).

Gillham, Nicholas W., *A Life of Sir Francis Galton: From African Exploration to the Birth of Eugenics* (New York: Oxford University Press, 2001).

Gillis, John R., Louise A. Tilly, and David Levine, eds., *The European Experience of Declining Fertility, 1850–1970: The Quiet Revolution,* (Cambridge, MA: Blackwell, 1992).

Glass, D. V., *Numbering the People: The Eighteenth Century Population Controversy and the Development of Census and Vital Statistics in Britain* (Farnbourough, Eng.: Saxon House, 1973).

Gofman, John W., *What We Do Know about Heart Attacks* (New York: Putnam's Sons, 1958).

Goldberg, Robert J., et al., "A Communitywide Perspective of Sex Differences and Temporal Trends in the Incidence and Survival Rates After Acute Myocardial Infarction and Out-of-Hospital Deaths Caused by Coronary Heart Disease," *Circulation* 87 (1993): 1947–53.

Goldberger, Emanuel, *Heart Disease: Its Diagnosis and Treatment* (Philadelphia: Lea and Febiger, 1951).

Goldbourt, Uri, and Shomit Yaari, "Cholesterol and Coronary Heart Disease Mortality: A 23–Year Follow-Up Study of 9902 Men in Israel," *Arteriosclerosis* 10 (1990): 512–19.

Goldstein, Michael S., *Alternative Health Care: Medicine, Miracle, or Mirage?* (Philadelphia, PA: Temple University Press, 1999).

———, *The Health Movement: Promoting Fitness in America* (New York: Twayne, 1992).

Gordis, Leon, "The Virtual Disappearance of Rheumatic Fever in the United States: Lessons in the Rise and Fall of Disease," *Circulation* 72 (1985): 1155–62.

Gordon, Tavia, "The Framingham Diet Study: Diet and the Regulation of Serum Cholesterol," Section 24, The Framingham Study: an Epidemiological Investigation of Cardiovascular Disease (Washington, DC: National Institutes of Health, 1970?).

Gordon, Tavia, et al., "Some Methodological Problems in the Long-Term Study of Cardiovascular Disease: Observations on the Framingham Study," *Journal of Chronic Diseases* 10 (1959): 186–206.

Gordon, Tavia, and William B. Kannel, "Premature Mortality from Coronary Heart Disease," *JAMA* 215 (1971): 1617–25.

Gordon, William H., Edward F. Bland, and Paul D. White, "Coronary Artery Disease Analyzed Post Mortem: With Special Reference to the Influence of Economic Status and Sex," *American Heart Journal* 17 (1939): 10–14.

Gori, Gio Batta, "The Regulation of Carcinogenic Hazards," *Science* 208 (1980): 256–61.

Gover, Mary, "Statistical Studies of Heart Disease: VII. Mortality from Eight Specific Forms of Heart Disease Among White Persons," *Public Health Reports* 65 (1950): 819–38.

Gradmann, Christoph, "Robert Koch and the Pressures of Scientific Research: Tuberculosis and Tuberculin," *Medical History* 45 (2001): 1–32.

Graham, Frank Jr., *Since Silent Spring* (Boston: Houghton Mifflin, 1970).

Graham, John D., Laura C. Green, and Marc J. Roberts, *In Search of Safety: Chemicals and Cancer Risk* (Cambridge, MA: Harvard University Press, 1988) .

Graham, John D., and Jonathan B. Wiener, eds., *Risk Versus Risk: Tradeoffs in Protecting Health and the Environment* (Cambridge, MA: Harvard University Press, 1995).

Graham, Loren R., *Between Science and Values* (New York: Columbia University Press, 1981).

Granshaw, Lindsay, "'Upon This Principle I have Based a Practice': The Development and Reception of Antisepsis in Britain, 1867–90," in *Medical Innovations in Historical Perspective*, ed. John V. Pickstone (New York: St. Martin's Press, 1992).

Grant, H. Roger, *Insurance Reform: Consumer Action in the Progressive Era* (Ames: Iowa State University Press, 1979).

Graunt, John, *Natural and Political Observations Mentioned in a Following Index and Made Upon the Bills of Mortality* (1662; New York: Arno Press, 1975) .

Greenwald, Maurine W., and Margo Anderson, eds., *Pittsburgh Surveyed: Social Science and Social Reform in the Early Twentieth Century* (Pittsburgh, PA: University of Pittsburgh Press, 1996).

Grimshaw, Margaret L., "Scientific Specialization and the Poliovirus Controversy in the Years Before World War II," *Bulletin of the History of Medicine* 69 (1995): 44–65.

Grob, Gerald N., *Edward Jarvis and the Medical World of Nineteenth Century America* (Knoxville: University of Tennessee Press, 1978).

———, *Mental Institutions in America: Social Policy to 1875* (New York: Free Press, 1973).

Groedel, Franz M., "Observations on the Circulatory System of Combatants During World War I," *Experimental Medicine and Surgery* 1 (1943): 94–102.

Gross, Cary P., et al., "The Relation Between Funding by the National Institutes of Health and the Burden of Disease," *New England Journal of Medicine* 340 (1999): 1881–87.

Grove, Robert D., and Alice M. Hetzel, *Vital Statistics Rates in the United States, 1940–1960* (Washington, DC: U.S. Department of Health, Education, and Welfare, 1968).

Gutman, Robert, *Birth and Death Registration in Massachusetts, 1639–1900* (New York: Milbank Memorial Fund, 1959).

Hacking, Ian, *The Emergence of Probability: A Philosophical Study of Early Ideas about Probability, Induction, and Statistical Inference* (London: Cambridge University Press, 1975).

———, *The Taming of Chance* (Cambridge: Cambridge University Press, 1990) .

Haines, Stephen J., "Randomized Clinical Trials in the Evaluation of Surgical Innovations," *Journal of Neurosurgery* 51 (1979): 5–11.

Hald, Anders, *A History of Probability and Statistics and Their Applications Before 1750* (New York: Wiley, 1990) .

"Haley Fiske and the Public Health," *Statistical Bulletin* 10 (Mar. 1929): 2–7.

Hamilton, Diane, "The Cost of Caring: The Metropolitan Life Insurance Company's Visiting Nurse Service, 1909–1953," *Bulletin of the History of Medicine* 63 (1989): 414–34.

Hamilton, Frank H., "Report on Deformities after Fractures: Part Third," *Transactions of the American Medical Association* 10 (1857): 299–307.

Hammond, E. Cuyler, "Smoking in Relation to Heart Disease," *American Journal of Public Health* 50, suppl. (Mar. 1960): 20–26.

———, "Smoking in Relation to Lung Cancer," *Connecticut State Medical Journal* 18 (1954): 3–9.

Hammond, E. Cuyler, and Daniel Horn, "The Relationship between Human Smoking Habits and Death Rates," *JAMA* 155 (1954): 1316–28.

Hammonds, Evelynn M., *Childhood's Deadly Scourge: The Campaign to Control Diphtheria in New York City, 1880–1930* (Baltimore, MD: Johns Hopkins University Press, 1999).

"Handicaps of Overweight" *Statistical Bulletin* 33 (Aug., 1952): 3–5.

Hankins, Frank H., *Adolphe Quetelet as Statistician* (New York: 1908).

Hapgood, Hutchins, *The Spirit of the Ghetto* (Cambridge, MA: Harvard University Press, 1967) .

Harlan, William R., and Jeoffrey K. Stross, "An Educational View of a National Initiative to Lower Plasma Lipid Levels" *JAMA* 253 (1985): 2087–90.

Harris, Marvin and Eric B. Ross, eds., *Food and Evolution: Toward a Theory of Human Food Habits* (Philadelphia: Temple University Press, 1987).

Hart, Julian T., *Hypertension: Community Control of High Blood Pressure,* 2nd ed. (Edinburgh: Churchill Livingstone, 1987).

Haughton, Betsy, Joan D. Gussow, and Janice M. Dodds, "An Historical Study of the Underlying Assumptions for United States Food Guides from 1917 Through the Basic Four Food Group Guide," *Journal of Nutrition Education* 19 (1987): 169–75.

Hausman, Patricia, *Jack Spratt's Legacy: The Science and Politics of Fat and Cholesterol* (New York: Marek, 1981).

Havlik, Richard J., and Manning Feinleib, eds., *Proceedings of the Conference on the Decline in Coronary Heart Disease Mortality* (Bethesda, MD: National Institutes of Health, 1978).

The Health of Women and Children (New York: Arno Press, 1977).

Healthy People: The Surgeon General's Report on Health Promotion and Disease Prevention, 1979 (Washington, DC: U.S. Department of Health, Education, and Welfare, 1979).

"Heart Disease and Socioeconomic Status" *Statistical Bulletin* 39 (March, 1958): 6–8.

Heart Disease Control Program, *Cardiovascular Disease: Data on Mortality, Prevalence and Control Activities* (Washington, DC: U.S. Public Health Service, 1955).

Henderson, Robert, "Insurance of Substandard Lives," *Annals of the American Academy of Political and Social Science,* 130 (March 1927).

Hibbs, Henry H., Jr., *Infant Mortality: Its Relation to Social and Industrial Conditions* (New York: Russell Sage, 1916).

Higgins, I. T. T., A. L. Cochrane, and A. J. Thomas, "Epidemiological Studies of Coronary Disease," *British Journal of Preventive and Social Medicine* 17 (1963): 153–65 .

Higgins, Millicent W., and Russell V. Luepker, eds., *Trends in Coronary Heart Disease Mortality: The Influence of Medical Care,* (New York: Oxford University Press, 1988).

Higginson, John, Calum S. Muir, and Nubia Munoz, *Human Cancer: Epidemiology and Environmental Causes* (Cambridge: Cambridge University Press, 1992).

Hill, A. Bradford, *Principles of Medical Statistics* (London: Lancet, 1937).

"Historical Highlights of ALIMD, 1889–1964," *Transactions of the Association of Life Insurance Medical Directors of America,* 73th Annual Meeting (New York: 1965), 279–85.

Hoag, Ernest B., and Lewis M. Terman, *Health Work in the Schools* (Boston: Houghton Mifflin, 1914).

Hoerder, Dirk, ed., *Labor Migration in the Atlantic Economies: The European and North American Working Classes During the Period of Industrialization* (Westport, CT: Greenwood, 1985).

Holt, L. Emmett, et al., "The Report of the American Pediatric Society's Collective Investigation into the Use of Antitoxin in the Treatment of Diphtheria in Private Practice," *Medical News* 69 (1896): 1–12.

Holt, W. Stull, *The Bureau of the Census: Its History, Activities, and Organization* (Washington: Brookings Institution, 1929).

Hopkins, Paul N., "Effects of Dietary Cholesterol on Serum Cholesterol: A Meta-analysis and Review," *American Journal of Clinical Nutrition* 55 (1992): 1060–70.

Howard, Martha C., "The Margarine Industry in the United States: Its Development Under Legislative Control" (Ph.D. Dissertation, Columbia University, 1951).

Hoy, Suellen, *Chasing Dirt: The American Pursuit of Cleanliness* (New York: Oxford University Press, 1995).

Hudnot, James M., *History of the New-York Life Insurance Company: 1895–1905* (New York: 1906).

Hunninghake, Donald B., et al., "The Efficacy of Intensive Dietary Therapy Alone or in Combination with Lovastatin in Outpatients with Hypercholesterolemia," *New England Journal of Medicine* 328 (1993): 1213–19.

Hunter, Arthur, "Selection of Risks from the Actuarial Standpoint," *Transactions of the Actuarial Society of America* 12 (1911): 1–17.

Hyman, Albert S., and Aaron E. Parsonnet, *The Failing Heart of Middle Life: The Myocardosis Syndrome, Coronary Thrombosis, and Angina Pectoris* (Philadelphia: Davis, 1932).

Hyman, Herbert H., *Taking Society's Measure: A Personal History of Survey Research* (New York: Russell Sage Foundation, 1991).

Hypertension Detection and Follow-up Program Cooperative Group, "Five-Year Findings of the Hypertension Detection and Follow-up Program," *JAMA* 242 (1979): 2572–77.

Imperato, Pascal J., *The Administration of a Public Health Agency: A Case Study of the New York City Department of Health* (New York: Human Sciences Press, 1983).

Ingle, Dwight J., ed., *Life and Disease: New Perspectives in Biology and Medicine,* (New York Basic Books: 1963).

Intersalt Cooperative Research Group, "Intersalt: An International Study of Electrolyte Excretion and Blood Pressure: Results for 24 Hour Urinary Sodium and Potassium Excretion," *British Medical Journal* 297 (1988): 319–28.

Institute of Medicine, *Improving America's Diet and Health: From Recommendations to Action* (Washington, DC: National Academy Press, 1991).

Irwin, Warren, Jr., and Alexander M. Burgess, Jr., "The Abuse of Bed Rest in the Treatment of Myocardial infarction," *New England Journal of Medicine* 243 (1950): 486–89.

James, George, Robert E. Patton, and A. Sandra Heslin, "Accuracy of Cause-of-Death Statements on Death Certificates," *Public Health Reports* 70 (1955): 39–51.

James, Marquis, *The Metropolitan Life: A Study in Business Growth* (New York: Viking, 1947).

Janeway, Theodore C., *The Clinical Study of Blood-Pressure: A Guide to the Use of the Sphygmomanometer* (New York: Appleton, 1904, 1910).

Jenks, Jeremiah W., W. Jett Lauck, and Rufus D. Smith, *The Immigration Problem: A Study of American Immigration Conditions and Needs,* 6th ed. (New York: Funk & Wagnalls, 1926).

Jones, David S., "Visions of a Cure: Visualization, Clinical Trials, and Controversy in Cardiac Therapeutics, 1968–98," *Isis* 91 (2000): 504–41.

Kannel, William B., "Contribution of the Framingham Study to Preventive Cardiology," *Journal of the American College of Cardiology* 15 (1990): 206–11.

———, "Hypertension: Relationship with Other Risk Factors," *Drugs* 31, suppl. 1 (1986): 1–11.

Kannel, William B., and Robert D. Abbott, "Incidence and Prognosis of Unrecognized Myocardial Infarction: An Update on the Framingham Study," *New England Journal of Medicine* 311 (1984): 1144–47.

Kannel, William B., and Paul R. Sorlie, "Some Health Benefits of Physical Activity: The Framingham Study," *Archives of Internal Medicine* 139 (1979): 857–61.

Kannel, William B., and Thomas J. Thom, "Declining Cardiovascular Mortality," *Circulation* 70 (1984): 331–36 .

Kannel, William B., et al., "Epidemiology of Coronary Heart Disease," *Geriatrics* 17 (1962): 675–90.

———, "Factors of Risk in the Development of Coronary Heart Disease: Six-Year Follow-up Experience: The Framingham Study," *Annals of Internal Medicine* 55 (1961): 33–50.

———, "Risk Factors in Coronary Heart Disease," *Annals of Internal Medicine* 61 (1964): 888–99.

Kaplan, George A. and Julian E. Keil, "Socioeconomic Factors and Cardiovascular Disease: A Review of the Literature," *Circulation* 88 no. 4 pt. 1 (Oct., 1993): 1973–98.

Kaplan, Norman M., *Clinical Hypertension* 6th ed. (Baltimore: Williams and Wilkens, 1994).

Keller, Morton, *The Life Insurance Enterprise, 1885–1910: A Study in the Limits of Corporate Power* (Cambridge, MA: Harvard University Press, 1963).

Kessler, Irving I. and Morton L. Levin, eds., *The Community as an Epidemiological Laboratory* (Baltimore: Johns Hopkins Press, 1970).

Keys, Ancel, "Atherosclerosis: A Problem in Newer Public Health," *Journal of the Mount Sinai Hospital New York* 20 (1953): 118–39.

———, [letter], *New England Journal of Medicine* 325 (1991): 584.

Keys, Ancel, Joseph T. Anderson, and Francisco Grande, "Prediction of Serum-Cholesterol Responses of Man to Changes in Fats in the Diet," *Lancet* 2 (1957): 959–66.

Keys, Ancel, et al., "Diet and Serum Cholesterol in Man," *Journal of Nutrition* 59 (1956): 39–56.

———, *Seven Countries: A Multivariate Analysis of Death and Coronary Heart Disease* (Cambridge, MA: Harvard University Press, 1980).

Keys, Ancel, ed., "Coronary Heart Disease in Seven Countries," *Circulation* 41, suppl. (April, 1970).

Killip, Thomas, "Twenty Years of Coronary Bypass Surgery," *New England Journal of Medicine* 319 (1988): 366–68.

Kirby, Jane, "Nutrition Education: A Food Editor's Perspective," *Nutrition Today* 29 (May–June 1994): 6–9.

Klag, Michael J., et al., "Serum Cholesterol in Young Men and Subsequent Cardiovascular Disease," *New England Journal of Medicine* 328 (1993): 313–18.

Kluger, Richard, *Ashes to Ashes: America's Hundred-Year Cigarette War, the Public Health, and the Unabashed Triumph of Philip Morris* (New York: Knopf, 1996).

Koch, Robert, *Essays of Robert Koch,* trans. K. Codell Carter (Westport, CT: Greenwood Press, 1987).

Kohn, Robert R., "Cause of Death in Very Old People," *JAMA* 247 (1982): 2793–97.

Kolata, Gina, "Heart Panel's Conclusions Questioned," *Science* 227 (1985): 40–41.

Koplik, Henry, "The History of the First Milk Depot or Gouttes de Lait with Consultations in America," *Journal of the American Medical Association* 63 (1914): 1574–75.

Koren, John, ed., *The History of Statistics: Their Development and Progress in Many Countries* (1918; New York: Burt Franklin, 1970).

Korner, P. O., et al., "Untreated Mild Hypertension: A Report by the Management Committee of the Australian Therapeutic Trial in Mild Hypertension," *Lancet* 1 (1982): 185–91.

Kraut, Alan M., *Silent Travelers: Germs, Genes, and the "Immigrant Menace"* (New York: Basic Books, 1994) .

Krimsky, Sheldon, and Dominic Golding, eds., *Social Theories of Risk* (Westport, CT: Praeger, 1992).

Kris-Etherton, Penny M., and Shaomei Yu, "Individual Fatty Acid Effects on Plasma Lipids and Lipoproteins: Human Studies," *American Journal of Clinical Nutrition* 65, suppl. (1997): 1628S–44S.

Kronmal, Richard A., "Commentary on the Published Results of the Lipid Research Clinics Coronary Primary Prevention Trial," *JAMA* 253 (1985): 2091–93.

Krüger, Lorenz, Lorraine J. Daston, and Michael Heidelberger, *The Probabilistic Revolution Vol. 1: Ideas in History* (Cambridge, MA: MIT Press, 1987).

Kuller, Lewis H., et al., "Sudden Death and the Decline in Coronary Heart Disease Mortality," *Journal of Chronic Diseases* 39 (1986): 1001–19.

Laffel, Glenn L., and Eugene Braunwald, "Thrombolytic Therapy: A New Strategy for the Treatment of Acute Myocardial Infarction," *New England Journal of Medicine* 311 (1984): I: 710–17, II: 770–76.

Laidlaw, Walter, *Population of the City of New York, 1890–1930* (New York: 1932).

Lancaster, H. O., *Expectations of Life: A Study of the Demography, Statistics, and History of World Mortality* (New York: Springer–Verlag, 1990).

Laragh, John H., ed., *Hypertension Manual* (New York: Yorke, 1974).

Lave, Lester B., "Health and Safety Risk Analyses: Information for Better Decisions," *Science* 236 (1987): 291–95.

Leavitt, Judith, *Typhoid Mary: Captive to the Public's Health* (Boston: Beacon Press, 1996).

"Lee K. Frankel (1867–1931): A Leader in Public Health," *Statistical Bulletin of the Metropolitan Life Insurance Company* 12 (July 1931): 3–4.

Leichter, Howard M., *Free to be Foolish: Politics and Health Promotion in the United States and Great Britain* (Princeton: Princeton University Press, 1991).

Lenfant, Claude, "A New Challenge for America: The National Cholesterol Education Program," *Circulation* 73 (1986): 855–56.

Levenstein, Harvey, *Paradox of Plenty: A Social History of Eating in Modern America* (New York: Oxford University Press, 1993).

Levine, Samuel A., *Clinical Heart Disease* (Philadelphia: Saunders, 1938).

———, *Clinical Heart Disease,* 4th ed. (Philadelphia: Saunders, 1951).

———, *Coronary Thrombosis: Its Various Clinical Features* (Baltimore: Williams and Wilkins, 1929).

Levy, Robert I., et al., eds., *Nutrition, Lipids, and Coronary Heart Disease: A Global View,* (New York: Raven, 1979).

Levy, Robert L., ed., *Diseases of the Coronary Arteries and Cardiac Pain* (New York: Macmillan, 1936).

Levy, Robert L., Howard G. Bruenn, and Dorothy Kurtz, "Facts on Disease of the Coronary Arteries, Based on a Survey of the Clinical and Pathologic Records of 762 Cases," *American Journal of the Medical Sciences* 187 (1934): 376–90.

Lew, Edward A., "Biostatistical Pitfalls in Studies of Atherosclerotic Heart Disease," *Federation Proceedings* 21 (4) pt. 2 (July–Aug. 1962): 62–70.

————, "Some Implications of Mortality Statistics Relating to Coronary Artery Disease," *Journal of Chronic Diseases* 6 (1957): 192–209.

Linder, Forrest E., and Robert D. Grove, *Vital Statistics Rates in the United States: 1900–1940* (Washington, DC: U.S. Government Printing Office, 1943).

Lipid Research Clinics Program, "The Lipid Research Clinics Coronary Primary Prevention Trial Results 1. Reduction in Incidence of Coronary Heart Disease," *JAMA* 251 (1984): 351–64.

Lipset, Seymour M., and William Schneider, *The Confidence Gap: Business, Labor, and Government in the Public Mind* (New York: Free Press, 1983).

Lloyd-Jones, Donald, et al., "Accuracy of Death Certificates for Coding Coronary Heart Disease as the Cause of Death," *Annals of Internal Medicine* 129 (1998): 1020–26.

Louis, Pierre Charles A., *Researches on the Effects of Bloodletting in some Inflammatory Diseases,* trans. C.G. Putnam (Boston: Hilliard, Gray, 1836).

"Lowering Blood Cholesterol to Prevent Heart Disease," *JAMA* 253 (1985): 2080–86.

Maclean, Joseph B., *Life Insurance* (New York: McGraw-Hill, 1929).

————, *Life Insurance,* 9th ed. (New York: McGraw-Hill, 1962) .

MacMahon, Stephen, et al., "Blood Pressure, Stroke, and Coronary Heart Disease," *Lancet* 335 (1990): 765–74.

McBride, Patrick E., et al., "Smoking Screening and Management in Primary Care Practices," *Archives of Family Medicine* 6 (1997): 165–72.

McConnell, R. B., K. C. T. Gordon, and Thelwall Jones, "Occupational and Personal Factors in the Aetiology of Carcinoma of the Lung," *Lancet* 2 (1952): 651–56.

McGrady, Pat, *The Savage Cell: A Report on Cancer and Cancer Research* (New York: Basic Books, 1964).

McIsaac, Warren J., David Naylor, and Antoni Basinski, "Mismatch of Coronary Risk and Treatment Intensity under the National Cholesterol Education Program Guidelines," *Journal of General Internal Medicine* 6 (1991): 518–23.

McNamara, J. Judson, et al., "Coronary Artery Disease in Combat Casualties in Vietnam," *JAMA* 216 (1971): 1185–87.

McNutt, Kristen, "Dietary Advice to the Public: 1957 to 1980," *Nutrition Reviews* 38 (1980): 353–60.

Madsen, T., and Sten Madsen, "Diphtheria in Denmark: I. Serum Therapy," *Danish Medical Journal* 3 (1956): 112–21.

Magee, John H., *Life Insurance,* 3rd ed. (Homewood, IL: Irwin, 1958).

Maistrov, L. E., *Probability Theory: A Historical Sketch* (New York: Academic Press, 1974).

Mann, Charles C., "Press Coverage: Leaving Out the Big Picture," *Science* 269 (1995): 166.

Mann, George V., ed., *Coronary Heart Disease: The Dietary Sense and Nonsense* (London: Janus, 1993).

Manton, Kenneth G., and Eric Stallard, *Recent Trends in Mortality Analysis* (Orlando, FL: Academic Press, 1984).

Marchand, Roland, *Advertising the American Dream: Making Way for Modernity, 1920–1940* (Berkeley: University of California Press, 1985).

————, *Creating the Corporate Soul: The Rise of Public Relations and Corporate Imagery in American Big Business* (Berkeley: University of California Press, 1998).

Markowitz, Milton, and Leon Gordis, *Rheumatic Fever,* 2nd ed. (Philadelphia: Saunders, 1972).

Marks, Harry M., *The Progress of Experiment: Science and Therapeutic Reform in the United States, 1900–1990* (Cambridge: Cambridge University Press, 1997).

Marmot, M. G., et al., "Employment Grade and Coronary Heart Disease in British Civil Servants," *Journal of Epidemiology and Community Health* 32 (1978): 244–49.

Marmot, Michael, and Paul Elliott, eds., *Coronary Heart Disease Epidemiology: From Aetiology to Public Health* (Oxford: Oxford University Press, 1992).

Martensen, Robert L., "The Effect of Medical Conservatism on the Acceptance of Important Medical Discoveries," *JAMA* 276 (1996): 1933.

Master, Arthur M., Simon Dack, and Harry L. Jaffe, "The Relation of Effort and Trauma," *Industrial Medicine* 9 (1940): 359–64.

Master, Arthur M., Charles I. Garfield, and Max B. Walters, *Normal Blood Pressure and Hypertension: New Definitions* (Philadelphia: Lea and Febiger, 1952).

Matthews, J. Rosser, *Quantification and the Quest for Medical Certainty* (Princeton: Princeton University Press, 1995).

Maulitz, Russell C., and Diana C. Long, eds., *Grand Rounds: One Hundred Years of Internal Medicine* (Philadelphia: University of Pennsylvania Press 1988).

Mayo, Deborah G., and Rachelle D. Hollander, eds., *Acceptable Evidence: Science and Values in Risk Management* (New York: Oxford University Press, 1991).

McCollum, J. H., "Section on Medicine," *Medical News* 63 (1896): 81–82.

Mead, Franklin B., "Substandard Insurance: Its Evolution and a Review of Some of its Principles," *Record of the American Institute of Actuaries* 11 (1922): 158–86.

Means, Richard K., *A History of Health Education in the United States* (Philadelphia: Lea and Febiger, 1962).

———, *Historical Perspectives on School Health* (Thorofare, NJ: Slack, 1975).

Meckel, Richard A., *Save the Babies: American Public Health Reform and the Prevention of Infant Mortality, 1850–1929* (Baltimore: Johns Hopkins University Press, 1990).

Medical Research Council Working Party, "MRC Trial of Treatment of Mild Hypertension: Principal Results," *British Medical Journal* 291 (1985): 97–104.

———, "Stroke and Coronary Heart Disease in Mild Hypertension: Risk Factors and the Value of Treatment," *British Medical Journal* 296 (1988): 1565–70.

Meltzer, Lawrence E., and Arend J. Dunning, eds., *Textbook of Coronary Care* (Philadelphia: Charles Press, 1972).

Merz, Beverly, "Low-Fat Diet May be Imprudent for Some, Say Opponents of Population-Based Cholesterol Control," *JAMA* 256 (1986): 2779–80.

The Metropolitan Life Insurance Company, *Educating for Longer Life* (New York: 1928).

———, *An Epoch in Life Insurance: A Third of a Century of Achievement,* 2nd ed. (New York: Metropolitan Life Insurance Company, 1924).

———, *Greater New York Directory: Metropolitan Visiting Nurse Service* (New York: 1940s?).

———, *The Metropolitan Life Insurance Company: Its History, Its Present Position in the Insurance World, Its Home Office Building and its Work Carried on Therein* (New York: Metropolitan Life Insurance Company, 1914).

———, *The Mortality from the Principal Cardiovascular-Renal Diseases: A Study of the Experience Among the Industrial Policyholders of the Metropolitan Life Insurance Company 1911 to 1930,* Monograph 4 (New York: Metropolitan Life Insurance Company, 1938?).

———, *Nursing Manual,* revised ed. (New York: Metropolitan Life Insurance Company, 1937).

"Metropolitan Life Insurance Company," *Fortune* 10 (Aug. 1934): 48ff.

"Metropolitan Life Makes Housing Pay," *Fortune* (April 1946): 133ff.

Meyer, Ernst C., *Infant Mortality in New York City* (New York: 1921).

Miall, W. E. and Gillian Greenberg, *Mild Hypertension: Is There Pressure to Treat?* (Cambridge: Cambridge University Press, 1987).

Michaels, L., "Aetiology of Coronary Artery Disease: An Historical Approach," *British Heart Journal* 28 (1966): 258–64.

Miles, Robert H., *Coffin Nails and Corporate Strategies* (Englewood Cliffs, NJ: Prentice-Hall, 1982).

Miller, David C., et al., "The Community Problem in Coronary Heart Disease: A Challenge for Epidemiologic Research," *American Journal of the Medical Sciences* n.s. 232 (1956): 329–59.

Miller, Genevieve, *The Adoption of Inoculation for Smallpox in England and France* (Philadelphia: University of Pennsylvania Press, 1957) .

Miller, Sanford A., and Marilyn G. Stephenson, "Scientific and Public Health Rationale for the Dietary Guidelines for Americans," *American Journal of Clinical Nutrition* 42 (1985): 739–45.

Mishler, Elliot G., et al., *Social Contexts of Health, Illness, and Patient Care* (Cambridge: Cambridge University Press, 1981).

Mitchell, J. R., "Anticoagulants in Coronary Heart Disease: Retrospect and Prospect," *Lancet* 1 (1981): 257–62.

Mitchell, Robert B., *From Actuarius to Actuary: The Growth of a Dynamic Profession in the Canada and the United States* (n.p.: Society of Actuaries, 1974).

Moch, Leslie P., *Moving Europeans: Migration in Western Europe Since 1650* (Bloomington: Indiana University Press, 1992).

Moore, Harry H., *Public Health in the United States* (New York: Harper, 1923).

Moore, Thomas J., "The Cholesterol Myth," *Atlantic Monthly* 264 (Sept. 1989): 37ff.

Moore, William W., *Fighting for Life: The Story of the American Heart Association 1911—1975* (n.p.: American Heart Association, 1983).

Morgan, A. D., "Some Forms of Undiagnosed Coronary Disease in Nineteenth Century England," *Medical History* 12 (1968): 344–58.

Morgan, W. Keith and Anthony Seaton, *Occupational Lung Diseases,* 3rd ed. (Philadelphia: Saunders, 1995).

Moriyama, Iwao M. "Development of the Present Concept of Cause of Death," *American Journal of Public Health* 46 (1956): 436–41.

———, "Factors in Diagnosis and Classification of Deaths from CVR Diseases," *Public Health Reports* 75 (1960): 189–95.

Moriyama, Iwao M., Dean E. Krueger, and Jeremiah Stamler, *Cardiovascular Diseases in the United States* (Cambridge, MA: Harvard University Press, 1971).

"Mortality Among Overweight Men," *Statistical Bulletin* 41 (Feb. 1960): 6–10 .

"Mortality Among Overweight Women," *Statistical Bulletin* 41 (Mar. 1960): 1–4.

"Mortality in the First Month of Life According to Nativity of Mother" *Statistical Bulletin* 4 (Dec. 1923): 7–8.

"Mortality of Overweights with Impairments," *Statistical Bulletin* 41 (May 1960): 3–6.

Multhauf, Robert P., *Neptune's Gift: A History of Common Salt* (Baltimore, MD: Johns Hopkins University Press, 1978).

Multiple Risk Factor Intervention Trial Research Group, "Mortality Rates after 10.5 Years for Participants in the Multiple Risk Factor Intervention Trial," *JAMA* 263 (1990): 1795–1801.

———, "Multiple Risk Factor Intervention Trial," *JAMA* 248 (1982): 1465–77.

Muntzel, Martin and Tilman Drueke, "A Comprehensive Review of the Salt and Blood Pressure Relationship," *American Journal of Hypertension* 5, suppl. (April 1992): 1S–42S.

Myers, Martin G., et al., "Recommendations from the Canadian Hypertension Society Consensus Conference on the Pharmacologic Treatment of Hypertension," *Canadian Medical Association Journal* 140 (1989): 1141–46.

National Center for Health Statistics, *Health United States* (Hyattsville, MD: various years).

National Heart and Lung Institute Task Force on Arteriosclerosis, *Arteriosclerosis* (Washington, DC: U.S. GPO, 1971).

National Research Council, *Science and Judgment in Risk Assessment* (Washington, DC: National Academy Press, 1994).

National Research Council, National Academy of Sciences, *The Role of Dietary Fat in Human Health* (Washington, DC, 1958).

National Research Council Committee on Diet and Health, *Diet and Health: Implications for Reducing Chronic Disease Risk* (Washington, DC: National Academy Press, 1989).

National Research Council Food and Nutrition Board, *Dietary Fat and Human Health* (Washington, DC: National Academy of Sciences, 1966).

Neaton, James D., et al., "Total and Cardiovascular Mortality in Relation to Cigarette Smoking, Serum Cholesterol Concentration, and Diastolic Blood Pressure Among Black and White Males Followed up for Five Years," *American Heart Journal* 108 (1984): 759–69.

———, "The Treatment of Mild Hypertension Study: Final Results," *JAMA* 270 (1993): 713–24.

Nestle, Marion, *Food Politics: How the Food Industry Influences Nutrition and Health* (Berkeley: University of California Press, 2002).

Neuberger, Maurine B., *Smoke Screen: Tobacco and the Public Welfare* (Englewood Cliffs, NJ: Prentice-Hall, 1963).

"The 1988 Report of the Joint National Committee on Detection, Evaluation, and Treatment of High Blood Pressure," *Archives of Internal Medicine* 148 (1988): 1023–38.

Nordenfelt, Lennart, and Ingemar B. Lindahl, eds., *Health, Disease, and Causal Explanations in Medicine* (Dordrecht: Reidel, 1984).

Norris, George W., *Blood-Pressure: Its Clinical Applications* (Philadelphia: Lea and Febiger, 1914).

Norris, George W., Henry C. Bazett, Thomas M. McMillan, *Blood-Pressure: Its Clinical Applications,* 4th ed. (Philadelphia: Lea and Febiger, 1927).

Norris, James D., *Advertising and the Transformation of American Society, 1865–1920* (New York: Greenwood Press, 1990).

Ockene, Ira S., and Judith K. Ockene, eds., *Prevention of Coronary Heart Disease* (Boston: Little, Brown, 1992).

O'Keefe, Colleen E., Donna F. Hahn, Nancy M. Betts, "Physicians' Perspectives on Cholesterol and Heart Disease," *Journal of the American Dietetic Association* 91 (Feb., 1991): 189–92.

Oliver, Michael, Michael Ashley-Miller, and David Wood, eds., *Screening for Risk of Coronary Heart Disease* (Chichester: Wiley, 1987).

Osler, William, *The Principles and Practice of Medicine*, 8th ed. (New York: Appleton, 1914).

"Overweight Shortens Life" *Statistical Bulletin* 32 (Oct. 1951): 1–4.

"Overweights Benefit from Weight Reduction," *Statistical Bulletin* 41 (Apr. 1960): 1–3.

Page, Irvine H., et al., "Atherosclerosis and the Fat Content of the Diet," *Circulation* 16 (1957): 163–78.

Park, William H., "The History of Diphtheria in New York City," *American Journal of Diseases of Children* 42 (1931): 1439–46.

Park, William H., and Alfred L. Beebe, "Diphtheria and Pseudo-Diphtheria," *Medical Record* 46 (1894): 385–401.

Parrish, Henry M., "Epidemiology of Ischemic Heart Disease Among White Males, II: Autopsy Incidence of Ischemic Heart Disease and Autopsy Prevalence of Coronary Atherosclerosis," *Journal of Chronic Diseases* 14 (1961): 326–38.

Patterson, James T., *The Dread Disease: Cancer and Modern American Culture* (Cambridge, MA: Harvard University Press, 1987).

Paul, John R., *The Epidemiology of Rheumatic Fever* (New York: Metropolitan Life Insurance Company, 1930).

———, *The Epidemiology of Rheumatic Fever*, 3rd ed. (New York: American Heart Association, 1957).

———, *A History of Poliomyelitis* (New Haven: Yale University Press, 1971).

Pearson, Karl, *The Fight Against Tuberculosis and the Death-rate from Phthisis* (London: Cambridge University Press, 1911).

Pell, Sidney, and C. Anthony D'Alonzo, "Acute Myocardial Infarction in a Large Industrial Population," *JAMA* 185 (1963): 831–38.

Pell, Sidney, and William Fayerweather, "Trends in the Incidence of Myocardial Infarction and in Associated Mortality and Morbidity in a Large Employed Population, 1957–1983," *New England Journal of Medicine* 312 (1985): 1005–11.

Perrot. Jean-Claude, and Stuart J. Woolf, *State and Statistics in France, 1789–1815* (Chur, Switzerland: Harwood Academic Publishers, 1984) .

Pickering, George W., *High Blood Pressure* (New York: Grune and Stratton, 1955) .

———, *The Nature of Essential Hypertension* (New York: Grune and Stratton, 1961).

———, "Normotension and Hypertension: The Mysterious Viability of the False," *American Journal of Medicine* 65 (1983): 561–63.

———, "Salt Intake and Essential Hypertension," *Cardiovascular Reviews and Reports* 1 (April 1980): 13–17.

Plunz, Richard, *A History of Housing in New York City: Dwelling Type and Social Change in the American Metropolis* (New York: Columbia University Press, 1990).

Pope, Daniel, *The Making of Modern Advertising* (New York: Basic Books, 1983).

Popkin, Barry M., Anna M. Siega-Riz, and Pamela S. Haines, "A Comparison of Dietary Trends Among Racial and Socioeconomic Groups in the United States," *New England Journal of Medicine* 335 (1996): 716–20.

Porter, Donna V., "Health Claims on Food Products: NLEA," *Nutrition Today* 31 (Jan.–Feb. 1996): 35–38.

Porter, Theodore M., *The Rise of Statistical Thinking: 1820–1900* (Princeton, NJ: Princeton University Press, 1986) .

————, *Trust in Numbers: The Pursuit of Objectivity in Science and Public Policy* (Princeton, NJ: Princeton University Press, 1995).

Presbrey, Frank, *The History and Development of Advertising* (1929; New York: Greenwood, 1968).

President's Commission on Heart Disease, Cancer and Stroke, *Report to the President: A National Program to Conquer Heart Disease, Cancer and Stroke,* 2 vols. (Washington, DC: US GPO, 1965).

Preventive Medicine USA (New York: Prodist, 1976).

Proctor, Robert N., *Cancer Wars: How Politics Shapes What We Know and Don't Know About Cancer* (New York: Basic Books, 1995).

Prospective Studies Collaboration, "Cholesterol, Diastolic Blood Pressure, and Stroke," *Lancet* 346 (1995): 1647–53.

Quetelet, Lambert A. J., *A Treatise on Man and the Development of His Faculties* (Gainesville, FL: Scholars' Facsimiles and Reprints, 1969) .

Rabkin, S. W., F. A. Mathewson, and R. B. Tate, "Relationship of Blood Pressure in 20–39–Year-Old Men to Subsequent Blood Pressure and Incidence of Hypertension over a 30–year Period," *Circulation* 65 (1982): 291–300.

Ragland, Kathleen E., Steve Selvin, and Deane W. Merrill, "The Onset of Decline in Ischemic Heart Disease Mortality in the United States," *American Journal of Epidemiology* 127 (1988): 516–31.

Ramsay, L. E., W. W. Yeo, P. R. Jackson, "Dietary Reduction of Serum Cholesterol Concentration: Time to Think Again," *British Medical Journal* 303 (1991): 953–57.

Ramsey, Lawrence E., et al., "Interpretation of Prospective Trials in Hypertension: Do Treatment Guidelines Accurately Reflect Current Evidence?" *Journal of Hypertension* 14, suppl. 5 (1996): S187–94.

"Rationale of the Diet-Heart Statement of the American Heart Association," *Arteriosclerosis* 2 (1982): 177–91.

Raucher, Alan R., *Public Relations and Business, 1900–1929* (Baltimore: Johns Hopkins Press, 1968).

Ravenel, Mazyck P., ed., *A Half Century of Public Health* (1921; New York: Arno Press, 1970).

Ravnskov, U., "Cholesterol Lowering Trials in Coronary Heart Disease: Frequency of Citation and Outcome," *British Medical Journal* 305 (1992): 15–19.

"Recent Trends in Mortality from Cardiovascular Diseases," *Statistical Bulletin* 60 (April–June 1979): 2–8.

"Recent Trends in Mortality from Heart Disease," *Statistical Bulletin* 56 (June 1975): 2–6 .

Reiser, Raymond, "A Commentary on the Rationale of the Diet-Heart Statement of the American Heart Association," *American Journal of Clinical Nutrition* 40 (1984): 654–58.

"A Report of a Study of the Effect of the Termination of Metropolitan Nursing Contracts," *Public Health Nursing* 43 (1951): 285–93.

"Report of the National Cholesterol Education Program Expert Panel on Detection, Evaluation, and Treatment of High Blood Cholesterol in Adults," *Archives of Internal Medicine* 148 (1988): 1023–38.

Report of the President's Committee on Health Education (New York, 1973).

"Rheumatic Fever a Major Health Problem Today," *Statistical Bulletin* 23 (Sept. 1942): 2–5.

Robbins, Jessica M., "Class Struggles in the Tubercular World: Nurses, Patients, and Physicians, 1903–1915," *Bulletin of the History of Medicine* 71 (1997): 412–34.

Roberts, James C., Jr., and Reuben Straus, eds., *Comparative Atherosclerosis* (New York: Hoeber, 1965).

Roberts, Peter, *The New Immigration* (1912; New York: Arno Press, 1970).

Robinson, Corinne H., et al., *Normal and Therapeutic Nutrition,* 17th ed. (New York: Macmillan, 1986).

Robinson Samuel C., and Marshall Brucer, "Range of Normal Blood Pressure" *Archives of Internal Medicine* 64 (1939): 409–44.

Rogot, Eugene, and Zdenek Hrubec, "Trends in Mortality from Coronary Heart Disease and Stroke Among U.S. Veterans, 1954–79," *Journal of Clinical Epidemiology* 42 (1989): 245–56.

Rosen, George. "Problems in the Application of Statistical Analysis to Questions of Health: 1700–1880," *Bulletin of the History of Medicine* 29 (1955): 27–45.

———, "Urbanization, Occupation and Disease in the United States, 1870–1920: The Case of New York City," *Journal of the History of Medicine* 43 (1988): 391–425.

Rosenblatt, Roger A., et al., "The Content of Ambulatory Care in the United States: An Interspecialty Comparison," *New England Journal of Medicine* 309 (1983): 892–97.

Rosner, David, ed., *Hives of Sickness: Public Health and Epidemics in New York City* (New Brunswick, NJ: Rutgers University Press, 1995).

Ross, Walter S., *Crusade: The Official History of the American Cancer Society* (New York: Arbor House, 1987).

Rothman, David, *Beginnings Count: The Technological Imperative in American Health Care* (New York: Oxford University Press, 1997).

Rothman, Kenneth J., "A Show of Confidence," *New England Journal of Medicine* 299 (1978): 1362–63.

Rothstein, William G., *American Medical Schools and the Practice of Medicine: A History* (New York: Oxford University Press, 1987).

Rushefsky, Mark E., *Making Cancer Policy* (Albany: State University of New York Press, 1986).

Ruskin, Arthur, ed., *Classics in Arterial Hypertension* (Springfield, IL: Thomas, 1956).

Rusnock, Andrea A., "The Quantification of Things Human: Medicine and Political Arithmetic in Enlightenment England and France" (Ph.D. dissertation, Princeton University, 1990).

Ryle, John A., and W. T. Russell, "The Natural History of Coronary Disease," *British Heart Journal* 11 (1949): 370–89.

Samet, Jonathan M., ed. *Epidemiology of Lung Cancer* (New York: Dekker, 1994).

Saywell, Robert M., Jr., et al., "Indiana Family Physician Attitudes and Practices Concerning Smoking Cessation," *Indiana Medicine* 89 (1996): 149–56.

Schucker, Beth, et al., "Change in Cholesterol Awareness and Action," *Archives of Internal Medicine* 151 (1991): 666–73.

———, "Change in Physician Perspective on Cholesterol and Heart Disease: Results from Two National Surveys," *JAMA* 258 (1987): 3521–26.

Segall, Harold N., "Quest for Korotkoff," *Journal of Hypertension* 3 (1985): 317–26.

Seltzer, Carl C., and Seymour Jablon, "Army Rank and Subsequent Mortality By Cause: 23-Year Follow-up," *American Journal of Epidemiology* 105 (1977): 559–66.

Shannon, Gary W., and Gerald F. Pyle, *Disease and Medical Care in the United States: A Medical Atlas of the Twentieth Century* (New York: Macmillan, 1993).

Shapiro, Sam, Edward R. Schlesinger, and Robert E. Nesbitt, Jr., *Infant, Perinatal, Maternal, and Childhood Mortality in the United States* (Cambridge, MA: Harvard University Press, 1968).

Shekelle, Richard B., et al., "Diet, Serum Cholesterol, and Death from Coronary Heart Disease: The Western Electric Study," *New England Journal of Medicine* 304 (1981): 65–70.

Shepherd, James, et al., "Prevention of Coronary Heart Disease with Pravastatin in Men with Hypercholesterolemia," *New England Journal of Medicine* 333 (1995): 1301–7.

Sherman, Debra L., and Thomas J. Ryan, "Coronary Angioplasty versus Bypass Grafting: Cost Benefit Considerations," *Medical Clinics of North America* 79 (1995): 1085–95.

Sherman, May, *Rheumatic Fever and Rheumatic Heart Disease: A Review of Research Grants Supported By the National Heart Institute 1949 to 1966* (Bethesda, MD: National Institutes of Health, 1966).

Sherry, Sol, "The Origin of Thrombolytic Therapy," *Journal of the American College of Cardiology* 14 (1989): 1085–92.

———, "Revisiting the Development of Thrombolytic Therapy: An Historical Perspective," *Transactions and Studies of the College of Physicians of Philadelphia,* ser. 5, vol. 11 (1989): 337–54.

Shevchenko, Yury L., and Joshua E. Tsitlik, "90th Anniversary of the Development By Nikolai S. Korotkoff of the Auscultatory Method of Measuring Blood Pressure," *Circulation* 94 (1996): 116–18.

Shils, Maurice E., James A. Olson, and Moshe Shike, eds., *Modern Nutrition in Health and Disease,* 8th ed. (Philadelphia: Lea and Febiger, 1994).

Siemiatycki, Jack, ed. *Risk Factors for Cancer in the Workplace* (Boca Raton, FL: CRC Press, 1991).

Sigurdsson, Emil, et al., "Unrecognized Myocardial infarction: Epidemiology, Clinical Characteristics, and the Prognostic Role of Angina Pectoris: The Reykjavik Study," *Annals of Internal Medicine* 122 (1995): 96–102 .

"The Sixth Report of the Joint National Committee on Detection, Evaluation, and Treatment of High Blood Pressure," *Archives of Internal Medicine* 157 (1997): 2413–46.

Skolbekken, John-Arne, "The Risk Epidemic in Medical Journals," *Social Science and Medicine* 40 (1995): 291–305.

Skyler, Jay. S., "Walter Kempner: A Biographical Note," *Archives of Internal Medicine* 133 (1974): 752–755.

Slattery Martha L., and D. Elizabeth Randall, "Trends in Coronary Heart Disease Mortality and Food Consumption in the United States Between 1909 and 1980," *American Journal of Clinical Nutrition* 47 (1988): 1060–7.

"The Slowness with Which Important Medical Discoveries are Generally Put to Practical Use," *JAMA* 276 (1996): 1932 [originally in *Journal of the American Medical Association* 27 (1896): 1210–11].

Smith, F. B., *The People's Health: 1830–1910* (New York: Holmes and Meier, 1979).

Smith, G. R., ed., Topley and Wilson's *Principles of Bacteriology, Virology and Immunology,* 7th ed. (Baltimore: Williams and Wilkens, 1983–84).

Smith, George D., et al., "Plasma Cholesterol Concentration and Mortality: The Whitehall Study," *JAMA* 267 (1992): 70–76.

Snow, John, *Snow on Cholera* (New York: Commonwealth Fund, 1936).

Solberg, Lars A., and Jack P. Strong, "Risk Factors and Atherosclerotic Lesions: A Review of Autopsy Studies," *Arteriosclerosis* 3 (1983): 187–98.

Solomon, Caren G., and JoAnne E. Manson, "Obesity and Mortality: A Review of the Epidemiologic Data," *American Journal of Clinical Nutrition* 66, suppl. (1997): 1044S–50S.

Solomon, Henry A., *The Exercise Myth* (San Diego: Harcourt Brace Jovanovich, 1984).

Spain, David M., and Victoria A. Bradess, "The Relationship of Coronary Thrombosis to Coronary Atherosclerosis and Ischemic Heart Disease," *American Journal of the Medical Sciences* 240 (1960): 701–10.

Speck, Reinhard S., "Cholera," in *The Cambridge World History of Human Disease,* ed. Kenneth F. Kiple (Cambridge: Cambridge University Press, 1993).

Spodick, David H., "Revascularization of the Heart: Numerators in Search of Denominators," *American Heart Journal* 81 (1971): 149–57.

Stallones, Reuel A., "Mortality Due to Ischemic Heart Disease: Observations and Explanations," *Atherosclerosis Reviews* 9 (1982): 43–52.

Stamler, Jeremiah, Rose Stamler, and Theodore N. Pullman, eds. *The Epidemiology of Hypertension* (New York: Grune and Stratton, 1967).

Stare, Frederick J., Robert E. Olson, and Elizabeth M. Whelan, *Balanced Nutrition: Beyond the Cholesterol Scare* (Holbrook, MA: Bob Adams, 1989).

Stead, Eugene A., "Walter Kempner: A Perspective," *Archives of Internal Medicine* 133 (1974): 756–57.

Stearns, Peter N., *Fat History: Bodies and Beauty in the Modern West* (New York: New York University Press, 1997).

Stella, Antonio, "The Effects of Urban Congestion on Italian Women and Children," *Medical Record* 73 (1908): 722–32.

Stephen, Alison M., and Nicholas J. Wald, "Trends in Individual Consumption of Dietary Fat in the United States, 1920–1984," *American Journal of Clinical Nutrition* 52 (1990): 457–69.

Stern, Paul C., and Harvey V. Fineberg, eds., *Understanding Risk: Informing Decisions in a Democratic Society* (Washington, DC: National Academy Press, 1996).

Stigler, Stephen M., *The History of Statistics: The Measurement of Uncertainty before 1900* (Cambridge, MA: Harvard University Press, 1986) .

Stillings, Bruce R., "Trends in Foods," *Nutrition Today* 29 (Sept.–Oct. 1994): 6–13.

Stollerman, Gene H., "Rheumatic Fever," *Lancet* 349 (1997): 935–42.

Strasser, Susan, *Satisfaction Guaranteed: The Making of the American Mass Market* (New York: Pantheon, 1989).

Strong, Jack P., "Coronary Atherosclerosis in Soldiers: A Clue to the Natural History of Atherosclerosis in the Young," *JAMA* 256 (1986): 2863–74.

Stroud, William D., ed., *The Diagnosis and Treatment of Cardiovascular Disease,* 4th ed. (Philadelphia: Davis, 1950).

Sullivan, Jay M., "Salt Sensitivity: Definition, Conception, Methodology, and Long-Term Issues," *Hypertension* 17 Supp. 1 (1991): I-61–68.

"Summary of 1993 World Health Organization-International Society of Hypertension Guidelines for the Management of Mild Hypertension," *BMJ* 307 (1993): 1541–46.

"Survivorship after Recovery from Disability Due to Heart Disease," *Statistical Bulletin* 35 (Feb. 1954): 4–6.

"Survivorship in Heart Disease," *Statistical Bulletin* 31 (Sept. 1950): 8–10 .

Susser, Mervyn, *Causal Thinking in the Health Sciences* (New York: Oxford University Press, 1973).

Swales, J. D., ed., *Platt Versus Pickering: An Episode in Recent Medical History* (n.p.: Keynes Press, 1985).

Swartout, H. O., and Robert G. Webster, "To What Degree Are Mortality Statistics Dependable?" *American Journal of Public Health* 30 (1940): 811–15.

Symonds, Brandreth, "The Blood Pressure of Healthy Men and Women," *Journal of the American Medical Association* 80 (1923): 232–36.

A Symposium on Essential Hypertension: An Epidemiologic Approach to the Elucidation of its Natural History in Man (Boston, 1951).

Tannahill, Reay, *Food in History,* 2rd ed. (New York: Crown, 1988).

Taranta, Angelo, and Milton Markowitz, *Rheumatic Fever,* 2rd ed. (Dordrecht: Kluwer, 1989).

Taylor, Peter, *The Smoke Ring: Tobacco, Money, and Multinational Politics* (New York: Pantheon, 1984).

Taylor, Philip, *The Distant Magnet: European Emigration to the U.S.A.* (New York: Harper and Row, 1971).

Taubes, Gary, "Looking for the Evidence in Medicine," *Science* 272 (1996): 22–24 .

Teaford, Jon C., *The Unheralded Triumph: City Government in America, 1870–1900* (Baltimore: Johns Hopkins University Press, 1984).

Tedlow, Richard S., *Keeping the Corporate Image: Public Relations and Business, 1900–1950* (Greenwich, CT: JAI Press, 1979).

Teller, Michael E., *The Tuberculosis Movement: A Public Health Campaign in the Progressive Era* (New York: Greenwood, 1988).

Thom, Thomas J., "International Mortality from Heart Disease: Rates and Trends," *International Journal of Epidemiology* 18, suppl. 1 (1989): S20–S28.

Thomas, William I., *Old World Traits Transplanted* (1921; Montclair, NJ: Patterson Smith, 1971).

Thompson, W. Gilman, *The Occupational Diseases: Their Causation, Symptoms, Treatment, and Prevention* (New York: Appleton, 1914).

Thorndike, Anne N., et al., "National Patterns in the Treatment of Smokers by Physicians," *JAMA* 279 (1998): 604–8.

Tobacco and the Clinician: Interventions for Medical and Dental Practice, Monograph no. 5 (n.p.: National Institutes of Health, 1994).

Treatment of Mild Hypertension Research Group, "The Treatment of Mild Hypertension," *Archives of Internal Medicine* 151 (1991): 1413–23.

Trowell H. C., and D. P. Burkitt, eds., *Western Diseases: Their Emergence and Prevention* (Cambridge, MA: Harvard University Press, 1981).

Truswell, A. Stewart, "Evolution of Dietary Recommendations, Goals, and Guidelines," *American Journal of Clinical Nutrition* 45 (1987): 1060–72.

"12 American Health Heroes," *Health Bulletin for Teachers,* 1943–46, Vols. 15, 16, 17.

Uemura, Kazuo, and Zbynek Pisa, "Trends in Cardiovascular Disease Mortality in Industrialized Countries Since 1950," *World Health Statistics Quarterly* 41 (1988): 155–78.

Ungerleider, Harry E., and Richard S. Gubner, *Life Insurance and Medicine: The Prognosis and Underwriting of Disease* (Springfield, IL: Thomas, 1958).

U.S. Bureau of the Census, *A Century of Population Growth: From the First Census of the United States to the Twelfth, 1790–1900* (Washington, DC: 1909) .

———, *Historical Statistics of the United States, Colonial Times to 1970* (Washington, DC: 1975).

————, *Mortality Statistics, 1907,* 8th Annual Report (Washington, DC: 1909).

————, *Mortality Statistics, 1908,* 9th Annual Report (Washington, DC: 1910).

U.S. Children's Bureau, *Birth Registration: An Aid in Protecting the Lives and Rights of Children; Necessity for Extending the Registration Area,* Monograph No. 1 (Washington, DC: 1913).

————, *Proceedings of Conference on Rheumatic Fever,* Publication No. 308 (Washington, DC: 1945).

U.S. Department of Labor, *Proceedings of Conference on Rheumatic Fever, 1943,* Children's Bureau Publication 308 (Washington, DC: 1944).

U.S. House of Representatives Committee on Energy and Commerce, Subcommittee on Health and the Environment, *Hearing on Cholesterol Education Program,* 101st Congress, 1st sess., Dec. 7, 1989, serial No. 101–107 (Washington, DC: 1990).

U.S. National Clearing House for Smoking and Health, *The Health Consequences of Smoking: A Public Health Service Review: 1967* (Washington, DC: U.S. Public Health Service, 1968).

————, *The Health Consequences of Smoking: A Public Health Service Review: 1968 supplement to the 1967 Public Health Service Review* (Washington, DC: U.S. Public Health Service, 1968).

————, *The Health Consequences of Smoking: A Report of the Surgeon General: 1971* (Washington, DC: U.S. Public Health Service, 1971).

U.S. Public Health Service, *The Health Consequences of Involuntary Smoking: A Report of the Surgeon General* (Rockville, MD: U.S. Public Health Service, 1986).

U.S. Senate Select Committee on Nutrition and Human Needs, *Dietary Goals for the United States,* 2nd ed. (Washington, DC: 1977).

————, *Dietary Goals for the United States–Supplemental Views,* 95th Congress, 1st sess. (Washington, DC: 1977).

————, *Hearings,* 90th Congress, 2nd sess., and 91st Congress, 1st sess. (Washington, DC: 1969).

U.S. Senate Subcommittee of the Committee on Labor and Public Welfare, *Hearings on National Heart Institute S.720 and S. 2215,* April 8–9, 1948, 80th Congress, 2d sess. (Washington, DC: 1948).

U.S. Surgeon General, *The Surgeon General's Report on Nutrition and Health, 1988* (Washington, DC: Public Health Service, 1988).

U.S. Surgeon General's Advisory Committee on Smoking and Health, *Smoking and Health* (Washington, DC: U.S. Department of Health, Education, and Welfare, 1964).

"Untreated Mild Hypertension: A Report by the Management Committee of the Australian Therapeutic Trial in Mild Hypertension," *Lancet* 1 (1982): 185–91.

van Stuyvenberg, J. H., ed., *Margarine: An Economic, Social and Scientific History 1869–1969* (Toronto: University of Toronto Press, 1969).

Verrett, Jacqueline, and Jean Carper, *Eating May be Hazardous to your Health* (Garden City, NY: Anchor, 1975).

Veterans Administration Cooperative Study Group on Antihypertensive Agents, "Effects of Treatment on Morbidity in Hypertension," *JAMA* 202 (1967): 116–22 .

————, "Effects of Treatment on Morbidity in Hypertension II," *JAMA* 213 (1970): 1143–52.

de Ville, Kenneth Allen, *Medical Malpractice in Nineteenth Century America: Origins and Legacy* (New York: New York University Press, 1990).

Vinikas, Vincent, *Soft Soap, Hard Sell: American Hygiene in an Age of Advertisement* (Ames: Iowa State University Press, 1992).

Wade, Nicholas, "Food Board's Fat Report Hits Fire," *Science* 209 (1980): 248–50.

Wagner, Susan, *Cigarette Country: Tobacco in American History and Politics* (New York: Praeger, 1971).

Walker, Charles, Leroy C. Gould, and Edward J. Woodhouse, eds., *Too Hot to Handle? Social and Policy Issues in the Management of Radioactive Wastes* (New Haven, CT: Yale University Press, 1983).

Ware, Caroline F., *Greenwich Village, 1920–1930* (1935; New York: Octagon, 1977).

Warner, Kenneth E., *Selling Smoke: Cigarette Advertising and Public Health* (Washington, DC: American Public Health Association, 1986).

———, "Tobacco Industry Scientific Advisors: Serving Society or Selling Cigarettes?" *American Journal of Public Health* 81 (1991): 839–42.

Watson, William T., "Personal Experience with Laryngeal Diphtheria," *Maryland Medical Journal* 36 (1897): 241–47.

Wechsler, Henry, et al., "The Physician's Role in Health Promotion: A Survey of Primary-Care Practitioners," *New England Journal of Medicine* 308 (1983): 97–100.

Weinblatt, Eve, et al., "Mortality after First Myocardial Infarction: Search for a Secular Trend," *JAMA* 247 (1982): 1576–81.

Weissler, Arnold M., Brian I. Miller, and Harisios Boudoulas, "The Need for Clarification of Percent Risk Reduction Data in Clinical Cardiovascular Trial Reports," *Journal of the American College of Cardiology* 13 (1989): 764–66.

Weisz, George "Academic Debate and Therapeutic Reasoning in Mid-19th Century France," in *Medicine and Change: Historical and Sociological Studies of Medical Innovation,* ed. Ilana Lowy (Paris: John Libby Eurotext, 1993), 287–315.

Wellford, Harrison, *Sowing the Wind* (New York: Bantam, 1973).

Whelan, Elizabeth M., *A Smoking Gun: How the Tobacco Industry Gets Away with Murder* (Philadelphia: Stickley, 1984).

White, Kerr L., *Healing the Schism: Epidemiology, Medicine, and the Public's Health* (New York: Springer-Verlag, 1991).

White, Paul Dudley, *Heart Disease* (New York: Macmillan, 1931).

———, *Heart Disease,* 3rd ed. (New York: Macmillan, 1944).

———, "The Incidence of Heart Disease in Massachusetts," *Boston Medical and Surgical Journal* 196 (1927): 689–93.

———, *My Life and Medicine: An Autobiographical Memoir* (Boston: Gambit, 1971).

Whiteside, Thomas, *Selling Death: Cigarette Advertising and Public Health* (New York: Liveright, 1971).

Wilkening, Virginia L., "FDA's Regulations to Implement the NLEA," *Nutrition Today* 31 (Sept.–Oct. 1993): 13–20.

Willcox, Walter F., *Studies in American Demography* (1940; New York: Russell and Russell, 1971).

Williams, David R., and Chiquita Collins, "U.S. Socioeconomic and Racial Differences in Health: Patterns and Explanations," *Annual Review of Sociology* 21 (1995): 349–86.

Willis, R. A., *Pathology of Tumours* (St. Louis, MO: Mosby, 1948).

Wilson, Martha D., and Lawrence L. Rudel, "Review of Cholesterol Absorption with Emphasis on Dietary and Biliary Cholesterol," *Journal of Lipid Research* 35 (1994): 943–55.

Wilson, May G., Wan N. Lim, and Ann M. Birch, "The Decline of Rheumatic Fever," *Journal of Chronic Diseases* 7 (1958): 183–94.

Winslow, C.-E. A., *The Health of the Worker: Dangers to Health in the Factory and Shop and How to Avoid Them* (New York: Metropolitan Life Insurance Company, 1913).

———, *The Life of Hermann M. Biggs: Physician and Statesman of the Public Health* (Philadelphia: Lea and Febiger, 1929).

Winslow, C.-E. A., and Savel Zimand, *Health under the "El"* (New York: Harper, 1937).

Winters, J. E., "Comment," in John W. Brannon, "Observations of Antitoxine in Diphtheria" *New York Medical Journal* 63 (1896): 222–24.

Witts, L. J., ed., *Medical Surveys and Clinical Trials,* 2nd ed. (London: Oxford University Press, 1964).

Wolinsky, Howard, and Tom Brune, *The Serpent on the Staff: The Unhealthy Politics of the American Medical Association* (New York: Putnam, 1994).

Woodbury, Robert M., *Causal Factors in Infant Mortality: A Statistical Investigation based on Investigations in Eight Cities,* U.S. Children's Bureau Publication No. 142 (Washington, DC: 1925).

Woolsley, Theodore D., and I. M. Moriyama, "Statistical Studies of Heart Disease: II. Important Factors in Heart Disease Mortality Trends," *Public Health Reports* 63 (1948): 1247–73.

Working Party of the British Cardiac Society, "Coronary Angioplasty in the United Kingdom," *British Heart Journal* 66 (1991): 325–31.

Wright, Carroll D., *The History and Growth of the United States Census* (1900; New York: Johnson Reprint Corp., 1966).

Wulff, Henrik R., *Rational Diagnosis and Treatment: An Introduction to Clinical Decision-Making,* 2nd ed. (Oxford: Blackwell, 1981).

Wyman, Mark, *Round-Trip to America: The Immigrants Return to Europe, 1880–1930* (Ithaca, NY: Cornell University Press, 1993).

Wynder, Ernst L. "Tobacco and Health: A Review of the History and Suggestions for Public Health Policy," *Public Health Reports* 103 (1988): 8–18.

———, "Tobacco as a Cause of Lung Cancer," *Pennsylvania Medical Journal* 57 (1954): 1073–83.

Wynder, Ernst L., and Evarts A. Graham, "Tobacco Smoking as a Possible Etiologic Factor in Bronchiogenic Carcinoma," *JAMA* 143 (1950): 329–36 .

Wysowski, Diane K., Dianne L. Kennedy, and Thomas P. Gross, "Prescribed Use of Cholesterol-Lowering Drugs in the United States 1978 through 1988," *JAMA* 263 (1990): 2185–88 .

Yans-McLaughlin, Virginia, *Immigration Reconsidered: History, Sociology, and Politics* (New York: Oxford University Press, 1990).

Yerushalmy, J., and Herman E. Hilleboe, "Fat in the Diet and Mortality from Heart Disease," *New York State Journal of Medicine* 57 (1957): 2343–54.

Yusuf, S., et al., "Intravenous and Intracoronary Fibrinolytic Therapy in Acute Myocardial Infarction," *European Heart Journal* 6 (1985): 556–85.

Zukel, William J., Oglesby Paul, and Harold W. Schnaper, "The Multiple Risk Factor Intervention Trial: 1. Historical Perspectives," *Preventive Medicine* 10 (1981): 387–401.

Zunz, Olivier, *Making America Corporate 1870–1920* (Chicago: University of Chicago Press, 1990).

INDEX

Printed and bound by CPI Group (UK) Ltd, Croydon, CR0 4YY

27/10/2024

14580347-0004